D1559048

Molecular Genetics
and the
Human Personality

Molecular Genetics and the Human Personality

Edited by

Jonathan Benjamin, M.D.
Richard P. Ebstein, Ph.D.
Robert H. Belmaker, M.D.

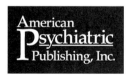

Washington, D.C.
London, England

Copyright © 2002 American Psychiatric Publishing, Inc.
ALL RIGHTS RESERVED
Manufactured in the United States of America on acid-free paper
06 05 04 03 02 5 4 3 2 1
First Edition

American Psychiatric Publishing, Inc.
1400 K Street, N.W.
Washington, DC   20005
www.appi.org

Library of Congress Cataloging-in-Publication Data

Molecular genetics and the human personality / edited by Jonathan Benjamin, Richard P. Ebstein, Robert H. Belmaker.
    p.; cm.
  Includes bibliographical references and index.
  ISBN 0-88048-755-0 (alk. paper)
    1. Personality. 2. Molecular genetics. 3. Genetic psychology. 4. Behavior genetics. I. Benjamin, Jonathan, 1950- II. Ebstein, Richard P., 1943-
III. Belmaker, Robert H.
    [DNLM: 1. Personality Disorders—genetics. 2. Genetics, Behavioral.
WM 190 M718 2002]
  QP402.M654 2002
  616.89'042—dc21   2001045792

British Library Cataloguing in Publication Data
A CIP record is available from the British Library.

For Miri, 1956–1996

J.B.

CONTENTS

Contributors   ix
Foreword   xiii
Irving I. Gottesman, Ph.D.

1   Principles and Methods in the Study of
    Complex Phenotypes   1
    D. C. Rao, Ph.D., and Chi Gu, Ph.D.

2   Relevance of Normal Personality for Psychiatrists   33
    C. Robert Cloninger, M.D.

3   Genetics of Personality:
    The Example of the Broad Autism Phenotype   43
    Joseph Piven, M.D.

4   Animal Models of Personality   63
    Jonathan Flint, M.D.

5   *DRD4* and Novelty Seeking   91
    Paolo Prolo, M.D., and Julio Licinio, M.D.

6   Serotonin Transporter, Personality, and Behavior:
    Toward Dissection of Gene-Gene and
    Gene-Environment Interaction   109
    *K. P. Lesch, M.D., B. D. Greenberg, M.D., Ph.D.,
    J. D. Higley, Ph.D., A. Bennett, Ph.D., and
    D. L. Murphy, M.D.*

7   Dopamine D4 Receptor and Serotonin Transporter
    Promoter Polymorphisms and Temperament
    in Early Childhood   137
    Richard P. Ebstein, Ph.D., and Judith G. Auerbach, Ph.D.

8   Personality, Substance Abuse, and Genes   151
    Richard P. Ebstein, Ph.D., and Moshe Kotler, M.D.

9   Role of *DRD2* and Other Dopamine Genes
in Personality Traits   165
David E. Comings, M.D., Gerard Saucier, Ph.D., and
James P. MacMurray, Ph.D.

10   Genetics of Sensation Seeking   193
Marvin Zuckerman, Ph.D.

11   Quantitative Trait Loci and General Cognitive Ability   211
Robert Plomin, Ph.D.

12   Genetic Polymorphisms and Aggression   231
Antonia New, M.D., Marianne Goodman, M.D.,
Vivian Mitropoulou, M.A., and Larry Siever, M.D.

13   Molecular Genetics of Temperamental
Differences in Children   245
Louis A. Schmidt, Ph.D., and Nathan A. Fox, Ph.D.

14   Genetics of Sexual Behavior   257
Dean H. Hamer, Ph.D.

15   From Phenotype to Gene and Back:
A Critical Appraisal of Progress So Far   273
David Goldman, M.D., and Chiara Mazzanti, Ph.D.

16   Human Correlative Behavioral Genetics:
An Alternative Viewpoint   293
Evan Balaban, Ph.D.

17   Genetics of Human Personality:
Social and Ethical Implications   315
Jon Beckwith, Ph.D., and Joseph S. Alper, Ph.D.

18   Genes for Human Personality Traits:
Endophenotypes of Psychiatric Disorders?   333
Jonathan Benjamin, M.D., Richard P. Ebstein, Ph.D., and
R. H. Belmaker, M.D.

Index   345

CONTRIBUTORS

Joseph S. Alper, Ph.D.
Department of Chemistry, University of Massachusetts, Boston, Massachusetts, United States

Judith G. Auerbach, Ph.D.
Department of Behavioral Sciences, Ben-Gurion University of the Negev, Beer Sheva, Israel

Evan Balaban, Ph.D.
The Neurosciences Institute, San Diego, California, United States

Jon Beckwith, Ph.D.
Department of Microbiology and Molecular Genetics, Harvard Medical School, Boston, Massachusetts, United States

Jonathan Benjamin, M.D.
Department of Psychiatry, Barzilai Medical Center, Ben Gurion University of the Negev, Beersheva, Israel

R. H. Belmaker, M.D.
Beersheva Mental Health Center, Ben Gurion University of the Negev, Beersheva, Israel

A. Bennett, Ph.D.
Laboratory of Clinical Studies, National Institute on Alcohol Abuse and Alcoholism, National Institutes of Health Primate Center, Poolesville, Maryland, United States

C. Robert Cloninger, M.D.
Departments of Psychiatry, Genetics, and Psychology, Washington University, St. Louis, Missouri, United States

David E. Comings, M.D.
Department of Medical Genetics, City of Hope Medical Center, Duarte, California, United States

Richard P. Ebstein, Ph.D.
Research Laboratory, S. Herzog Memorial Hospital, Jerusalem, Israel

ix

Jonathan Flint, M.D.
Wellcome Trust Center for Human Genetics, Oxford, United Kingdom

Nathan A. Fox, Ph.D.
Institute for Child Study, University of Maryland, College Park,
Maryland, United States

David Goldman, M.D.
National Institute on Alcohol Abuse and Alcoholism, Rockville,
Maryland, United States

Marianne Goodman, M.D.
Mount Sinai School of Medicine, New York, New York, United States

Irving I. Gottesman, Ph.D.
University of Minnesota Medical School and Department of Psychology,
University of Minnesota, Minneapolis, Minnesota, United States

B. D. Greenberg, M.D., Ph.D.
Laboratory of Clinical Science, National Institute of Mental Health,
Bethesda, Maryland, United States

Chi Gu, Ph.D.
Division of Biostatistics, Washington University School of Medicine, St.
Louis, Missouri, United States

Dean H. Hamer, Ph.D.
Laboratory of Biochemistry, National Cancer Institute, National Institutes
of Health, Bethesda, Maryland, United States

J. D. Higley, Ph.D.
Laboratory of Clinical Studies, National Institute on Alcohol Abuse and
Alcoholism, National Institutes of Health Primate Center, Poolesville,
Maryland, United States

Moshe Kotler, M.D.
Beersheva Mental Health Center, Faculty of Health Sciences, Ben Gurion
University of the Negev, Beersheva, Israel

K. P. Lesch, M.D.
Department of Psychiatry, University of Würzburg, Würzburg, Germany

Julio Licinio, M.D.
Department of Psychiatry and Biobehavioral Sciences, University of
California, Los Angeles, United States

James P. MacMurray, Ph.D.
Department of Psychiatry, Loma Linda University School of Medicine, Loma Linda, California, United States

Chiara Mazzanti, Ph.D.
National Institute on Alcohol Abuse and Alcoholism, Rockville, Maryland, United States

Vivian Mitropoulou, M.A.
Mount Sinai School of Medicine, New York, New York, United States

D. L. Murphy, M.D.
Laboratory of Clinical Science, National Institute of Mental Health, Bethesda, Maryland, United States

Antonia New, M.D.
Mount Sinai School of Medicine, New York, New York, United States

Joseph Piven, M.D.
North Carolina Mental Retardation and Developmental Disabilities Research Center, University of North Carolina, Chapel Hill, North Carolina, United States

Robert Plomin, Ph.D.
Social, Genetic, and Developmental Psychiatry Research Centre, Institute of Psychiatry, King's College, London, United Kingdom

Paolo Prolo, M.D.
Department of Psychiatry and Biobehavioral Sciences, University of California, Los Angeles, United States

D. C. Rao, Ph.D.
Division of Biostatistics and Departments of Psychiatry and Genetics, Washington University School of Medicine, St. Louis, Missouri, United States

Gerard Saucier, Ph.D.
Department of Psychology, University of Oregon, Eugene, Oregon, United States

Louis A. Schmidt, Ph.D.
Department of Psychology, McMaster University, Hamilton, Ontario, Canada

Larry Siever, M.D.
Mount Sinai School of Medicine, New York, New York, United States

Marvin Zuckerman, Ph.D.
Department of Psychology, University of Delaware, Newark, Delaware, United States

FOREWORD

Genes, Temperament, and Personality: Past and Prospect

Irving I. Gottesman, Ph.D.

A solid precedent exists for the concern of the field of psychopathology with persons who behave in an "abnormal" way although they themselves are neither psychotic nor mentally retarded. Such prescientific, often degrading, terms as *moral insanity, affectionless, weak-willed, asthenic, hyperthymic, insecure (sensitives and anankasts) psychopaths,* and *constitutional inferiors,* peppered the language and writing of nineteenth- and early twentieth-century psychopathologists (Berrios 1991; Hirsch and Shepherd 1974; Slater and Roth 1969). Pure descriptive psychiatry slowly gave way to ideas that lent themselves more readily to quantification, and pressures from both industry and the military for efficient selection of vast numbers of humans for specific tasks led to the development of inventories and tests for assessment of personality traits (Bernreuter 1933; Eysenck 1947; Hathaway and McKinley 1940). A scientific nomenclature developed (Allport 1937) in connection with test development, and it was used to identify traits and personality types, often with the aid of factor analysis (Cattell 1946; Guilford and Guilford 1936), but not necessarily (Murray 1938).

The intellectual debt owed by these early personologists to numerous European lines of thought are quite clear and often explicit. Such grand figures of psychopathology as Jaspers (1913/1963), Kretschmer (1921/1925), Schneider (1923/1958), Pavlov (1927), and Essen-Moller (1979) directly and indirectly inspired the study of personality as a bridge, with or without steps or stages, to the better understanding of severe mental disorders and personality disorders (cf. Crow 1998; DiLalla et al. 1993). All were willing to give serious consideration to aspects of continuity in the etiologies of the mental disorders; all were willing to take as an article of faith that constitutional, biological, and hereditary factors somehow played a major role—a role awaiting acceptable scientific proof.

Bill of Fare

The author-editors of the current volume have boldly assembled a gourmet's intellectual feast of facts, conjectures, hopes, and misgivings for students of psychopathology bold enough to hold in abeyance their understandable misgivings about the conjunction of molecular genetics and human personality. Mavens enlisted to prepare and to present the courses are world-class theoreticians, empiricists—spanning the strategies required from integrationism to reductionism—clinicians, developmentalists, and statisticians. Although the disciplinary backgrounds of the authors are heavily weighted toward formal training as psychiatrists, physicians, geneticists, or psychologists, other disciplines are represented as well, and many of them comfortably wear two or more hats, including those of ideologically fired critics. All in all, you are about to have a most satisfying and memorable encounter—one that will stick not to the ribs, but to the neurons in long-term memory. You will not find much stonewalling or pontification here—the subject matter, in various stages of development and far from definitive, does not lend itself to such obfuscation. The contributions do celebrate remarkable progress over a very short period of time, using tools and technologies from molecular genetics that are themselves still novel (Collins 1999; http://www.Lexgen.com/ [for guides to 60,000 knockout mouse clones as well as 60,000 embryonic stem cell clones]) and not expressly designed for application to behavioral traits/syndromes. The editors, to their credit, expose us to work-in-progress, based on initial findings and promise for the near future; they also, perhaps reflecting their confidence about the merits of the corpus of research and their insight about its potential for abuse and misuse (cf. Gottesman and Bertelsen 1996; Proctor 1988; http://www.bioethics.net), have invited two chapters of sometimes stinging criticisms from fellow biological scientists who are not willing to join the celebration of the findings about molecular genetics and human personality. Lest there be irrational exuberance, or a risk of intoxication with the substantive and the tenuous-but-heady research, the critics provide a built-in dose of Antabuse. Concerns and cautions about premature applications of the information generated in this volume in the policy arena are reasonable (cf. Chapters 15–17) (Pokorski 1997; Rothstein 1997).

Throughout this volume there is a general appreciation of the fact that the kinds of information generated by research programs into the (molecular and population) genetics of complex traits or diseases will be used probabilistically and not to abet an obsolete determinism (Gottesman 1994, 1997; Sing et al. 1996). The chapter (Chapter 1) on principles and methods that follows is so user-friendly and Socratic as to melt most "fears of computing"; it, like the chapters on animal models for personality (Chapter 4) and human intelligence as a model for personality (Chapter 11) skillfully and masterfully prepare you for appreciating the remaining empirical findings on human personality qua personality. Afficionados will discover (Chapter 1) a less-Draconian superego for acceptable levels of statistical significance in whole-genome scanning than the one currently in practice (Lander and Kruglyak 1995), and they will be guided to the important roles for the phenomenon of epistasis (gene by gene interactions) in personality genetics (Cheverud and Routman 1995; Rao and Province 2000). A welcome and essential emphasis on the neurodevelopmental and ontogenetic aspects of personality is provided by many of the chapters (Chapters 6, 7, 9, 11, 13). Child psychiatrists will take special pleasure from the integrative overview of the broad autism phenotype (Chapter 3), and there is much to enlighten experts in drug and alcohol abuse (Chapters 5, 8, 10). Variation in sexuality has a place in the feast (Chapter 14) as a main course or as dessert, depending on your preferences. Adding balance and mature perspectives on how all the chapters complement and sometimes challenge one another are the contributions of Cloninger (Chapter 2), a major figure in the renaissance of the relevance to psychopathology of both genetics and personality (1986, 1999), Goldman and Mazzanti (Chapter 15) with their informed critical appraisal of the state of the art, and the editors themselves (Chapter 18), judiciously contemplating what they have wrought. A major emphasis in this volume on the receptors and transporters for the neurotransmitters dopamine and serotonin is a rational starting point, but the future will bring the field many other candidate genes that today cannot even be imagined, given our ignorance of the genes involved in the prenatal development of the central nervous system.

The use of the term *endophenotype* in the title of the last chapter gives me particular personal pleasure. It is a concept that Shields and I (Gottesman 1997; Gottesman and Shields 1972) discovered in the world of insect genetics and quickly adapted for use in psychiatric genetics as a concept that mediated the genes-to-behavior pathway. The endophenotype concept facilitates thinking and research about complex traits or diseases that involve many genes, many environmental factors—prenatal, perinatal, and postnatal—and variable "doses" of chaotic and stochastic contributions in both idiographic and nomothetic ways (cf. Petronis et al. 1999; Woolf 1997).

Developments in Genetics and Feasibility

In 1957 when I began my own studies into the heritability of personality traits, in normal adolescents, that were likely to be related to psychopathology (DiLalla et al. 1996; Gottesman 1962, 1963), I often felt as if I were a lonely voice in the wilderness. Bold, but naïve in retrospect, attempts to broach the molecular genetics of personality were undertaken by Cohen and Thomas (1962) who examined the distribution of ABO and Rh blood groups in smokers and nonsmokers; Cattell et al. (1964) used an analysis of covariance in a search for associations between blood groups and personality trait factors. Neither effort was taken seriously although similar strategies for duodenal ulcer were accepted. My first efforts were rejected by editors as anachronistic and as an attempt to resurrect the defunct nature versus nurture battles of the 1920s and 1930s; the achievements and continuing promise in the present volume give me the liberty to say, "I told you so." The yields revealed in this volume are only the beginning of a new era, an era made possible by the electrifying pace of discovery and innovation in the fields of molecular genetics. The processes of evolution have guaranteed that virtually any genetic polymorphism discovered in *Drosophila* or mouse that causes brain malfunctions may be of vital interest to the domain covered here. Some 41,000 DNA markers are now available to point our way on the physical map of the human genome, a count that was as low as 16,000 in 1996. Collins (1999) and Wall Street predict with confidence that the rough draft sequencing of the human genome will be available for 90% of the genome as this chapter is being written, and the smooth version will be finished in 2003. It takes an internet address to keep up with progress: http://www.ncbi.nlm.nih.gov/ is provided by the (U.S.A.) National Center for

Biotechnology Information. It is too easy to suppress the facts that our species has an estimated 50,000 to 140,000 genes, that the length of one chromosome contains between 2,000 and 9,000 genes, and that the entire genome contains some 3 billion base pairs. As scientists and as citizens we are compelled to continuously distinguish between overselling our knowledge with its attendant raising of false hopes, and a dyspeptic skepticism with its attendant raising of despair. I recommend a mind-set of cautious optimism to the consumers of this forward-looking volume.

References

Allport GW: Personality: A Psychological Interpretation. New York, Holt, Rinehart, and Winston, 1937

Bernreuter RG: The theory and construction of the personality inventory. J Social Psychol 4:387–405, 1933

Berrios GE: British psychopathology since the early twentieth century, in One-Hundred-Fifty Years of British Psychiatry, 1841–1991. Edited by Berrios GE, Freeman H. Washington DC, American Psychiatric Press, 1991, pp 232–244

Cattell RB: The Description and Measurement of Personality. New York, Harcourt, Brace, and World, 1946

Cattell RB, Young HB, Hundleby JD: Blood groups and personality traits. Am J Hum Genet 16:397–402, 1964

Cheverud J, Routman EJ: Epistasis and its contribution to genetic variance components. Genetics 139:963–971, 1995

Cloninger CR: A unified biosocial theory of personality and its role in the development of anxiety states. Psychiatric Development 4:167–226, 1986

Cloninger CR (ed): Personality and Psychopathology. Washington DC, American Psychiatric Press, 1999

Cohen BH, Thomas CB: Comparison of smokers and non-smokers, II: the distribution of ABO and Rh(D) blood groups. Bulletin of the Johns Hopkins Hospital 110:1–7, 1962

Collins FS: Shattuck lecture: medical and societal consequences of the human genome project. N Engl J Med 341:28–37, 1999

Crow TJ: From Kraepelin to Kretschmer leavened by Schneider: the transition from categories of psychosis to dimensions of variation intrinsic to *Homo Sapiens*. Arch Gen Psychiatry 55:502–504, 1998

DiLalla DL, Gottesman II, Carey G: Assessment of normal personality traits in a psychiatric sample: dimensions and categories. Progress in Experimental Personality and Psychopathology Research 16:137–162, 1993

DiLalla DL, Carey G, Gottesman II, et al: Heritability of MMPI indicators of psychopathology in twins reared apart. J Abnorm Psychol 105:491–499, 1996

Essen-Moller E: Aspects of continuity in the aetiology of mental disorder, in Psychiatry, Genetics and Pathography: A Tribute to Eliot Slater. Edited by Roth M, Cowie V. London, Gaskell Press, 1979, pp 45–61

Eysenck HJ: Dimensions of Personality. London, Routledge and Kegan Paul, 1947

Gottesman II: Differential inheritance of the psychoneuroses. Eugenics Quarterly 9:223–227, 1962

Gottesman II: Heritability of personality: a demonstration. Psychol Monogr 77(9, Whole Nr. 572), 1963

Gottesman II: Complications to the complex inheritance of schizophrenia. Clinical Genetics 46:116–123, 1994

Gottesman II: Twins: en route to QTLs for cognition. Science 276:1522–1523, 1997

Gottesman II, Bertelsen A: Legacy of German psychiatric genetics. Am J Med Genet 67:317–322, 1996

Gottesman II, Shields J: Schizophrenia and Genetics: A Twin Study Vantage Point. New York, Academic Press, 1972

Guilford JP, Guilford RB: Personality factors S, E, and M, and their measurement. J Psychol 2:109–127, 1936

Hathaway SR, McKinley JC: A multiphasic personality schedule (Minnesota), I: construction of the schedule. J Psychol 10:249–254, 1940

Hirsch SR, Shepherd M: Themes and Variations in European Psychiatry. Charlottesville, University Press of Virginia, 1974

Jaspers K: General Psychopathology (1913). Translated by Hoenig J, Hamilton MW. Manchester, Manchester University Press, 1963

Kretschmer E: Physique and Character: An Investigation of Constitution and of the Theory of Temperament (1921). Translated by Sprott WJH. New York, Harcourt, Brace, 1925

Lander E, Kruglyak L: Genetic dissection of complex traits: guidelines for interpreting and reporting linkage results. Nat Genet 11:241–247, 1995

Murray HA: Explorations in Personality. New York, Oxford University Press, 1938

Pavlov IP: Conditioned Reflexes. Translated by Anrep GV. London, Oxford University Press, 1927

Petronis A, Paterson AD, Kennedy JL: Schizophrenia: an epigenetic puzzle? Schizophr Bull 25:639–656, 1999

Pokorski RJ: Insurance underwriting in the genetic era. Am J Hum Genet 60:205–216, 1997

Proctor RN: Racial Hygiene: Medicine Under the Nazis. Cambridge, MA, Harvard University Press, 1988

Rao DC, Province MA (eds): Genetic Dissection of Complex Traits: Challenges for the Next Millennium. San Diego, CA, Academic Press, 2000

Rothstein MA (ed): Genetic Secrets: Protecting Privacy and Confidentiality in the Genetic Era. New Haven, CT, Yale University Press, 1997

Schneider K: Psychopathic Personalities (1923). Translated by Hamilton MW. Springfield, IL, Charles C Thomas, 1958

Sing CF, Haviland MB, Reilly SL: Genetic architecture of common multifactorial diseases, in Variation in the Human Genotype. Edited by Cardew G. Chichester, John Wiley, 1996, pp 211–232

Slater E, Roth M: Mayer-Gross Slater and Roth Clinical Psychiatry. London, Bailliere, Tindall, and Cassell, 1969

Woolf CM: Does the genotype for schizophrenia often remain unexpressed because of canalization and stochastic events during development? Psychol Med 27:659–668, 1997

CHAPTER ONE

Principles and Methods in the Study of Complex Phenotypes

D. C. Rao, Ph.D
Chi Gu, Ph.D.

Genetic dissection of complex traits has been difficult, and often even large-scale investigations give frustrating results. Investigators experienced in genetic investigations of complex traits realize that numerous genes and environmental factors interact to produce the traits. Not surprisingly, simple-minded approaches have largely failed to identify any genes for complex traits. Sometimes, what appear to be conflicting results may not actually be conflicting in the sense that different genes may segregate in different study populations. When this is true, mandating replication studies may render far too many false negatives (i.e., missing real genes). However, this should not be used as an escape clause to explain away all conflicting results.

Complex traits do not likely result from genes with big effects. The effect sizes of any of the multiple etiological factors are likely to be modest. Therefore, methodologies meant for detecting genes with large effects

This work was partly supported by a grant from the National Institute of General Medical Sciences (GM 28719) of the National Institutes of Health. We are grateful to Drs. R. C. Elston and M. A. Province for insightful discussions and comments.

(major genes) are unlikely to be successful with complex traits, as the experience of recent years has shown. Most likely, complex traits are oligogenic (a few genes each with a moderately large effect) and may even be polygenic (many genes each with a small effect). As the number of trait genes increases and their individual effects decline, the distinction between oligogenic and polygenic effects becomes blurred. Even though the individual gene effects may be small, interactions among the genes and environments could make a substantial contribution to the final manifestation of the trait. Failure to recognize and accommodate such interactions may often mask the effects of the individual genes. Therefore, we must pay attention to all relevant aspects of gene finding, including study design, optimal methods of analysis, and interpretation of the results. The brute force of very large sample size alone may not achieve the desired goal, although sufficiently large sample sizes are necessary.

A common approach to enhance the power of any study is to utilize larger sample sizes. The concept of multicenter genetic studies (e.g., Begleiter et al. 1995; Higgins et al. 1996) is rapidly evolving as a means of generating large samples of standardized family data. The motivation is to provide an adequate sample for relatively rare traits as well as for relatively common traits where the effect size of any individual etiological factor is likely to be modest (e.g., schizophrenia). Even in preplanned collaborations of this sort where common protocols are used and data collection is standardized, one must remember that the frequency and distribution of risk factors—both genetic and environmental—may well be different among the study centers. To pool data from studies that were conducted independently encompasses even greater challenges because there may be considerable differences in the sampling strategy, the phenotypic measurement, the particular genetic markers that were typed, or the ancillary information available for classification or phenotypic adjustment. Some of these issues have been considered in the development of meta-analytical methods for pooling results from multiple linkage studies (e.g., Gu et al. 1998c; Li and Rao 1996).

Study Design

Study design is perhaps the single most important consideration in the planning of any genetic study. Statistical power, cost-effectiveness, and feasibility all depend critically on the design. It is important that available knowledge about the disease/trait (physiology, etiology, etc.) be fully used in devising sampling schemes, selecting sampling units, and choosing analytical methods. More information should lead to better designs.

Definition and Refinement of Phenotype

Although definition of the phenotype may at first seem to be a trivial issue, some thought should be given to whether the current definition of the phenotype, however expertly done originally, is still the right one to use in gene finding studies. After all, our goal is to find the trait genes, not to follow a traditional or a revolutionary approach. Different definitions of the phenotype do lead to different results. Certain definitions tend to dwarf the signal, whereas others might have the potential to sharpen, and relatively enhance, the signal. The fundamental idea behind our general approach to gene finding is one of looking for correlation between the degree of phenotypic similarity and genotypic similarity among relatives. This correlation is weakened if either type of similarity (phenotypic or genotypic) is underestimated. In particular, to avoid underestimating the phenotypic similarity, or at least to minimize the extent of underestimation, we must require that the phenotype be reasonably reproducible. If, for example, a certain questionnaire-derived phenotype tracks poorly over a matter of just a few weeks, the phenotypic similarity among relatives will be severely compromised if different relatives are "measured" at different times. Multiple administrations of the same instrument and/or using other pertinent information (e.g., age at onset, severity of the disease, family history) can lead to considerably refined phenotypes and may result in drastic reduction of the necessary sample size. For quantitative traits, the average of multiple measurements represents a good phenotype (e.g., Rao 1998). Finally, for phenotypes that are not highly reproducible, it would seem desirable to study them in smaller family units rather than in extended pedigrees.

Sampling Unit

Several features of any genetic study are highly interdependent. The most critical among them are the sampling unit, the sampling method, and the sample size. One should not be decided independently of the other two. For genetic studies of complex traits, sib pairs of one type or another are commonly used in conjunction with model-free methods of analysis. When using sib pairs, the total number of participants needed in a study can be minimized by sampling larger sibships, as opposed to sampling independent sib pairs (Todorov et al. 1997). In typical cases, one can reduce sample size by one-third by sampling sib trios rather than independent sib pairs.

Other more powerful sampling units such as extremely discordant (ED) sib pairs (Eaves 1994; Risch and Zhang 1995) or extremely discordant and extremely concordant (EDAC) sib pairs (Gu et al. 1996) can reduce the sample size even more. Sampling some sibs from above the ninetieth percentile of a trait distribution and other sibs from below the thirtieth percentile appears to provide an optimum strategy. This includes ED sib pairs, sib pairs above the ninetieth percentile (high concordant), and sib pairs below the thirtieth percentile (low concordant). High concordance sampling is analogous to the affected sib-pair (ASP) method. However, for discrete diseases, an affected individual and an unaffected sib do not constitute an ED sib pair; they would represent a discordant sib pair, not necessarily an extremely discordant sib pair. Sampling simply discordant sib pairs does not constitute a good design.

Selective Sampling

Selective sampling optimizes study designs by enhancing power, cutting down the cost, or both. The ASP method is a good example. If we consider only random samples, we will have greatly reduced power to detect genetic linkage, because the difference in the observed and expected identical-by-descent (IBD) sharing between the sibs would be quite small. By sampling ASPs, we magnify the difference in the IBD sharing of an affected sib pair (Risch 1990b; Suarez et al. 1978), which leads to greatly increased power.

For discrete diseases/traits, the ASP (and ASP-like) method is a good sampling approach. One may also select on severity of the disease if such a thing exists. For quantitative traits, one may select on extreme trait values (Carey and Williamson 1991; Eaves 1994). For example, Risch and Zhang (1995) used an extreme selection scheme on the trait values of a quantitative trait (the ED sib-pair method) and showed a dramatic increase in power.

As noted earlier, the sampling method has an important bearing on the cost of a genetic study. For example, Gu et al. (1997) investigated cost-effectiveness when sampling extreme sib pairs. Sampling high-risk individuals and screening for their extreme siblings to form extreme sib pairs (ESP) was shown to be an effective design. We also showed that combining all available extreme concordant (EC) sib pairs—including high-high sib pairs analogous to the ASPs as well as low-low sib pairs—with ED pairs is more economical than pursuing ED pairs alone. However, genotyping all available EC pairs (especially the low concordant) may not be an optimal strategy for reducing cost. In general, to make optimal use of EC pairs, one should apply an optimal selection scheme for genotyping so that the least possible number of EC pairs are genotyped in combination with all the ED pairs to produce the desired statistical power (Gu and Rao 1997a, 1997b).

Genotyping Issues

A lot of attention has been paid to which types of markers to use, the number of markers to use (density), and whether to genotype all relatives, especially the parents (e.g., Elston 1992; Elston et al. 1996; Holmans 1993). With the advent of large-scale genotyping using automated robotics, we should be more careful about data management and quality control issues (e.g., Rao 1998; Weber and Broman, 2001). In general, genotyping errors can have a significant effect on the power of a study. For example, a 10% genotypic (not allelic) error rate requires a sample of 250 ED sib pairs to yield the same 80% power as would a sample of 190 ED sib pairs with a zero genotypic error rate when the marker involves eight alleles (Rao 1998). Note that the difference of 60 ED sib pairs is huge, and that the situation is a lot worse for markers with fewer alleles. Weber and Broman (2001) reviewed issues surrounding the quality of genotyping and their implications for genomewide scans.

Linkage Versus Association

Although there is not a clear consensus as to what precisely constitutes a linkage study or an association study, it is commonly recognized that a linkage study analyzes the cosegregation of two genetic loci (some may be latent, such as a disease locus) in families, whereas an association study investigates the coexistence (nonindependence) of two loci in individuals. However, the premise of a genetic association is based on the hope that association induced by linkage disequilibrium will lead us to the gene, and spurious association will be excluded by other means of study (such as using family-based controls).

It is commonly believed that linkage studies have a limited genetic resolution of about 1 cM, and therefore, although linkage studies can narrow down genomic regions, fine tuning requires other approaches. On the other hand, association studies, notorious for false positives, have a much finer resolution because the recombination history is in a sense used in the calculation. The transmission disequilibrium test alleviates the false-positive problem caused by population admixture (Spielman and Ewens 1998; Spielman et al. 1993).

Two-Stage Designs (Linkage in Stage 1 and Association in Stage 2)

Elston (1992) was the first to propose a two-stage strategy as a cost-effective way of designing genomic scans; a relatively sparse marker map is used in the first stage to generate linkage signals, followed by a second stage with a denser marker map around the suggested signals. Most recently, Elston et al. (1996) has investigated the properties and performance of the one-stage and two-stage strategies, concluding that a two-stage procedure could halve the cost of a study as compared with a one-stage procedure. In such designs, it is critical that the first stage have excellent power, well over the usual 80%, because the second stage cannot recover any linkages missed in the first stage. Also, use of the same sample for both stages may not be helpful in terms of pruning false positives. It is desirable to use independent samples of relative pairs in each stage. Two-stage strategies are in general more attractive as long as one is willing to accept a trade-off between false negatives and false positives, exchanging a lower rate of false negatives for a slight increase in the rate of false positives (Todorov and Rao 1997).

As noted, sometimes the same sample is used for both stages of a genome scan. Such a choice appears to result in cost savings but may not carry other optimal properties (Elston et al. 1996). The question arises as to how often the second stage is able to prune out (or validate) signals detected in the first stage. Perhaps a better two-stage design is one where the first stage carries out a linkage analysis using a relatively dense map and identifies (and narrows down using fine structure mapping) potential regions to be assessed in the second stage with association studies. The effect of using the same sample in such a design is unclear; however, we would recommend using separate samples for the two stages. Finally, the cost-effectiveness of such a design warrants further study.

Sample Size and Power

For a given significance level, the power (ability to detect true genes) increases with sample size. Likewise, for a given sample size (which holds after a study has been carried out) the power increases with the significance level. Unfortunately, false positives also increase with the significance level. It is important to note that, in earlier days, the real cost of a false positive was unaffordably high, and accordingly, the emphasis was on keeping false positives to a minimum. False positives were minimized by choosing small significance levels. Unfortunately, this resulted in low power, thus missing true linkages. This was not a big problem because linkage analysis was used primarily to map disease genes that were already known to exist. Now, we use linkage analysis of complex traits to first prove that such genes exist and, in the process, to map them. Therefore in the current situation, we cannot afford to miss genes, rendering the issue of sample size and power even more important.

It is well known that even the first detection of complex trait genes is difficult, and replication of a particular linkage finding is even more difficult, especially under genetic heterogeneity (e.g., Suarez et al. 1994). The need to detect genes for increasingly complex traits prompted several investigations of optimal sampling because the sample size alone cannot be indefinitely increased. Nonrandom sampling delivers a lot more power for the same sample size (e.g., Carey and Williamson 1991). The ED sib pair strategy was developed to provide more power with much smaller samples sizes (Risch and Zhang 1995).

For most psychiatric illnesses, investigators commonly use the ASP method. In Table 1–1, we provide the power of the method under a variety of situations corresponding to a range of sample sizes. This may be useful when designing new genome scans. Three choices of population prevalence (K_p = 1%, 5%, and 10%), three levels of locus-specific heritability (h^2 = 10%, 15%, and 20%), two levels of residual sibling correlation due to other genetic and familial environmental effects (ρ = 0.1 and 0.3), and five choices of sample size (ASPs = 200, 400, 600, 800, and 1000) were considered. Power is reported corresponding to each of two significance levels. Both were based on the same discrete map of 400 markers but on different rates of false positives: α = 0.00009 corresponding to one expected false positive in 20 genome scans as suggested by Lander and Kruglyak (1995), and α = 0.00227 corresponding to one expected false positive per genome scan (Rao and Province 2000; see also "Interpretation of Results" in this chapter). These significance values were computed using the theory of Feingold et al. (1993). It should be noted that whereas Lander and Kruglyak (1995) recommended an α = 0.000022 corresponding to continuous marker density, we have translated their value to α = 0.00009 corresponding to a marker density with 400 markers (using the approximations given by Feingold et al. [1993]).

TABLE 1–1　Power under various genetic models using an affected sib-pair study design

		Number of affected sib pairs				
K_p	h^2	200	400	600	800	1000
		$\rho = 0.10$				
1%	10%	**87.9**/59.3	**99.8**/97.3	**100.0**/99.9	**100.0**/100.0	**100.0** /100.0
1%	15%	**99.8**/97.4	**100.0**/100.0	**100.0**/100.0	**100.0**/100.0	**100.0**/100.0
1%	20%	**100.0**/100.0	**100.0**/100.0	**100.0**/100.0	**100.0**/100.0	**100.0**/100.0
5%	10%	**31.7**/8.2	**69.7**/34.4	**89.9**/64.0	**97.2**/84.1	**99.3**/94.1
5%	15%	**73.8**/38.5	**98.2**/88.0	**99.9**/98.9	**100.0**/99.9	**100.0**/100.0
5%	20%	**95.0**/75.9	**100.0**/99.5	**100.0**/100.0	**100.0**/100.0	**100.0**/100.0
10%	10%	**12.1**/1.9	**31.9**/8.3	**52.6**/19.8	**69.8**/34.6	**82.0**/50.1
10%	15%	**36.1**/10.1	**75.4**/40.8	**93.2**/71.5	**98.5**/89.3	**99.7**/96.7
10%	20%	**65.4**/29.8	**96.1**/79.8	**99.8**/97.0	**100.0**/99.7	**100.0**/100.0
		$\rho = 0.30$				
1%	10%	**64.3**/28.8	**95.7**/78.5	**99.7**/96.6	**100.0**/99.6	**100.0**/100.0
1%	15%	**97.2**/83.5	**100.0**/99.9	**100.0**/100.0	**100.0**/100.0	**100.0**/100.0
1%	20%	**100.0**/99.2	**100.0**/100.0	**100.0**/100.0	**100.0**/100.0	**100.0**/100.0
5%	10%	**17.7**/3.3	**44.9**/14.9	**68.6**/33.4	**84.2**/53.5	**92.8**/70.6
5%	15%	**52.1**/19.2	**89.8**/63.6	**98.6**/90.0	**99.9**/98.1	**100.0**/99.7
5%	20%	**83.9**/52.4	**99.5**/95.3	**100.0**/99.8	**100.0**/100.0	**100.0**/100.0
10%	10%	**7.1**/0.9	**18.5**/3.5	**32.4**/8.6	**46.6**/15.9	**59.5**/25.1
10%	15%	**22.7**/4.8	**55.0**/21.4	**78.7**/45.2	**91.3**/67.2	**96.9**/82.8
10%	20%	**48.0**/16.5	**86.9**/57.9	**97.8**/86.4	**99.7**/96.8	**100.0**/99.4

Note. Three choices each of the population prevalence (K_p) and trait heritability (h^2) are considered, together with five choices of the sample size (N) and two choices of the residual sibling correlation (ρ). Power is reported as **x**/y corresponding to two significance levels, each with a discrete map of 400 markers: For **x**, we used $\alpha = 0.00227$, corresponding to one false positive (on average) per scan (power displayed in **bold**); for y, we used $\alpha = 0.00009$, corresponding to one false positive in 20 scans.

Table 1–2 provides the power under a variety of situations for the ED sib-pair design. The organization of Table 1–2 is identical to that of Table 1–1 except for the sample size. Here we consider a different range of the sample sizes (50, 75, 100, 150, and 200 ED sib pairs). Note that although an affected sib and an unaffected sib constitute a discordant sib pair, extreme discordance requires that the sibs be in the two tails of a distribution and not merely on either side of a threshold.

Cost-Benefit Analysis

No matter what an investigator wishes to pursue, in the end, a fixed budget and practical constraints determine the type of study. Especially when

TABLE 1–2   Power under various genetic models using an extremely discordant sib-pair study design

K_p	h^2	Number of extremely discordant sib pairs				
		50	75	100	150	200
				$\rho = 0.10$		
1%	10%	**12.5**/1.9	**22.5**/4.6	**33.5**/8.8	**55.1**/21.3	**72.5**/37.1
1%	15%	**43.0**/12.9	**67.5**/30.9	**83.7**/51.2	**97.0**/82.2	**99.6**/95.3
1%	20%	**80.9**/45.2	**96.1**/78.0	**99.4**/93.7	**100.0**/99.7	**100.0**/100.0
5%	10%	**6.5**/0.7	**11.3**/1.6	**17.0**/3.0	**30.0**/7.4	**43.6**/14.0
5%	15%	**21.1**/4.1	**37.2**/10.3	**53.0**/19.5	**77.4**/42.6	**90.6**/64.9
5%	20%	**48.0**/15.6	**73.1**/36.4	**88.0**/58.4	**98.3**/87.5	**99.8**/97.4
10%	10%	**2.9**/0.2	**4.7**/0.5	**6.8**/0.8	**11.8**/1.8	**17.7**/3.3
10%	15%	**8.4**/1.1	**14.9**/2.5	**22.5**/4.6	**39.1**/11.5	**55.0**/21.2
10%	20%	**20.1**/3.8	**35.7**/9.6	**51.2**/18.2	**75.7**/40.4	**89.6**/62.5
				$\rho = 0.30$		
1%	10%	**35.1**/9.2	**57.7**/22.6	**75.2**/39.6	**93.3**/71.0	**98.6**/89.3
1%	15%	**82.6**/47.7	**96.8**/80.3	**99.6**/94.7	**100.0**/99.8	**100.0**/100.0
1%	20%	**99.0**/89.5	**100.0**/99.4	**100.0**/100.0	**100.0**/100.0	**100.0**/100.0
5%	10%	**18.3**/3.3	**32.6**/8.3	**47.2**/15.8	**71.5**/35.8	**86.6**/57.0
5%	15%	**53.5**/19.0	**78.4**/42.9	**91.5**/65.9	**99.1**/91.9	**99.9**/98.7
5%	20%	**86.4**/53.4	**98.0**/85.1	**99.8**/96.8	**100.0**/99.9	**100.0**/100.0
10%	10%	**7.0**/0.8	**12.2**/1.8	**18.4**/3.4	**32.5**/8.4	**46.8**/15.8
10%	15%	**21.9**/4.3	**38.5**/10.9	**54.7**/20.6	**78.9**/44.6	**91.6**/67.1
10%	20%	**47.7**/15.3	**72.8**/36.0	**87.9**/58.1	**98.3**/87.4	**99.8**/97.4

Note. Three choices each of the population prevalence (K_p) and trait heritability (h^2) are considered, together with five choices of the sample size *(N)* and two choices of the residual sibling correlation (ρ). Power is reported as **x**/*y* corresponding to two significance levels, each with a discrete map of 400 markers: For **x**, we used $\alpha = 0.00227$, corresponding to one false positive (on average) per scan (power displayed in **bold**); for *y*, we used $\alpha = 0.00009$, corresponding to one false positive in 20 scans.

proposing an ED or EDAC sib-pair approach, we have to be realistic in terms of how feasible or how impractical a proposed sample size is. The EDAC approach was developed primarily to render the extreme sib-pair studies more feasible (Gu et al. 1996). A simple method may allow a quick assessment of the cost versus the benefit (e.g., Gu and Rao 1997b). For example, let the cost be C_p for phenotyping and C_G for genotyping of one person. If we have to screen *N* sib pairs to get a certain number (n_{ED}) of ED sib pairs for genotyping, the total cost of the study is $2NC_p + 2n_{ED}C_G$. The total cost for a corresponding EDAC study would be $2N_1C_p + 2(n_{ed} + n_{lc} + n_{hc})C_G$, where N_1 is the total number of sib pairs needing to be screened to obtain a smaller number (n_{ed}) of ED pairs *and* ($n_{lc} + n_{hc}$) extremely concordant sib pairs of both types. Clearly, $N_1 < N$ and $n_{ed} < n_{ED}$. Therefore, the EDAC study is not only more feasible compared with an ED study, it is also less expensive so long as $C_G \leq C_P(N - N_1)/(n_{ed} + n_{lc} + n_{hc} - n_{ED})$. Gu and Rao (1997b) have provided detailed guidelines for cost-benefit analysis.

Methods of Analysis

A rich arsenal of analytical tools has been developed and enhanced over the years. Because the early methods were developed primarily for Mendelian traits, these methods are good for mapping loci with large effects and may not be as effective for mapping complex trait genes. Recent extensions and improvements to these methods have made them more applicable for mapping complex traits. We briefly review these methods and point out their advantages and pitfalls when applied to complex traits.

There are two stages when analytical methods may be chosen: at the stage of study design or at the stage of actual data analysis (i.e., after completion of data collection). It is desirable to choose the analytical methods at the design stage, because the method should be an integral part of a design that affects the power and cost-effectiveness of a study.

Methods for Linkage Analysis

Genetic linkage is the phenomenon where alleles at different loci coseg-regate in families. The strength of this cosegregation is measured by the recombination fraction θ, the probability of an odd number of crossovers. Under special cases, the rate of recombination may be counted directly by observing recombinants in a sample of families; but, in most cases, because of unknown phase and other limitations, the value of θ needs to be estimated and tested statistically using appropriate methods. Three classes of methods are most commonly used today for linkage analysis: the classical lod score method, which is generally regarded as a parametric or a model-based method, so called because the method is based on assumptions about the disease model; the nonparametric or model-free relative pair methods, so called because these generally do not assume a disease inheritance model; and finally what might be called hybrid variance components methods, so called because they do not make strong assumptions about the disease inheritance model but do involve some relatively weaker assumptions.

The lod Score (Model-Based) Method

In his seminal paper, Morton (1955) presented a powerful method using Barnard's (1949) lod score (Z) as a measure of the linkage effect and gave a sequential procedure to determine the acceptance or rejection of linkage. He proposed two thresholds: $Z \geq 3$ to accept and $Z \leq -2$ to exclude the hypothesis of linkage. These thresholds have become the gold standard in the field and are still in use worldwide.

Under any given genetic model (θ, gene frequencies, penetrances, etc.), the lod score is calculated as the logarithm of the ratio of the likelihoods under the alternative hypothesis (under which the recombination fraction $\theta < 1/2$) and under the null hypothesis of no linkage (under which the recombination fraction $\theta = 1/2$):

$$Z(\theta) = \log_{10} [L(\theta)/L(\theta = 0.5)]$$

Computer implementations of this simple yet most powerful method benefited immensely from advances in the general pedigree likelihood algorithms developed by Elston and Stewart (1971). For example, the LIPED computer program (Ott 1974) became an instant success, as did the subsequent and more general implementations such as LINKAGE (Lathrop et al. 1984). When the disease/trait model specified is close to the true model, the lod score method is unquestionably more powerful than any of the nonparametric alternatives (see, e.g., a recent review by Wijsman and Amos [1997]). However, the method does suffer when the disease model is misspecified, and the false-positive rate could also be inflated when the lod score is maximized over all possible models (Clerget-Darpoux et al. 1986; Risch and Giuffra 1992; Weeks et al. 1990). A correction was proposed by Ott (1989) when the lod score is maximized over all models, and its applicability was later validated by Weeks et al. (1990). According to these guidelines, when a lod score is maximized over n models, the traditional threshold of 3 should be increased to $3 + \log(n)$. For example, if a lod score is maximized over 10 possible models, a more appropriate threshold would be 4, and if it is based on 100 models, the threshold should be 5 (instead of the traditional 3).

Multipoint analysis evaluates linkage of a group of loci jointly and can therefore compensate for information loss due to uninformative markers and missing marker information (which is perhaps more relevant for model-free methods). However, multipoint linkage analysis is far more challenging and involves certain assumptions relating to interference and mapping functions. In any case, it can be particularly useful when estimating the exact location of a trait locus after linkage has been detected. Faster algorithms developed by Lander and Green (1987) and later implemented by Lander and Kruglyak (1995) make it possible to carry out multipoint analysis on a genomewide scale, although the size of pedigree is still somewhat limited.

Strengths of the lod score method lie in its ability to model and test for interactions, its ability to get better estimates of gene location via multipoint analysis, and its poolability across studies. In many ways, the lod score method provides a method for meta-analysis. Given these strengths and the fact that the method is sensitive to model misspecification, the lod score method may be especially useful as a refinement tool at later stages of mapping quantitative trait loci (QTLs), after some gene(s) have been detected.

Model-Free (Nonparametric) Methods

Especially for complex traits, one usually lacks reasonable trait models, and therefore the classical lod score method is not particularly attractive. This realization has given rise to the development of alternative methods that are not based on strong assumptions about the trait inheritance. It is natural to reason that the existence of a susceptibility gene should lead to an elevated probability that a pair of affected siblings would inherit the same gene(s) from their parents. From this observation, a class of nonparametric methods, or more generally, model-free methods, has been developed based on IBD allele sharing among relative pairs (Blackwelder and Elston 1985; Penrose 1935; Suarez et al. 1978). The IBD distribution was well characterized by Suarez et al. (1978) using population prevalence and additive and dominance variances. Risch (1990a) later gave a rigorous characterization of the IBD distribution using a parameter called the relative-risk ratio (λ) for various types of affected relative pairs. The values of λ are estimable, based on which the strength of a linkage signal, the power of a study, and the possibility of the existence of a multilocus model can be deduced (Risch 1990b) (see next section for extensions to QTL mapping).

One problem with the sib-pair method is that at times the IBD score is ambiguous for a particular sib pair, or at a particular marker position, especially in a genomewide scan. Various types of imputation schemes have been proposed (e.g., Sandkuyl 1989; Terwilliger and Ott 1993). These methods use either the family structure (conditional on affection status) or information at adjacent markers. Gu et al. (1995) proposed a

IBD = identity by descent

multipoint method incorporating interference and showed how linkage information at the nearby markers can be used to infer missing IBD information at a particular marker. Weeks and Lange (1988) used identity by state (IBS) instead of IBD, and proposed the affected-pedigree member method, for which gene frequencies need to be used as a compensation for the loss of information. The problem with this method (and any IBD imputation method that uses gene frequencies) is that it can be sensitive to the misspecification of gene frequencies and can result in inflated false-positive rates (Gu et al. 1998a). More recently, Kruglyak and Lander (1995) extended Green's algorithm and gave a fast algorithm for realization of distribution of transmission vectors, which can be used for rapid imputation of relative IBD values. They later proposed a unified treatment of the lod score method and the nonparametric (model-free) method, in which a nonparametric linkage method extended the affected-pedigree member method and used the IBD sharing of all affected relative pairs in a pedigree. Kong and Cox (1997) gave a semiparametric extension of this method using a single parameter to characterize the IBD sharing effect.

Although the sib-pair method is likely less powerful than the lod score method when the model specified is close to the true model, the simplicity of its execution and robustness to model misspecification makes it an attractive analytical tool for early-stage screening in the mapping of complex traits. After genes are first detected, parametric models of transmission involving interactions can be introduced to fine-tune the location. As we pointed out earlier, these model-free methods all require knowledge of IBD sharing. Although various imputation schemes are available, they may be sensitive to misspecification of gene frequencies when they are used. This, in some cases, could limit the application of such model-free methods. For a review of model-free methods of linkage analysis, see Elston and Cordell (2001).

Methods for Quantitative Traits

For quantitative traits, the first insightful method was presented by Haseman and Elston (1972), who took the squared difference of trait values of a sib pair as the outcome variable and regressed it on the proportion of IBD genes shared by the sib pair using the model $E(Y_j | \pi_j) = \beta_0 + \beta_1 \pi_j$. A significantly negative regression coefficient β_1 implies genetic linkage to the marker. Goldgar (1990) and Amos (1994) used the maximum likelihood method to model directly the covariance structure of sib pairs and arrived at a variance components method that is often more powerful than the original Haseman-Elston method. Fulker and Cardon (1994) extended the Haseman-Elston method to estimate the location of a QTL using flanking markers by applying the interval mapping method of Goldgar (1990). As a hybrid of the model-based and model-free methods, the variance components method combines the strengths of both methods and seems to perform well. These methods are called model-free because the effects of trait genes are not modeled except for the assumption of their existence somewhere in the genome. These methods use all the data available within a pedigree, without abandoning subjects with partially missing information or producing redundancy in the statistics by counting all relative pairs.

Blangero and colleagues (Blangero and Almasy 1996) have generalized the method and presented an excellent implementation of the variance components approach (SOLAR). Province et al. (in press) have developed a multipurpose package (SEGPATH) that can also perform variance components linkage analysis with the flexibility of modeling structural relationships among the variables. More recently, Elston and colleagues have extended the Haseman-Elston method using the mean-corrected cross product in place of the squared trait difference and have shown that the improved Haseman-Elston method is as powerful as the variance components method (Elston et al. 2000). All these methods can deal with multilocus models and multivariate phenotypes.

An alternative treatment of quantitative traits is via polychotomization. We generalized Risch's concept of relative risk ratio (λ) to sib pairs with various quantitative trait outcomes and developed a scheme for optimizing study designs using estimates of the generalized λ values and the EDAC design (Gu and Rao 1997a). We showed that with the help of these λ values and a knowledge of the trait heritability, it is possible to choose trait thresholds and combinations of types of extreme sib pairs to optimize the chances of finding QTLs (Gu and Rao 1997b).

One advantage of the variance components method is its enhanced power compared with model-free methods. However, modeling of the phenotypic distribution is still mandatory, although normality is not always required. Its sensitivity to outliers, to distributional departures, and to ascertainment methods needs further exploration. The significance of the test may become less tractable when the trait distribution assumption is violated, and ascertainment correction may become necessary although may not be always possible because of obscure or unspecified ascertainment.

Methods for Association Analysis

also inbreeding

In the absence of disturbing forces such as selection, mutation, or migration that would change gene frequencies over time, random mating in a large population leads to equilibrium with respect to a single locus in one generation, and one should then observe the so-called Hardy-Weinberg proportions for the genotypic frequencies: $P_{uu} = p^2_u$, $P_{vv} = p^2_v$, and $P_{uv} = 2p_u p_v$. Similar equilibrium can also be reached jointly for more than one locus, but the rate of approach to equilibrium depends also on the number of generations and the recombination fractions between loci. Departure from such Hardy-Weinberg equilibrium is called Hardy-Weinberg disequilibrium, which signals certain violations of the above conditions. When other conditions are satisfied except for the independence of two loci, we can infer that any significant disequilibrium is linkage induced and that the two loci are closely linked. This is the basis of genetic association analysis. There has been considerable debate regarding what association analysis is capable of revealing (Hodge 1993; Spielman et al. 1994; Suarez and Hampe 1994). It is worth noting that association studies, when correctly designed, should be capable of detecting linkage disequilibrium, thus leading the investigator to finding the disease genes. Whenever possible, spurious associations should be ruled out by the very design.

Case-Controlled Studies

Let M denote the "hot allele" and m all other alleles, and let A denote the affected cases, and $\bar{A}$ the controls. The nonindependence between M and the disease may be described by a 2 × 2 table with the four probability values defining the odds ratio:

$$P(M|A) \quad P(m|\bar{A})$$
$$P(m|A) \quad P(M|\bar{A})$$

It is easy to see that if population estimates are used in the above formula in place of controls, it gives a measure of relative risk (Elston 1998). If there are more than two alleles, we have an $m \times 2$ table or m 2 × 2 tables (classified by "hot" and "other" alleles). Although a Pearson's χ^2 test of $m - 1$ df is a reasonable choice to test for the overall nonindependence, investigators often choose specific alleles and perform 1 df tests over a few 2 × 2 tables and achieve greater power even with Bonferroni-type corrections.

The above is a simple design for association studies. If a genetic model is assumed/given, one can derive/estimate haplotype probabilities conditional on affection status as well as other population parameters (effective population size, generation of disease mutation, etc.). A maximum likelihood scheme and the resulting likelihood ratio test can then be used to make an inference on the linkage equilibrium (Kaplan et al. 1995; Terwilliger 1995; Weir 1990). With such refinement, more parameters can be incorporated in the model and the method can be used for mapping of complex traits. For example, the likelihood method proposed by Terwilliger (1995) should work for multiple alleles and many marker loci. Certain factors in such a simple design are often out of the control of the investigators, resulting in spurious associations. For example, nongenetic causes such as population stratification by admixture and/or nonrandom mating may manifest a false association in the population.

Transmission Disequilibrium Test and Other Family-Based Methods

To remedy the problem of spurious association, Falk and Rubinstein (1987) proposed using untransmitted genotypes that did not pass to a case as a matched control and presented a haplotype relative risk test statistic. This design ensures that the controls are from the same subpopulation as the cases and therefore eliminates spurious associations caused by admixture. Ott and colleagues constructed tests using the marginals of the 2 × 2 table (haplotype-based haplotype relative risk test) and used McNemar's statistic (Ott 1989; Terwilliger and Ott 1992). A more general treatment using the contingency test was later proposed, called the affected family-based controls method (Thomson 1995). Spielman and colleagues (Spielman et al. 1993) showed that the transmission disequilibrium test (TDT), based on the matched design of Falk and Rubinstein, is a valid test of linkage in the presence of association (even if it was not linkage induced). They also showed that it is also a valid test of association given that only simplex families (trio families consisting of parents and an affected child) are used for the calculation (Spielman and Ewens 1996). For multiplex families, the test is unnecessarily conservative. Various extensions of the TDT to multiple marker alleles (Rice et al. 1995; Sham and Curtis 1995), sibship data (Speilman and Ewens 1998), discordant sib pairs (Boehnke and Langefeld 1998), and pedigrees (George et al. 1999) have been proposed.

Genomic Linkage Disequilibrium Scan

The enhanced power of the TDT method was shown by Risch and Meri-kangas (1996), who demonstrated dramatic differences in the sample sizes required by a linkage design and an association design using the TDT. These observations led to the concept of genomewide linkage disequilib-rium (LD) scans. When large numbers of single nucleotide polymorphisms (SNPs) are available throughout the genome, such a design may be at-tractive for the mapping of complex traits.

However, the glamour seems to be fading as people have more closely examined the design and discovered that the power of the LD method decreases quickly as the LD effect deviates from its maximum (i.e., the marker is not really close to the trait locus, or the marker allele frequency is different from that of the disease allele; see Abel and Müller-Myshok [1998]). Another problem comes from the overwhelmingly large number of repeated tests, because an association scan requires very large numbers of SNPs. How to control for false positives is still an open question. More-over, SNPs are not evenly distributed along the genome, and it is not clear how that should be reflected in an LD study design. For other issues per-taining to genomewide association scans with SNPs, see Weber and Bro-man (2001).

One possible solution is to employ a two-stage design: in the first stage a linkage scan is used to identify promising regions and then narrow them down by means of dense mapping; in the second stage partial association scans are performed in the candidate regions identified in the first stage. To do this, however, we first need to address the following issues: 1) How many polymorphic markers or diallelic SNPs are necessary for the second-stage detailed scanning of the hit regions? 2) How does the magnitude of LD between markers and that between a marker and the trait locus affect the power of a two-stage design? 3) What marker characteristics (hetero-zygosity, spacing, etc.) are most important in such a design? It may be desirable to confine the second stage to only the positional candidate genes in the regions identified in the first stage. With careful attention to these issues, the two-stage design may become attractive for mapping complex traits.

When the trait in question is quantitative, a polychotomization method was proposed by Allison (1997) as an extension of the TDT. Also, George et al. (1999) presented a TDT-like procedure for quantitative traits in ped-igrees using multiple regression. Methods testing linkage and association effects jointly have also been proposed. The MASC method of Clerget-

Darpoux et al. (1988) considers marker association and segregation jointly with the disease. More recently, Fulker et al. (1999) proposed a method of regression where the linkage effect is modeled according to the variance components formulation and the LD effect is modeled in the means; they showed an appreciable enhancement of the power to detect QTLs. A similar extension of the SEGPATH method has recently been presented (Gu et al. 1999b).

Meta-Analysis

The application of meta-analytical techniques to genetic studies began only recently (Gu et al. 1998c; Li and Rao 1996; Rice 1998). The term *meta-analysis* is used for a wide variety of statistical procedures developed for quantitative reviews of summary statistics from clinical trials and epidemiological studies (see Olkin [1995] for a review). For continuous outcomes, methods analogous to the traditional analysis of variance may be employed to estimate the grand mean and the standard error. In short, meta-analysis treats summary statistics from primary studies as raw data and pools quantitative effect sizes across multiple studies.

In general, meta-analysis involves a preanalysis procedure where the literature on the subject is collected and its quality is assessed. The analysis step then defines a certain common effect, which is extracted from the primary studies, and statistical models are constructed and tested on these effects; then possible trends in effect sizes are examined. Finally, a postanalysis procedure interprets the final results, resolving the source of any heterogeneity across studies and formulating and testing new hypotheses. We want to emphasize the importance of the preanalysis procedure to the success of any meta-analysis study. As a rule of thumb, assessment of possible publication bias should always be performed prior to synthesizing results.

For meta-analysis of linkage results, we proposed using the proportion of IBD genes shared at a marker locus by a sib pair with specified trait outcomes as a common effect variable for pooling, and we gave a procedure for extracting and combining the common linkage effects from linkage studies employing nonparametric sib-pair methods (Gu et al. 1998c). A random effects model was used to characterize the among-study variability in the effect, and a weighted estimate of the overall effect and the variance components were given using the weighted least squares method. A heterogeneity test was also provided to assess variability among studies. Gu et al. (1998c) also presented detailed discussion of the meta-analysis methodology, design issues, and practical issues on its application to mapping disease genes. Recently, we extended this model to incorporate study-specific covariates using a mixed effects model that enables explanation of possible heterogeneity among studies (Gu et al. 1999a).

Multivariate Methods

Another characteristic of complex traits is that clinical disease often manifests in a battery of correlated traits that need appropriate methods of multivariate analysis. Todorov et al. (1998) proposed a treatment of multiple traits using structural relationships among multiple phenotypes to differentiate direct causal effects from intermediate influence of genes. The multivariate analysis methods such as principal component analysis and factor analysis are often used to reduce the dimensionality of data (e.g., Bartholomew 1987). With respect to genetic studies, the principal component analysis method can be used to construct a few summary phenotypes (explaining most of the variance) from a large number of correlated traits, which can be used in turn for genetic analysis (e.g., Gu et al. 1998b). Alternatively, the method of latent factor analysis can be used to select a group of latent factors that could explain the observed correlation structure in the multivariate phenotypic data (Neuman et al. 1999). The ideal case would be that the latent factors selected coincide well with the actual underlying genetic loci responsible for the observed multiple traits, so that although all relationships are not detected, most if not all the loci and their major effects are reconstructed. One essential question about such reduction methods is how genetic variance is reflected in the orthogonalized components. Because the dimension of data that carries most of the variance may not coincide with that associated with genetic sources, linkage analysis of major principal components may produce only false negatives, and the linkage signals may be found in secondary components (Goldin and Chase 1999; Olson et al. 1999). Further investigation of such reduction methods is needed to study the effect on decomposition of complex diseases. Whenever possible, full multivariate methods employing multilocus models, such as in SOLAR and SEGPATH, should continue to be used.

Subgroup Analyses

Although analysis of aggregate samples employing sophisticated models has the potential to uncover complex trait genes, sometimes we have to rethink the way we analyze data. Subgroup analyses may offer added comfort in terms of getting the most from the data and for interpreting the overall performance of these methods.

Context Dependency

It is generally recognized that complex traits are derived from the inter-actions among many genes and nongenetic determinants. It is increasingly believed that the genes contributing to complex traits do not have the same effect across all times or across all environments. In general, context-dependent effects may be more likely to be detected when the contexts are explicitly considered (Cheverud and Routman 1995; Kardia 2000; Turner et al. 1999). When exploring the relationships between genetic variation and phenotypic variation, it is therefore instructive to carry out some of the analyses within particular contexts. The most important spe-cific contexts seem to be age, sex, and family history. Additional contexts may also be warranted depending on the trait of interest, such as general body size when dealing with cardiovascular and fitness related traits. Like-wise, socioeconomic factors might provide an additional context when dealing with diagnoses based on assessments.

Classification and Regression Trees

Another approach is to subdivide the data into potentially more homo-geneous subgroups, with the expectation that a simpler model with very few interacting determinants might suffice for analyses of individual sub-groups. The classification and regression trees (CART) methodology offers one promising way to subdivide the data (Breiman et al. 1984). The CART approach provides a purpose-oriented methodology for partitioning a data set into relatively homogeneous subgroups that give a gradient of risk to an outcome.

An inherent attraction of the CART methodology is that it assumes that interactions among the independent variables (the predictors) are more the rule than the exception, which appears to be the case with complex traits. The CART methods typically partition the data through a series of binary splits using one predictor at a time. In genetic studies, the CART methods can be used to focus attention on those families where the signal is the greatest. This could be done by using relevant covariate information to identify clinically and/or biologically more homogeneous subgroups, within each of which the disease etiology may be expected to be more homogeneous. Applications of this methodology for linkage studies are in the early stages (Province et al. 2001; Rao 1998; Shannon et al. 2001).

Interpretation of Results

As more and more markers become available and are used in genomewide scans, the ensuing analyses give rise to the problem of multiple testing. Therefore, some correction for multiple testing is necessary before declaring a result as a failure or a success. Failure to correct for multiple testing will inevitably yield far too many positive results, many of which would be false. Likewise, overcorrection for multiple testing will inevitably lead to far fewer positive results, thus missing some or even most of the very signals we seek in the first place. Perhaps some reasonable guidelines need to be followed so as to minimize both types of error (false positives that cannot be replicated and false negatives that remain undetected). It should be clarified that linkage analysis was used in earlier days for localizing genes that were already known to exist. Therefore, one could afford to use relatively more stringent criteria (such as a lod score of 3) because failure to localize a gene (which was known to exist) was acceptable. However, falsely mapping a gene to a wrong location had dire consequences in terms of the cost associated with following up on false positives. In stark contrast, linkage analysis of complex traits now serves a dual purpose: proving the very existence of a trait gene and finding its location on the gene map. Therefore, errors in inference have a different meaning and value now, although pursuing false positives still continues to be costly. This puts an extra degree of burden on the analyst when trying to interpret the results.

Significance Levels

It is important to note that a significance level merely indicates one's tolerance for inferring a false result. Choice of appropriate significance levels for genomewide scans has been a thorny issue (Lander and Kruglyak 1995; Morton 1998; Rao 1998; Risch 1991; Thomson 1994). Although everyone agrees that reporting false positives is both undesirable and misleading, the issue of false negatives (i.e., missing true signals) has not received the attention it deserves. For example, Lander and Kruglyak (1995) have recommended that the genomewide significance level α_g be set at 0.05, and that the pointwise (nominal) significance level α for an individual test with each marker be determined approximately from the equation $\alpha_g = (23 + 132T_\alpha^2)\alpha$, where T_α is the standard normal deviate corresponding to the nominal significance level of α (Feingold et al. 1993; Lander and Kruglyak 1995). For example, $\alpha_g = 0.05$ yields $\alpha = 0.000022$.

Although the desire to practically eliminate false positives is commendable, one should evaluate the implications of both false positives and false negatives before adopting such a stringent significance level.

The equation for computing the nominal α was based on an assumption of continuous marker density. Relaxing this assumption so as to correspond to actual practice (with a density of about 400 markers per genome scan) gives rise to a less stringent significance level (which can be computed from the approximations given by Feingold et al. [1993]). Finally, the total genome length is assumed to be 34 M, which may be slightly different from the assumptions that others have made. See Thomson (2001) and Cheverud (2001) for the most recent discussions on significance levels in genome scans. Finally, see Province (2000, 2001) for new methods of analysis and interpretation of genome scan data. These sequential methods hold a lot of promise and bypass the problem of multiple testing.

Trade-Off Between False Positives and False Negatives

It is highly desirable to strike a balance between the false positives and false negatives without neglecting or dismissing either. This is even more important for complex traits because the effect of any one gene is likely to be modest, which makes it that much more difficult to detect even with more moderate significance thresholds. We simply cannot afford to miss real signals.

Lander and Kruglyak (1995) have essentially recommended that we accept, on average, one false positive in 20 genome scans ($\alpha_g = 0.05$, which corresponds to a nominal α of 0.000022 and a lod score of 3.63). To safeguard against missing real linkages, Rao (1998) suggested relaxing the threshold so as to tolerate, on average, one false positive per genome scan (which also corresponds closely to the recommendation of Thomson [1994] to use $\alpha = 0.001$). Under continuous marker density, this corresponds to a nominal $\alpha = 0.00071$ (corresponding to a lod score of 2.21). If the marker density is adjusted to a total of 400 markers, this nominal α increases further to 0.0023 (which corresponds to a lod score of 1.75) (Rao and Province 2000), and Lander-Kruglyak's nominal α also increases from 0.000022 (corresponding to a lod score of 3.63) to 0.000090 (corresponding to a lod score of 3.05, which is remarkably the same as Morton's time-tested value). Although a nominal α of 0.0023 as suggested by Rao and Province (2000) produces on average one false positive per genome scan, it leads to impressive gains in power, thus minimizing nondetection of signals.

On balance, for genetic dissection of complex traits, it seems advisable to use the less stringent significance level of $\alpha = 0.0023$ for the purpose of identifying which genomic regions may be pursued further. In this case, other approaches should be developed for discriminating between false positives and real positives. On the other hand, when dealing with large samples and especially when major gene effects are expected, it is desirable to use the more stringent significance level of $\alpha = 0.00009$. In such cases, the more stringent criteria provide ample protection against false positives. See Rao and Gu (2001) for additional discussion of this subject.

Discussion

The study of human disease has fully arrived in the molecular age. Progress of the Human Genome Project has provided molecular tools necessary for the genetic dissection of human diseases and disorders. Yet, significant challenges remain, especially in understanding complex traits, which include such entities as coronary heart disease, hypertension, and most psychiatric disorders. Many complex traits are also common in the population, accounting for a significant proportion of the public health burden. In contrast to Mendelian traits, one seeks to identify the genes that influence *predisposition* to complex diseases rather than those that *cause* them, which is a considerably more daunting task that mandates newer and more imaginative approaches.

This is an exciting time to be a genetic epidemiologist, with unprecedented new opportunities unfolding that we could only dream of a few short years ago. Although we know that complex traits arise from interactions among multiple genes and environments, we have done little to date to reflect that realization. Most studies investigating the genetic basis of complex traits routinely ignore the interactions. We are only beginning to realize that complex traits need to be handled more thoughtfully if we are to discover their genes and begin to understand the way genes and environments work together. It is this realization that prompts investigators to come up with more innovative approaches for dealing with the outstanding challenges of the passing millennium. We begin the new millennium with challenges, but with it come enormous opportunities.

A genetic epidemiologist can hardly be overequipped with tools, and a tool that works in one case may not work in the next. So long as our primary objective is to find genes for complex diseases and disease-related traits, we should be willing to consider alternative strategies. In particular, we believe that a combination of lumping and splitting strategies can be useful. The lumping strategies include pooling data and/or results from multiple studies. Although pooling data may sometimes introduce greater heterogeneity, and therefore may at first seem counterintuitive, it can result in substantially more power, especially if the analytical methods can accommodate complications of heterogeneity. Alternatively, one may consider pooling the results from different studies using meta-analysis methods. Both approaches to lumping have their strengths and drawbacks, and one may be preferable over the other in a given context.

Splitting strategies involve subdividing the aggregate data into multiple homogeneous subgroups, and this may be done through the CART methodology or through other multivariate clustering techniques. In this case, separate analyses within subgroups may actually come with inherently more power. These strategies are particularly useful if, for example, different trait genes or subsets thereof operate within the subgroups.

Perhaps even more importantly, both lumping and splitting may be pursued at the same time. For example, data from multiple studies may all be pooled first. With the luxury of a much larger aggregate sample size, one may then undertake splitting the pooled data into multiple homogeneous subgroups, which could yield reasonably large sample sizes even within subgroups. This assumes that no single study may be capable of successfully dissecting the genetic architecture of a given complex trait/disease. There is tremendous opportunity for meaningful collaborations, and this may be the limiting factor in whether we succeed. For such collaborations to be productive, one must go beyond a mere willingness to share data. After all, the question is not whether there are genes, only when and how they might be found.

References

Abel L, Müller-Myshok B: Maximum-likelihood expression of the transmission/disequilibrium test and power considerations. Am J Hum Genet 63:664–667, 1998

Allison BB: Transmission-disequilibrium tests for quantitative traits. Am J Hum Genet 60:676–690, 1997

Amos CI: Robust variance-components approach for assessing genetic linkage in pedigrees. Am J Hum Genet 54:535–543, 1994

Barnard GA: Statistical inference. Journal of the Royal Statistical Society B11:115–139, 1949

Bartholomew DJ: Latent Variable Models and Factor Analysis. New York, Oxford University Press, 1987

Begleiter H, Reich T, Hasselbrock V, et al: The collaborative study on the genetics of alcoholism. Alcohol Health Research 19:228–236, 1995

Blackwelder WC, Elston RC: A comparison of sib-pair linkage tests for disease susceptibility loci. Genet Epidemiol 2:85–97, 1985

Blangero J, Almasy L: SOLAR: Sequential Oligogenic Linkage Analysis Routines (Technical Notes). San Antonio, TX, Southwest Foundation for Biomedical Research, Population Genetics Laboratory, 1996

Boehnke M, Langefeld CD: Genetic association mapping based on discordant sib pairs: the discordant-allele test. Am J Hum Genet 62:950–961, 1998

Breiman L, Friedman JH, Olshen RA, et al: Classification and Regression Trees. Belmont, CA, Wadsworth International Group, 1984

Carey G, Williamson JA: Linkage analysis of quantitative traits: increased power by using selected samples. Am J Hum Genet 49:786–796, 1991

Cheverud J: A simple correction for multiple comparisons in interval mapping genome scans. Heredity 87:52–58, 2001

Cheverud J, Routman EJ: Epistasis and its contribution to genetic variance components. Genetics 139:963–971, 1995

Clerget-Darpoux F, Bonaçti-Pellié C, Hochez J: Effects of misspecifying genetic parameters in lod score analysis. Biometrics 42:393–399, 1986

Clerget-Darpoux F, Babron MC, Prum B, et al: A new method to test genetic models in HLA associated diseases: the MASC method. Ann Hum Genet 52:247–258, 1988

Eaves LJ: Effect of genetic architecture on the power of human linkage studies to resolve the contribution of quantitative trait loci. Heredity 72:175–192, 1994

Elston RC: Designs for the global search of the human genome by linkage analysis, in Proceedings of the XVIth International Biometric Conference, Hamilton, New Zealand, 1992, pp 39–51

Elston RC: Linkage and association. Genet Epidemiol 15:565–576, 1998

Elston RC, Cordell H: Overview of model-free methods for linkage analysis. In Genetic Dissection of Complex Traits. Edited by Rao DC, Province MA. San Diego, CA, Academic Press, 2001

Elston RC, Stewart J: A general model for genetic analysis of pedigree data. Hum Hered 21:523–542, 1971

Elston RC, Guo X, Williams LV: Two-stage global search designs for linkage analysis using pairs of affected relatives. Genet Epidemiol 13:535–558, 1996

Elston RC, Buxbaum S, Jacobs KB, et al: Haseman and Elston revisited. Genet Epidemiol 19:1–17, 2000

Falk CT, Rubinstein P: Haplotype relative risks: an easy reliable way to construct a proper control sample for risk calculations. Ann Hum Genet 51:227–233, 1987

Feingold E, Brown PO, Siegmund D: Gaussian models for genetic linkage analysis using complete high-resolution maps of identity-by-descent. Am J Hum Genet 53:234–251, 1993

Fulker DW, Cardon LR: A sib-pair approach to interval mapping of Quantitative Trait Loci. Am J Hum Genet 54:1092–1103, 1994

Fulker DW, Cherny SS, Sham PC, et al: Combined linkage and association sib-pair analysis for quantitative traits. Am J Hum Genet 64:259–267, 1999

George V, Tiwari HK, Zhu X, et al: A test of transmission/disequilibrium for quantitative traits in pedigree data, by multiple regression. Am J Hum Genet 65:236–245, 1999

Goldgar D: Multipoint analysis of human quantitative genetic variation. Am J Hum Genet 47:957–967, 1990

Goldin LR, Chase GA: Comparison of two linkage inference procedures for genes related to the P300 component of the ERP. Genet Epidemiol 17:S163–S167, 1999

Gu C, Rao DC: A linkage strategy for detection of human quantitative trait loci, I: generalized relative risk ratios and power of sibpairs with extreme trait values. Am J Hum Genet 61:200–210, 1997a

Gu C, Rao DC: A linkage strategy for detection of human quantitative trait loci, II: optimization of study designs based on extreme sibpairs and generalized relative risk ratios. Am J Hum Genet 61:211–222, 1997b

Gu C, Suarez BK, Reich T, et al: A chromosome-based method to infer IBD scores for missing and ambiguous markers. Genet Epidemiol 12:871–876, 1995

Gu C, Todorov AA, Rao DC: Combining extremely concordant sibpairs with extremely discordant sibpairs provides a cost-effective way to linkage analysis of QTL. Genet Epidemiol 13:513–533, 1996

Gu C, Rice T, Pérusse L, et al: Principal component analysis of morphological measures in the Québec Family Study: familial correlation. American Journal of Human Biology 9:725–733, 1997

Gu C, Miller MA, Reich T, et al: The affected-pedigree-member method revisited under population stratification, in Statistical Methods in Genetics (The IMA Volumes in Mathematics and Its Applications, Vol 112). Springer-Verlag, New York, 1998a, pp 165–180

Gu C, Province MA, Rao DC: A meta-analysis methodology for combining results of family based genetic association studies. Paper presented at the seventh annual meeting of the International Genetic Epidemiology Society, Archachon, France, September 1998b

Gu C, Province MA, Todorov AA, et al: Meta-analysis methodology for combining non-parametric sibpair linkage results: genetic homogeneity and identical markers. Genet Epidemiol 15:609–626, 1998c

Gu C, Province MA, Rao DC: A meta-analysis approach for pooling sibpair linkage studies with study-specific covariates: mixed effects models. Genet Epidemiol 17:S599–604, 1999a

Gu C, Province MA, Rao DC: Precision mapping of human QTLs by combined linkage/disequilibrium analysis. Genet Epidemiol 17:227, 1999b

Haseman JK, Elston RC: The investigation of linkage between a quantitative trait and a marker locus. Behav Genet 2:3–19, 1972

Higgins M, Province MA, Heiss G, et al: The NHLBI Family Heart Study: objectives and design. Genet Epidemiol 143:1219–1228, 1996

Hodge SE: Linkage analysis versus association analysis: distinguishing between two models that explain disease-marker associations. Am J Hum Genet 53:367–384, 1993

Holmans P: Asymptotic properties of affected sibpair linkage analysis. Am J Hum Genet 52:362–374, 1993

Kardia SLR: Context-dependent effects in hypertension. Curr Hypertens Rep 2(1):32–38, 2000

Kaplan NL, Hill WG, Weir B: Likelihood methods for locating disease genes in nonequilibrium populations. Am J Hum Genet 56:18–32, 1995

Kong A, Cox NJ: Allele-sharing models: lod scores and accurate linkage tests. Am J Hum Genet 61:1179–1188, 1997

Kruglyak L, Lander E: Complete multipoint sib-pair analysis of qualitative and quantitative traits. Am J Hum Genet 57:439–454, 1995

Lander E, Green P: Construction of multilocus genetic linkage maps in humans. Proc Natl Acad Sci U S A 84:2363–2367, 1987

Lander E, Kruglyak L: Genetic dissection of complex traits: guidelines for interpreting and reporting linkage results. Nat Genet 11:241–247, 1995

Lathrop GM, Lalouel JM, Julier C, et al: Strategies for multilocus linkage analysis in humans. Proc Natl Acad Sci U S A 81:3443–3446, 1984

Li Z, Rao DC: A random effect model for meta-analysis of multiple quantitative sibpair linkage studies. Genet Epidemiol 13:377–383, 1996

Morton NE: Sequential tests for the detection of linkage. Am J Hum Genet 7:277–318, 1955

Morton NE: Significant levels in complex inheritance. Am J Hum Genet 62:690–697, 1998

Neuman RJ, Todd RD, Heath AC, et al: Evaluation of ADHD typology in three contrasting samples: a latent class approach. J Am Acad Child Adolesc Psychiatry 38:25–33, 1999

Olkin I: Statistical and theoretical consideration in meta-analysis. J Clin Epidemiol 48:133–146, 1995

Olson JM, Rao S, Jacobs K, et al: Linkage of chromosome 1 markers to alcoholism-related phenotypes by sibpair linkage analysis of principal components. Genet Epidemiol 17:S271–276, 1999

Ott J: Estimation of the recombination fraction in human pedigrees: efficient computation of the likelihood for human linkage studies. Am J Hum Genet 26:588–597, 1974

Ott J: Statistical properties of the haplotype relative risk. Genet Epidemiol 6:127–130, 1989

Penrose LS: The detection of autosomal linkage in data which consists of brothers and sisters. Annals of Eugenics 6:133–138, 1935

Province MA: A single, sequential, genome-wide test to simultaneously identify all promising areas in a linkage scan. Genet Epidemiol 19(4):301–322, 2000

Province MA: Linkage and association with structural relationships, in Genetic Dissection of Complex Traits. Edited by Rao DC, Province MA. San Diego, CA, Academic Press, 2001, pp 183–190

Province MA, Rice T, Borecki IB, et al: A multivariate and multilocus variance components approach using structural relationships to assess quantitative trait linkage via SEGPATH. Genet Epidemiol (in press)

Province MA, Shannon WA, Rao DC: Classification methods, in Genetic Dissection of Complex Traits. Edited by Rao DC, Province MA. San Diego, CA, Academic Press, 2001, pp 273–286

Rao DC: CAT scans, PET scans, and genomic scans. Genet Epidemiol 15:1–18, 1998

Rao DC, Gu C: False positives and false negatives in genomic scans, in Genetic Dissection of Complex Traits. Edited by Rao DC, Province MA. San Diego, CA, Academic Press, 2001, pp 487–498

Rao DC, Province MA: The future of path analysis, segregation analysis, and combined models for genetic dissection of complex traits. Hum Hered 50:34–42, 2000

Rice JP: The role of meta-analysis in linkage studies of complex traits. Am J Med Genet 74:112–114, 1998

Rice J, Neuman R, Hoshaw S, et al: TDT tests with covariates and genomic screens with mod scores: their behavior on simulated data. Genet Epidemiol 12:659–664, 1995

Risch N: Linkage strategies for genetically complex traits, I: multilocus models. Am J Hum Genet 46:222–228, 1990a

Risch N: Linkage strategies for genetically complex traits, II: the power of affected relative pairs. Am J Hum Genet 46:229–241, 1990b

Risch N: A note on multiple testing procedures in linkage analysis. Am J Hum Genet 48:1058–1064, 1991

Risch N, Giuffra L: Model misspecification and multipoint linkage analysis. Hum Hered 42:77–92, 1992

Risch N, Merikangas K: The future of genetic studies of complex human diseases. Science 273:1516–1517, 1996

Risch N, Zhang H: Extreme discordant sibpairs for mapping quantitative trait loci in humans. Science 268:1584–1589, 1995

Sandkuyl LA: Analysis of affected sib pairs using information from extended families. Progress in Clinical Biological Research 329:117–122, 1989

Sham PC, Curtis D: An extended transmission/disequilibrium test (TDT) for multi-allele marker loci. Ann Hum Genet 59:323–336, 1995

Shannon WD, Province MA, Rao DC: Tree-based recursive partitioning methods for subdividing sibpairs into relatively more homogeneous subgroups. Genet Epidemiol 20:293–306, 2001

Spielman RS, Ewens WJ: The TDT and other family based tests for linkage disequilibrium and association (invited editorial). Am J Hum Genet 59:983–989, 1996

Spielman RS, Ewens WJ: A sibship test for linkage in the presence of association: the sib transmission/disequilibrium test. Am J Hum Genet 62:450–458, 1998

Spielman RS, McGinnis RE, Ewens WJ: Transmission test for linkage disequilibrium: the insulin gene region and insulin-dependent diabetes mellitus (IDDM). Am J Hum Genet 52:506–516, 1993

Spielman RS, McGinnis RE, Ewens WJ: The transmission/disequilibrium test detects cosegregation and linkage (letter to the editor). Am J Hum Genet 54:559–560, 1994

Suarez BK, Hampe CL: Linkage and association (letter to the editor). Am J Hum Genet 54:554–559, 1994

Suarez BK, Rice JP, Reich T: The generalized sib pair ibd distribution: its use in the detection of linkage. Ann Hum Genet 42:87–94, 1978

Suarez BK, Hampe CL, Van Eerdewegh P: Problems of replicating linkage claims in psychiatry, in Genetic Approaches to Mental Disorders. Edited by Gershon ES, Cloninger CR. Washington, DC, American Psychiatric Press, 1994, pp 23–46

Terwilliger JD: A powerful likelihood method for the analysis of linkage disequilibrium between trait loci and one or more polymorphic marker loci. Am J Hum Genet 56:777–787, 1995

Terwilliger JD, Ott J: A haplotype-based "haplotype relative" risk approach to detect allelic associations. Hum Hered 42:337–346, 1992

Terwilliger JD, Ott J: A novel polylocus method for linkage analysis using lod-score or sib-pair method. Genet Epidemiol 10:477–482, 1993

Thomson G: Identifying complex disease genes: progress and paradigms. Nat Genet 8:108–110, 1994

Thomson G: Mapping disease genes: family based association studies. Am J Hum Genet 57:487–498, 1995

Thomson G: Significance levels in genomic scans, in Genetic Dissection of Complex Traits. Edited by Rao DC, Province MA. San Diego, CA, Academic Press, 2001, pp 475–486

Todorov AA, Rao DC: Trade-off between false positives and false negatives in the linkage analysis of complex traits. Genet Epidemiol 14:453–464, 1997

Todorov AA, Province MA, Borecki IB, et al: Trade-off between sibship size and sampling scheme for detecting quantitative trait loci. Hum Hered 47:1–5, 1997

Todorov AA, Vogler GP, Gu C, et al: Testing causal hypotheses in multivariate linkage analysis of quantitative traits: general formulation and application to sibpair data. Genet Epidemiol 15:263–278, 1998

Turner ST, Boerwinkle E, Sing CF: Context-dependent associations of the ACE I/D polymorphism with blood pressure. Hypertension 34(part 2):773–778, 1999

Weber J, Broman K: Human whole genome polymorphism scans: past, present and future, in Genetic Dissection of Complex Traits. Edited by Rao DC, Province MA. San Diego, CA, Academic Press, 2001, pp 77–96

Weeks DE, Lange K: The affected-pedigree-member method of linkage analysis. Am J Hum Genet 42:315–326, 1988

Weeks DE, Lehner T, Squires-Wheeler E, et al: Measuring the inflation of the lod score due to its maximization over model parameter values in human linkage analysis. Genet Epidemiol 7:237–243, 1990

Weir B: Genetic Data Analysis: Methods for Discrete Population Genetic Data. Sunderland, MA, Sinauer Associates, 1990

Wijsman EM, Amos CI: Genetic analysis of simulated oligogenic traits in nuclear families and extended families. Genet Epidemiol 14:719–735, 1997

CHAPTER TWO

Relevance of Normal Personality for Psychiatrists

C. Robert Cloninger, M.D.

Psychiatrists are expected to be able to understand and predict human behavior as well as to offer prevention and treatment of the disorders that arise in everyday life. At least for complex behaviors that involve emotion, cognition, and voluntary action, we need to begin such an understanding with the description of an individual's usual ways of feeling, thinking, and acting. This means that we need to describe and understand personalities of others. Recent research on personality, including its psychometrics, psychobiology, and genetics, has led to several major findings that cast a new light on the importance of normal personality for the practice of psychiatry. First, human personality has the same multidimensional structure in the general population and in clinical samples. This suggests that there are no sharp natural demarcations between what we choose to distinguish as normal and abnormal personality traits. Second, individual differences in multidimensional profiles of quantitative personality traits permit definitions of personality disorder that agree with traditional categorical distinctions. This suggests that personality disorders are extremes of quantitative variables with no natural boundaries between what is normal and what is abnormal. Third, individual differences in these same quantitative personality traits are associated with differences in the risk of the full range of psychopathology from neurosis to psychosis. This suggests that severe psychopathology emerges from vulnerabilities that can be quantified in terms of premorbid personality traits. Fourth, personality traits are the strongest predictors of response to treatment with both drugs and psychotherapy. This suggests that assessment of personality is essential for efficiency and effectiveness of treatment planning. Fifth, individual differences in patterns of lifestyle choice about diet, drinking, smoking, exercise, health care, and stress management—which are notoriously resistant to change—are strongly related to individual differences in personality. This suggests that noncompliance with public health recommendations, as well as personality disorders, may be understood as maladaptive behaviors related to individual differences in personality.

A comprehensive bibliography regarding these major findings is beyond the scope of this chapter. Instead, I describe the seminal studies that led to these conclusions using the Temperament and Character Inventory (TCI) and its forerunner, the Tridimensional Personality Questionnaire (Cloninger 1987; Cloninger et al. 1993). Additional information has been reviewed in more detail in other articles that are cited to guide interested readers (Cloninger 1999b; Cloninger et al. 1994, 1998a). This work has been carried out in order to provide a comprehensive model of human personality to guide hypothesis testing, as well as to provide reliable, easy-to-use assessment instruments that can be used in both psychobiological research and clinical practice.

The Structure of Human Personality

The first major finding about the relevance of normal personality for psychiatry is the observation that human personality has the same multidimensional structure in the general population and in samples of psychiatric outpatients or inpatients (Cloninger 1999b). Factor analytic studies of descriptors of behavior in natural language show that there are seven dimensions (Waller 1999). Earlier work with selected lists of descriptors had suggested that there are five dimensions, but these excluded terms of negative and positive valence relevant to psychiatry (Waller 1999). There are at least two major systems of learning and memory in humans, including procedural learning of habits and skills and propositional learning of goals and values (Cloninger 1994). These differences are preserved in the TCI by distinguishing between temperament and character traits.

Temperament is defined in terms of behaviors that can be understood in terms of individual differences in habit learning by reward and punishment. Character is defined in terms of goals and values, or what we make of ourselves intentionally.

The TCI measures four dimensions of temperament: Harm Avoidance (anxious vs. calm), Novelty Seeking (impulsive vs. reflective), Reward Dependence (warm vs. aloof), and Persistence (steadfast vs. fickle). It also measures three dimensions of character: Self-Directedness (resourceful vs. helpless), Cooperativeness (empathic vs. hostile), and Self-Transcendence (self-forgetful vs. acquisitive). Advocates of alternative assessment inventories may partition personality according to different variables, but these are well explained in terms of weighted combinations of the seven TCI dimensions (Cloninger et al. 1994).

When the TCI is administered to samples of psychiatric patients, the same multidimensional structure is observed as when it is administered to samples representative of the general population (Bayon et al. 1996; Cloninger 1991, 1994; Svrakic et al. 1993) on five different continents. The mean values of some traits may differ between patients and normal subjects, but the variability of each trait and the correlations among the traits are the same regardless of the presence of psychopathology. All personality varies quantitatively along multiple dimensions that are independent or weakly correlated. If personality profiles also predict the type of psychopathology (as shown in a later section), then this means that personality traits are either the defining characteristics or at least vulnerability indicators for psychiatric disorder.

General Criteria for Personality Disorders

Our current official system for classifying personality disorders, DSM-IV-TR (American Psychiatric Association 2000), has several serious problems, all related to the basic assumption that personality disorders are composed of multiple discrete categories of illness. There is no evidence for natural boundaries separating one category of personality disorder from another, so individuals who satisfy criteria for one category often satisfy criteria for multiple categories (Svrakic et al. 1993).

The absence of natural boundaries suggests that the basic assumption of discrete categories is in error. On the one hand, individuals who meet criteria for a disorder in the erratic (B) cluster often also meet criteria for a disorder in the anxious (C) cluster (Svrakic et al. 1993). On the other hand, there is extensive heterogeneity within categories of personality disorder. This is a consequence of the use of a long list of weakly correlated items to diagnose each category; individuals may qualify for a diagnosis by means of different items and have few or no items in common.

In recent clinical research, I have found that it is possible to understand the variation between and within categories in terms of profiles of multiple dimensions of personality. Specifically, individuals with any personality disorder are low in certain traits of character as measured by the TCI (Cloninger et al. 1993). For example, all categories of personality disorder are distinguished by low TCI Self-Directedness regardless of the cluster or category of personality disorder (Cloninger et al. 1993; Svrakic et al. 1993). Low Self-Directedness is defined by poor impulse control or weak ego strength as described by being irresponsible, purposeless, helpless, and low in self-acceptance. Likewise, most individuals with personality disorders are low in Cooperativeness, which is defined by poor interpersonal functioning as described by being intolerant, narcissistic, hostile or disagreeable, revengeful, and opportunistic. The core features of personality disorder can be rated in terms of severity from mild to severe (Cloninger 2000).

Research with the TCI by multiple independent groups has shown that different clusters are associated with different dimensions of temperament that are roughly independent (Svrakic et al. 1993). Specifically, Cluster C (anxious) disorders are characterized by high TCI Harm Avoidance, that is, being pessimistic, fearful, shy, anxious, and fatigable. Cluster B (impulsive) disorders are characterized by high TCI Novelty Seeking, that is, being easily bored, impulsive, quick-tempered, extravagant, and disorderly. Cluster C (aloof) disorders are characterized by low TCI Reward Dependence, that is, being aloof, independent, cold, insensitive, and unsentimental. In principle, this means that subtypes can be defined in a mutually exclusive fashion by their profile with regard to individual differences (high vs. low) along these three dimensions.

These findings have been replicated independently in several countries and indicate that personality disorders may be well defined in terms of individual differences in quantitative personality traits (Battaglia et al. 1996; Fossati et al. 1999; Mulder and Joyce 1997; Svrakic et al. 1993). The multidimensional structure of personality can be interpreted in terms of neurobiology, cognitive psychology, or psychodynamics, thereby allowing communication among practitioners with different training backgrounds (Mulder et al. 1996). Furthermore, independent replication of findings means that the causes of personality disorders can be discovered by studying personality as it varies quantitatively in the general population, which greatly increases the opportunities for molecular genetics research.

Comorbidity of Personality Disorders and Psychopathology

Extensive research using the TCI in samples of psychiatric patients and in the general population has revealed that different personality profiles are systematically associated with different forms of psychopathology (Battaglia et al. 1996; Bayon et al. 1996; Cloninger et al. 1994). This can be illustrated by the personality correlates of eating disorders. Patients with bulimia nervosa differ from those with anorexia nervosa: those with bulimia are high in both Novelty Seeking and Harm Avoidance, whereas those with anorexia are high in Persistence and Harm Avoidance (Brewerton et al. 1993; Kleifield et al. 1994). The binge-purge cycle in bulimia can be understood as a particular expression of the approach-avoidance conflict of individuals who are high in both Novelty Seeking (leading to bingeing) and Harm Avoidance (leading to purging). The high Harm Avoidance in both disorders is consistent with the anxiety-proneness of patients with eating disorders.

Likewise, the differences between patients with anxiety disorders and those with personality disorders are well understood in studies of personality (Bayon et al. 1996; Cloninger et al. 1994). High Harm Avoidance predisposes people to be low in Self-Directedness, so these two traits are moderately correlated. However, individuals with anxiety disorders are consistently high in Harm Avoidance but may or may not be low in Self-Directedness. In contrast, individuals with personality disorders are consistently low in Self-Directedness but may be high in Harm Avoidance (e.g., cluster C disorders) or low in Harm Avoidance (e.g., antisocial personality disorder). Individuals with substance dependence are usually high in Novelty Seeking and low in Self-Directedness (Cloninger 1999a; Cloninger et al. 1994). This is true of individuals with alcohol dependence, especially those with early onset and/or associated antisocial behavior.

Individuals with frequent somatization are usually high in Harm Avoidance and low in Self-Directedness (Cloninger et al. 1996). In other words, somatization involves both anxiety-proneness and immaturity.

Patients with major depressive disorders and dysthymia are also often high in Harm Avoidance and/or low in Self-Directedness. There is so much heterogeneity among those with depression that it may be more useful to describe them in terms of their underlying profile of temperament and character traits than in terms of subtypes that have been proposed on the basis of depressive symptoms and course. As described in the next section, the personality traits are more useful in treatment planning and predicting response to treatment than is any other clinical feature including severity and pattern of depressive symptoms (Joyce et al. 1994).

Personality as a Predictor of Treatment Response

A major finding about personality that has profound implications for clinical practice has been the importance of personality in predicting response to treatment for depression. Several independent studies now show that low TCI Harm Avoidance and high TCI Self-Directedness predict a rapid and good response to antidepressants, including both tricyclics and selective serotonin reuptake inhibitors (Joffe et al. 1993; Joyce et al. 1994; Tome et al. 1997). In contrast, individuals who are high in Harm Avoidance and low in Self-Directedness have a slow and poor response to such antidepressants. These personality traits explain from 35% to 50% of the variance in response to antidepressants (Joyce et al. 1994), whereas other features explain only a few percent of the variance.

Furthermore, differential response to particular antidepressants and other drugs may be predicted by other aspects of personality. For example, depressed individuals who are high in Novelty Seeking respond more rapidly and better to pindolol as an adjunct to paroxetine than do those who are low in Novelty Seeking.

In addition, personality is a crucial variable in predicting the response to cognitive-behavioral therapy. When patients with bulimia are treated with cognitive-behavioral therapy, those who are high in Self-Directedness respond rapidly and remain well after 1 year, whereas those who are low in Self-Directedness respond slowly and frequently relapse by one year (Bulik et al. 1998, 1999). Likewise, the TCI is useful in identifying the emotional conflicts and personality traits underlying problem areas in interpersonal psychotherapy (Luty et al. 1998). It is interesting that Harm Avoidance is not a significant predictor of response to cognitive therapy as it is with antidepressants, suggesting that Self-Directedness is more closely related to the features required for response to cognitive therapy.

These observations mean that an initial comprehensive personality assessment is a crucial part of an initial psychiatric evaluation (Cloninger and Svrakic 1997). Such improvement in efficiency and effectiveness is increasingly important in providing care with modern constraints on frequency and duration of visits.

Personality and Lifestyle Choice

Despite the advances in understanding of the important role of lifestyle on mental and physical health, physicians in all specialties have made little progress in achieving compliance with recommended lifestyle practices. The important lifestyle choices that are so resistant to preventative guidance include diet, weight, exercise, smoking, drinking, and stress management. Recent work has shown that individual differences in lifestyle choice are substantially predicted by personality traits. In fact, unhealthy lifestyle choices, such as eating fried foods, exercising little, smoking and drinking excessively, and not having regular sleep and relaxing recreation, are related to the same personality traits that define personality disorder. In other words, an unhealthy lifestyle may be a mild form of what psychiatrists call immaturity or personality disorder; this is not surprising because personality disorders are inflexible maladaptive lifestyle choices. Thus the problems in preventative medicine regarding noncompliance with recommendations about healthy lifestyle choices overlap with those of psychiatry in facilitating healthy character development. The assessment of personality is therefore a crucial aspect of public health efforts for prevention of both mental and physical disorders.

Discussion

The relations between normal personality traits and vulnerability to psychopathology are moderately strong except for personality disorders, where they are definitive. That means that understanding of psychopathology requires consideration of influences on human behavior beyond the genes and neurochemical events contributing to personality (Cloninger et al. 1997). The complexity of the genetics of personality and the incompleteness of personality as an explanation of psychopathology mean that we should not think in a narrow reductionistic manner about genetic engineering. The genes for personality are likely to provide molecular targets that will assist in therapeutics, but the gene-gene and gene-environmental interactions are too complex to allow the design of human personalities in the way fantasized by some critics of psychiatric genetics. We have shown in gene mapping studies of human personality that the broad heritability of personality is about 50%, but about half of this (25%) is due to epistasis, or gene-gene interactions (Cloninger et al. 1998b). The number of interacting genes and nongenetic influences is such that exact prediction of human personality and psychopathology by genetic engineering is unlikely to be a fruitful goal. However, the understanding of molecular genetic events associated with individual differences in personality development is likely to contribute in an important way to a rational understanding of psychobiological disorders and their treatment.

References

American Psychiatric Association: Diagnostic and Statistical Manual of Mental Disorders, 4th Edition, Text Revision. Washington, DC, American Psychiatric Association, 2000

Battaglia M, Przybeck TR, Bellodi L, et al: Temperament dimensions explain the comorbidity of psychiatric disorders. Compr Psychiatry 37:292–298, 1996

Bayon C, Hill K, Svrakic DM, et al: Dimensional assessment of personality in an outpatient sample: relations of the systems of Millon and Cloninger. J Psychiatr Res 30:341–352, 1996

Brewerton TD, Hand LD, Bishop ER Jr: The Tridimensional Personality Questionnaire in eating disorder patients. Int J Eat Disord 14:213–218, 1993

Bulik CM, Sullivan PF, Joyce PR, et al: Predictors of 1-year treatment outcome in bulimea nervosa. Compr Psychiatry 39:206–214, 1998

Bulik CM, Sullivan PF, Carter FA, et al: Predictors of rapid and sustained response to cognitive-behavioral therapy for bulimea nervosa. Int J Eat Disord 26:137–144, 1999

Cloninger CR: A systematic method for clinical description and classification of personality variants. Arch Gen Psychiatry 44:573–588, 1987

Cloninger CR: The Tridimensional Personality Questionnaire: U.S. normative data. Psychol Rep 69:1047–1057, 1991

Cloninger CR: Temperament and personality. Curr Opin Neurobiol 4:266–273, 1994

Cloninger CR: Genetics of substance abuse, in The APP Textbook of Substance Abuse Treatment, 2nd Edition. Edited by Galanter M, Kleber HD. Washington, DC, American Psychiatric Press, 1999a, pp 59–66

Cloninger CR (ed): Personality and Psychopathology. Washington, DC, American Psychiatric Press, 1999b

Cloninger CR: A practical way to diagnose personality disorder: a proposal. J Personal Disord 14:99–108, 2000

Cloninger CR, Svrakic DM: Integrative psychobiological approach to psychiatric assessment and treatment. Psychiatry 60:120–141, 1997

Cloninger CR, Svrakic DM, Przybeck TR: A psychobiological model of temperament and character. Arch Gen Psychiatry 50:975–990, 1993

Cloninger CR, Przybeck TR, Svrakic DM, et al: The Temperament and Character Inventory (TCI): A Guide to Its Development and Use. St. Louis, MO, Washington University, Center for Psychobiology of Personality, 1994

Cloninger CR, Svrakic DM, Bayon C, et al: Personality disorder, in Washington University Adult Psychiatry. St. Louis, MO, Mosby, 1996, pp 301–318

Cloninger CR, Svrakic NM, Svrakic DM: Role of personality self-organization in development of mental order and disorder. Dev Psychopathol 9:881–906, 1997

Cloninger CR, Bayon C, Svrakic DM: Measurement of temperament and character in mood disorders: a model of fundamental states as personality types. J Affect Disord 51:21–32, 1998a

Cloninger CR, Van Eerdewegh P, Goate A, et al: Anxiety proneness linked to epistatic loci in genome scan of human personality traits. Am J Med Genet 81:313–317, 1998b

Fossati A, Baudanza P, Crisci MA, et al: Temperament and character in DSM-IV personality disorders, in Proceedings of the Sixth

International Congress on Disorders of Personality, Geneva, Switzerland, 1999, pp 67–68

Joffe RT, Bagby RM, Levitt AJ, et al: The Tridimensional Personality Questionnaire in major depression. Am J Psychiatry 150:959–960, 1993

Joyce PR, Mulder RT, Cloninger CR: Temperament predicts clomipramine and desipramine response in major depression. J Affect Disord 30:35–46, 1994

Kleifield EI, Sunday S, Hurt S, et al: The Tridimensional Personality Questionnaire: an exploration of personality traits in eating disorders. J Psychiatr Res 28:413–423, 1994

Luty SE, Joyce PR, Mulder RT, et al: Relationship between interpersonal psychotherapy problem areas with temperament and character: a pilot study. Depress Anxiety 8:154–159, 1998

Mulder RT, Joyce PR: Temperament and the structure of personality disorder symptoms. Psychol Med 27:99–106, 1997

Mulder RT, Joyce PR, Sellman JD, et al: Towards an understanding of defense style in terms of temperament and character. Acta Psychiatr Scand 93:99–104, 1996

Svrakic DM, Whitehead C, Przybeck TR, et al: Differential diagnosis of personality disorders by the seven-factor model of temperament and character. Arch Gen Psychiatry 50:991–999, 1993

Tome MB, Cloninger CR, Watson JP, et al: Serotonergic autoreceptor blockade in the reduction of antidepressant latency: personality variables and response to paroxetine and pindolol. J Affect Disord 44:101–109, 1997

Waller NG: Evaluating the structure of personality, in Personality and Psychopathology. Edited by Cloninger CR. Washington, DC, American Psychiatric Press, 1999, pp 155–200

CHAPTER THREE

Genetics of Personality

The Example of the Broad Autism Phenotype

Joseph Piven, M.D.

Spectrum of Autistic Behavior

More than 50 years ago Leo Kanner provided the first description of what has since come to be referred to as autistic disorder (Kanner 1943). This severe, lifelong behavioral syndrome is defined in DSM-IV-TR (American Psychiatric Association 2000) by the presence of behavioral characteristics in three domains of behavior: 1) marked communication abnormalities such as language delay, echolalia, and deficits in the pragmatic use of language; 2) significant social deficits ranging from an absence of interest in interacting with others to a limited ability to engage in reciprocal social interactions; and 3) an excess of stereotyped, ritualistic, and repetitive behaviors, such as upset with minor changes in routine or changes in the environment, unusual preoccupations, and repetitive questioning. Although the severity, abnormal quality, and co-occurrence of the symptoms that make up this behavioral syndrome place it squarely in the category of a medical condition, the boundary between where autism ends and the

This research was supported by NIMH Grants MH55284 and MH101568.

abnormal dimensions of personality begin is not so clear. In 1987, DSM-III-R (American Psychiatric Association 1987) introduced the concept of a subthreshold diagnostic category referred to as a pervasive developmental disorder, not otherwise specified (PDD-NOS). As with autism, this condition is associated with substantial impairment in functioning; however, it differs from autism in that affected individuals do not quite meet the threshold for a diagnosis of autism in all three domains. Although classical autism, as originally and more narrowly defined by Kanner, is estimated to occur in roughly 2 children per 10,000 (Lotter 1967) and DSM-IV-TR autistic disorder, which is somewhat more broadly defined, is estimated to occur in approximately 5–10 children per 10,000 (Fombonne et al. 1999), the occurrence of PDD-NOS is estimated to be as high as 14–18 children per 10,000 in the population (Fombonne et al.). In addition to this widening of the criteria for diagnosing an autistic-like condition, increasing data on the natural progression of the childhood symptoms of the pervasive developmental disorders suggest that some of the traditional distinctions made in the diagnosis in childhood are not always as straightforward in adults. Not uncommonly, adults who met criteria for high-functioning (i.e., IQ > 80) autism or a pervasive developmental disorder as children, when viewed cross-sectionally at later ages, no longer meet criteria for a pervasive developmental disorder. Though impairment related to their social deficits or rigid behaviors is still present, these individuals often appear instead to meet criteria for a diagnosis of a personality disorder (e.g., schizoid, avoidant personality, and/or compulsive personality disorder) (Piven et al. 1996). Clearly the appropriate approach to diagnosis in these adults requires inquiry into childhood history where other aspects of the PDD-NOS syndrome will be identified, allowing these individuals to be correctly classified as having the adult manifestations of a childhood pervasive developmental disorder. Unfortunately little is currently known about the natural history of autistic behaviors in adults with a pervasive developmental disorder in childhood. Further blurring the boundaries of the behaviors between pervasive developmental disorders and the dimensions of personality are recent data suggesting that the underlying genetic liability for autism may be expressed in non-autistic relatives of autistic individuals, in personality and language characteristics that are milder and qualitatively similar to those seen in autism. Together these characteristics have been referred to as comprising a broad autism phenotype. In this chapter I review the concept of the broad autism phenotype and explore its relevance to current and future studies of the genetics of personality.

Genetic Factors in Autism

The importance of hereditary factors in the etiology of autism is now well recognized. The recurrence risk for autism following the birth of an autistic child is approximately 100 times the population base rate (Smalley et al. 1988), and three epidemiologically based twin studies have reported concordance rates for autism among monozygotic twins that range from 36% to 91%, as compared with zero concordance among dizygotic twins (the actual dizygotic concordance in a larger sample would be expected to approximate the recurrence risk for autism of approximately 3%–6%) (Bailey et al. 1995; Folstein and Rutter 1977; Steffenburg et al. 1989). These monozygotic concordance rates suggest that the heritability of autism may be greater than 90% (Bailey et al. 1995). The high relative risk ratio (λ_s) in autism (i.e., recurrence risk/population risk) of 75–150, together with the estimates of heritability, have stimulated a number of affected sib-pair genome screen studies to search for susceptibility genes underlying this disorder. Currently there is converging evidence for a possible susceptibility locus on chromosome 7q (Barrett et al. 1999; IMGSAC 2001), identified through several genome screen studies of affected sib pairs, as well as a possible locus on chromosome 15q11–13. The chromosome 15 locus has been suggested by the numerous reports of interstitial duplications and tetrasomies in this region, along with high rates of microduplications and deletions that appear to be due to maternal and paternal transmission, respectively (Baker et al. 1994; Barrett et al. 1999; Cook et al. 1997).

Although the evidence clearly establishes the importance of genetic factors in autism, no particular mode of inheritance underlying this disorder has been identified. Based on the differences in concordance rates for autism between mono- and dizygotic twins of greater than 4:1, and the absence of a pattern consistent with Mendelian inheritance for the full syndrome of autism, the most likely genetic mechanism underlying autism is considered to be oligogenic inheritance. Further complicating the search for susceptibility genes in autism is the presence of etiologic heterogeneity underlying this syndrome. Approximately 10% of individuals with autism have a co-occurring medical condition that is presumed to play an etiologic role in their autism. For example, autism has been detected in more than 20% of individuals with tuberous sclerosis (Baker et al. 1998), an autosomal dominant neurocutaneous disorder associated with benign brain lesions (tubers) and epilepsy; and approximately 3% of autistic individuals carry the full fragile X mutation (Piven et al. 1991).

Evidence for the Existence of a Broad Autism Phenotype

In his original description of the syndrome of infantile autism, along with the detailed accounts of the behavior of children with autism, Kanner made several astute observations about the behavioral characteristics of the parents of some of the affected children. Parents were often described as serious-minded, perfectionistic individuals, with an intense interest in abstract ideas, who appeared to lack a genuine interest in developing relationships with others (Kanner 1943). These early observations, however, were misinterpreted to mean that somehow parental personality and child-rearing practices resulted in the occurrence of autism. Numerous studies examining parent-child interactions have consistently failed to support this hypothesis (summarized by Cantwell et al. [1976]). However, although the notion that the family environment plays a role in the etiology of autism has clearly been laid to rest, there is increasing evidence that Kanner's observations about parental behavior were correct. Recent family and twin studies of autism suggest that the spectrum of behaviors related to autism may include personality and language characteristics expressed in nonautistic relatives of autistic probands, which are milder but qualitatively similar to the defining features of autism. This phenomenon, referred to recently as the broad autism phenotype (BAP), may provide a useful model for examining the genetic determinants of personality.

Twin Studies

Although Kanner provided the first detailed observations of the personality and behavior of parents through his anecdotal reports, it was Folstein and Rutter's twin study that provided the first systematic evidence that Kanner's observations may have been correct. In their study of 21 same-sex twin pairs in England, Folstein and Rutter (1977) reported that in addition to a higher monozygotic than dizygotic concordance rate for autism, the nonautistic co-twins in the monozygotic pairs also had elevated rates of a more broadly defined phenotype, defined as either autism or a milder cognitive deficit (e.g., severe reading disorder, language delay, mental retardation, or severe articulation disorder) when compared with the nonautistic dizygotic co-twins. Whereas concordance for autism was 36% and 0% in monozygotic and dizygotic twins, respectively, expanding the definition of affected to include either autism or a cognitive disorder resulted in concordance of 82% in monozygotic versus 10% in dizygotic twin pairs. In all cases, the cognitive deficit involved some type of speech or language abnormality, typically characterized as a delay in the development of useful speech. In three of the five nonautistic monozygotic co-twins, significant social deficits were also noted. However, given the difficulties in systematically characterizing social deficits in children, this observation was largely ignored for several years until several family studies using systematic assessment methods began to reveal similar abnormalities in the parents and adult relatives of autistic probands. In summary, Folstein and Rutter's twin study provided evidence that behavioral deficits that were milder but qualitatively similar to those found in autism might also be present at elevated rates in relatives of autistic probands. This observation led to the hypothesis that perhaps what is inherited in families of autistic individuals is not necessarily autism, but a milder, forme fruste of the full syndrome that might include a milder cognitive or social deficit.

In a recent follow-up of the original autism twin study, Bailey et al. (1995) reexamined subjects from the first British twin study and ascertained a second epidemiological sample of autistic twins in England. The cognitive and behavioral characteristics were assessed using the Autism Family History Interview, a semistructured family history interview developed specifically to examine hypotheses about potential aspects of the more broadly defined autism phenotype assessed in this study, defined as the presence of either social or cognitive deficits. In the combined sample (a total of 27 monozygotic and 20 dizygotic twins), 92% of the monozygotic pairs were concordant for autism or a more broadly defined phenotype including milder cognitive and social deficits, versus 10% of the dizygotic pairs, further extending the findings of the original Folstein and Rutter twin study of autism.

Family History Studies

Again using the Autism Family History Interview and interviewing an informant, Bolton et al. (1994) examined the relatives in a large sample of families of autistic and Down syndrome individuals. Relatives were coded as having communication, social, and/or stereotyped behavior deficits based on the presence of one definite or two probable abnormalities within each of the three defining behavioral domains in autism. First-degree relatives from autism families had higher rates of abnormalities from all three behavioral domains—social and communication deficits, and stereotyped-repetitive behaviors—than relatives from Down syndrome families, and Bolton et al. referred to this phenomenon as the BAP. For subsequent analyses, relatives were grouped into two categories of affected status: one based on a narrow definition, which meant having deficits in any two of the three behavioral domains examined; and one based on a broad definition, which meant having deficits in one of the domains. Using this approach they noted that proband verbal IQ was significantly associated with familial aggregation of both the broad and narrow definitions of the BAP. In the subset of autistic probands with speech, an association was also noted between the presence of the BAP in relatives and the number of ICD-10 autism symptoms present in probands. These analyses thus provide converging evidence for the validity (or genetic meaning) of the BAP, by not only showing differences in rates between cases and controls, but by showing a possible relationship between proband characteristics and the presence of the BAP in relatives.

Using a modified version of the Autism Family History Interview, Palmer and Piven (in press) compared rates of the BAP in multiple- and single-incidence autism and Down syndrome families in the Iowa Autism Family Study. They hypothesized that multiple-incidence autism families, ascertained through the presence of two autistic probands, would presumably carry a higher genetic liability for autism than single-incidence autism families, who presumably carry a higher genetic liability for autism than Down syndrome families. The latter can be assumed to reflect the genetic liability for autism present in the general population. Results revealed that rates of the BAP in relatives ascertained through multiple-incidence probands were indeed higher than those found in single-incidence autism families. The rates of the BAP in relatives from single-incidence families were, in turn, found to be significantly higher than the rates found in Down syndrome families. The results of this study suggest that the increasing genetic liability to autism, going from families ascertained through Down syndrome to single-incidence autism to multiple-incidence autism, is associated with increasing genetic liability for the BAP in relatives. Given the more common occurrence of the BAP in multiple-incidence autism families, as well as the likelihood that families ascertained through two autistic probands are likely to have fewer phenocopies than those ascertained through a single affected individual, multiple-incidence families offer an important, high-risk group for genetic studies of the BAP.

Defining the Nature and Boundaries of the BAP

Although family history studies have convincingly demonstrated high rates of the BAP in the nonautistic twins and family members of autistic individuals, the family history method provides only a relatively crude measure of this milder aspect of the phenotype. For studies that aim to go beyond the simple demonstration of differences in case-control or concordance rates of the BAP, to examine the biological significance of the BAP, it is likely that a more detailed understanding of the nature and boundaries of the BAP is warranted. This more detailed description of the manifestations of the BAP requires the direct assessment of individuals.

Personality Characteristics

The Modified Personality Assessment Schedule, Revised (M-PAS-R) was originally adapted from the Personality Assessment Schedule (Tyrer 1988; Tyrer and Alexander 1979; Tyrer et al. 1983), a semistructured interview for the assessment of personality disorder. A modified version of this instrument (M-PAS) was created for use in the cross-national Baltimore-London Autism Family Studies (Murphy et al. 2000; Piven et al. 1994) that included a subset of 18 personality characteristics that were thought to possibly be components of the BAP. Preliminary use of this instrument (Piven et al. 1994) revealed that 1) there was substantial overlap among the items; 2) adequate interrater reliability could not be achieved on several of the items; 3) several characteristics were infrequently endorsed; and 4) several items did not appear to be useful in distinguishing characteristics in relatives of those with autism. As a result, in a subsequent study, the Iowa Autism Family Study, only eight items were retained (and one item, rigidity, was substantially modified), in a version referred to as the Modified Personality Assessment Schedule, Revised (M-PAS-R) (Piven et al. 1997b).

Subjects (parents of autistic individuals) and informants (usually spouses) were interviewed using the M-PAS-R as part of a lengthy interview that began with examination of the subject's life story, including questions about family, school and work history, and relationships. M-PAS-R characteristics were rated separately in the subject interview and the informant interview, as present or absent, based on specific behavioral examples (not subjective impressions of the interviewer) given by the subject or informant. A single, blind, best-estimate rating was made from combin-ing data from the videotaped responses of both the subject and the informant for each characteristic. With the exception of the item *un-demonstrative* (kappa = 0.48), interrater reliability was found to be good to excellent for the items (Piven et al. 1997b).

Twenty-five mothers and 23 fathers from 25 multiple-incidence autism families and 30 mothers and 30 fathers from 30 Down syndrome families were examined. After correction for multiple comparisons, autism parents were found to be significantly more likely to be rated as aloof (23% autism vs. 3% Down syndrome), rigid (49% autism vs. 5% Down syndrome); anxious (26% autism vs. 5% Down syndrome), and hypersensitive to criticism (28% autism vs. 3% Down syndrome) than parents of Down syndrome probands. On the M-PAS-R, *rigid* is defined as having little interest in and/or difficulty adjusting to change; *aloof* is defined as having a lack of interest in or enjoyment from being with people; *anxious* is defined as nervousness not amounting to an anxiety state or phobic disorder; and *hypersensitivity to criticism* is defined as excessive distress at comments or behavior of others that is felt to be critical or insensitive. For these four characteristics the relative odds (RO) (including the 95% confidence interval [CI]) of being rated as affected if the subject was an autism parent were as follows: aloof, RO = 8.4 (CI: 1.7, 41.3); rigid, RO = 10.1 (CI: 3.3, 30.6); anxious, RO = 6.3 (CI: 1.6, 24.7); and hypersensitive to criticism, RO = 11.0 (CI: 2.3, 53.0). There was no evidence of gender-specific differences, except for the characteristic anxious, which was rated more commonly in autism versus Down syndrome fathers (35% vs. 0%, respectively) but showed no significant difference in frequency between autism and Down syndrome mothers (28% vs. 10%, respectively).

In order to more fully understand the meaning of the M-PAS-R personality characteristics detected at elevated rates in autism parents, Piven et al. (1997b) examined the relationship of these characteristics to those assessed in a well-known measure of the five-factor model of personality, the NEO Personality Inventory, Revised. An analysis of the correlation of items from the M-PAS-R and those of the NEO Personality Inventory, Revised, revealed a significant negative correlation between the aloof characteristic and two facets of extroversion, Warmth (E1) ($r = -0.31$, $P < 0.01$) and Gregariousness (E2) ($r = -0.32$, $P < 0.01$). The M-PAS-R Rigid characteristic was also significantly negatively correlated with O4 of the Openness dimension ($r = -0.30$, $P < 0.01$) and Agreeableness ($r = -0.32$, $P < 0.01$). Individuals who score low for O4 are characterized by a preference for routine and familiar experiences, an unwillingness to try new activities, and an avoidance of novelty. The presence of both (negative) openness and (negative) agreeableness is thought to describe an individual who is more than just closed to changes in experience (as expected by the O4 characteristic), and in addition displays what has been referred to as *interpersonal rigidity*). This suggests an additional social aspect of this characteristic that is consistent with an overall conceptualization of the BAP as involving both social deficits and rigidity. Finally, and as expected, the M-PAS-R items *anxious* and *hypersensitive to criticism* were significantly correlated with several facets of the Neuroticism dimension (anxiety and depression), whereas hypersensitivity to criticism was additionally correlated significantly with hostility, self-consciousness, and vulnerability.

Number and Quality of Friendships: A Simple Measure of Social Behavior

Recognizing the limitations of the measure of personality used in the characterization of the BAP (e.g., the M-PAS-R requires substantial training and effort to obtain reliable and meaningful data), several studies sought to characterize the social deficits seen in individuals thought to show evidence of the BAP, using simpler approaches. The Friendship Interview was developed as part of the Baltimore Autism Family Study to provide a reliable and relatively easy to administer measure of one aspect of social behavior: the quality and number of an individual's friendships. Two studies have been conducted using this instrument and have reported that parents of autistic individuals have fewer friendships that involve emotional support and confiding than do parents of Down syndrome individuals (Piven et al. 1997b). In the study by Piven et al., 46% of parents with multiple autistic children scored at least 1.5 standard deviations. beyond the mean of the control group on this measure, for an effect size of 1.1 (CI: $0.7 - 1.6$). The Friendship Interview score was also correlated significantly with the Pragmatic Language score ($r = 0.57$, $P < 0.001$) (see the section "Communication: At the Interface of Cognition and Personality") and aloof personality ($r = 0.43$, $P < 0.001$), demonstrating agreement across different measures for characterizing behaviors in the social domain.

Cognitive Deficits

Cognitive deficits, although not considered a defining feature of the disorder, are almost uniformly present in autistic individuals. Seventy-five percent of autistic individuals have an IQ that places them in the mentally retarded range, and language delay or the absence of the development of useful language is typical.

Deficits in particular cognitive functions have also been identified, resulting in a variety of explanatory theories about the cognitive basis of this disorder. So, for example, executive function deficits have been detected in a number of studies and are thought to possibly underlie a range of behavioral and other cognitive deficits seen in autism (Ozonoff et al. 1994). Particular patterns on subtests of the Wechsler IQ test (e.g., strengths in block design) have led others to suggest that the fundamental deficit in autism is in "central cohesion" (Happe and Frith 1996), or an overfocus on the relationship between parts of a whole with a relative deficit in ability to appreciate the overall gestalt.

A qualitatively similar pattern of deficits in some cognitive areas has been observed in relatives. The most clear-cut example comes from three independent studies demonstrating deficits in executive function on the Tower of Hanoi and one showing deficits on the intradimensional/extradimensional set shifting task, in siblings of autistic individuals (Ozonoff et al. 1993) and in their parents (Hughes et al. 1997; Piven et al. 1997b). Similarly, relatives of autistic individuals have high rates of deficits in communication-related abilities (e.g., language delay, rapid automatized naming, and reading comprehension) (Piven et al. 1997b). The finding of cognitive deficits in family members of autistic individuals provides a convergence of evidence supporting the validity of the concept of the BAP and suggests possible mechanisms that may underlie these behaviors in autistic individuals and their relatives.

Communication: At the Interface of Cognition and Personality

Social behavior in autism encompasses a complex array of behaviors that range from obvious (e.g., little interest in others) to more subtle (e.g., limited ability to appreciate social cues or the to and fro aspects of a social conversation) characteristics. In addition to deficits in social aspects of personality, as characterized by the rating of aloofness and friendship on the M-PAS-R and Friendship Interview, some parents of autistic individuals show more subtle deficits in the social aspects of their communication. Both deficits in pragmatic language (i.e., social use of language) and narrative discourse (i.e., the ability to tell a story) have been reported in autism parents and parallel similar, more severe deficits seen in autism. Landa et al. (1992) developed an observational measure of social use of language (the Pragmatic Language Scale), composed of 19 abnormal pragmatic behaviors in three categories: 1) disinhibited social communication (including being overly talkative, overly detailed, preoccupied with particular topics, giving confusing accounts, abruptly changing topics, and being overly candid); 2) awkward or inadequate expression (including inadequate clarification when asked to give more detail about a particular point; and terse, vague accounts with insufficient background for the listener); and 3) odd verbal interactions (including inappropriate topics, odd humor, limited to and fro conversation, and being overly formal or informal). In two family studies comparing blind ratings of the parents of autistic individuals and controls, autism parents showed significantly higher rates of pragmatic language deficits (Landa et al. 1992; Piven et al. 1997b). In the study by Piven et al. (1997b) the greatest differences were observed on a subset of items—giving accounts that were too detailed, failure to give proper references during the conversation, vague and disorganized accounts, failure to adequately clarify information when questioned further about it—that all pertained to the clarity and relevance of the message. Similarly, the most striking abnormalities in autism parents in the Landa et al. (1992) study fell into the category or factor of inadequate expression. Landa et al. (1992) hypothesized that this set of abnormal pragmatic behaviors in parents might be the result of using a rigid linguistic rule system that affects expression and comprehension of the message, indicating a possible convergence of deficits in the social and stereotyped-repetitive domains, which is reflected in characteristic patterns of language use.

Inadequate expression was also detected in studies by Landa et al. (1991), where parents of autistic individuals were found to have deficits in their abilities to tell a novel, coherent story (i.e., a deficit in narrative discourse ability). In the most recent study (R. Landa, J. Piven, unpublished data, 2001), autism parents produced longer stories with more reformulations and perspective taking errors (e.g., restatement of ideas, and expression of ambiguous, irrelevant, and redundant information) than controls (parents of Down syndrome individuals). Number of reformulations by autism parents was also significantly correlated with a nonverbal test of planning (the four-ring Tower of Hanoi), suggesting that deficits in narrative discourse may be the result of an impairment of executive function, and in particular in planning, in these individuals. These findings parallel similar hypotheses where executive function deficits, and more specifically, a rigid cognitive style, have been thought to underlie many of the behavioral abnormalities in autism.

In summary, these results suggest that the genetic liability for autism is expressed in nonautistic relatives in complex and broad ranging characteristics typically seen as falling within the construct of personality. Some of these broad ranging characteristics, such as social deficits in personality, are likely to be the end result of a complex interaction between abnormalities in social cognition, pragmatic language, and narrative discourse that eventually may be explained by more fundamental, underlying cognitive abnormalities such as deficits in executive function.

Psychiatric Disorder and the BAP

The observation that particular personality characteristics are common in relatives of autistic individuals raises the question of whether these characteristics are associated with impairment. Piven et al. (unpublished data) examined the parents from 25 multiple-incidence autism families and 30 Down syndrome families using the Structured Interview for DSM-III-R Personality Disorder (SIDP-R) (Pfohl et al. 1989). Although four autism and none of the control parents were found to have an avoidant personality disorder (Fisher's exact, $P = 0.045$), for the most part, the majority of autism parents did not have evidence of personality disorder or impairment related to the presence of particular personality characteristics such as aloof or rigid personality.

Axis I psychiatric disorders have also been examined in the nonautistic relatives of autistic individuals. Four studies employing structured psychiatric interviews have found elevated rates of recurrent major affective disorder (MAD) in parents of autistic individuals (Bolton et al. 1998; Piven and Palmer 1999; Smalley et al. 1995). Two of these studies examined the relationship of MAD to the BAP and failed to find an association. The most recent study by Piven and Palmer (1999) found preliminary evidence to suggest that high rates of MAD in parents of autistic individuals may be the result of assortative mating of parents with MAD for spouses with the BAP. Both the study by Smalley et al. (1995) and the study by Piven and Palmer (1999) also found elevated rates of social phobia in autism parents. Although Piven and Palmer (1999) failed to detect an association in individuals between the presence of social phobia and the presence of traits of the BAP, clearly social phobia is conceptually related to the aloof and anxious personality characteristics detected in autism parents.

Importance of the BAP for Genetic Studies of Autism and Personality

A Complex Phenotype

As with other complex neurobehavioral syndromes, much of the work aimed at disentangling the underlying pathogenesis in autism has, in the past, been based on the premise that there is a single underlying etiology or set of etiologies (i.e., simple patterns of inheritance) and a single, underlying mechanism in the brain. Although this concept may be a logical place to begin thinking about the pathogenesis of relatively unidimensional conditions such as hypertension and diabetes (and even these disorders have now clearly been linked to more complex underlying mechanisms), the complex phenotype of autism could hardly be expected to yield to such simple truths as those inherent in finding a unitary brain lesion or a single explanatory gene. To begin with, the defining features of autism alone encompass three qualitatively distinct domains of behavior: social deficits, communication deficits. and stereotyped-repetitive behaviors. Each of these domains overlaps phenomenologically with more narrowly defined disorders that are themselves the subject of studies aimed at uncovering their underlying genetic basis (e.g., specific language disorder, schizoid and avoidant personality disorder, and obsessive-compulsive disorder). So, for example, without the additional presence of the other features of the full syndrome of autism, the language deficits alone of autism could be viewed as constituting a specific language impairment. Similarly, the stereotyped-repetitive behaviors have much in common phenomenologically with the symptoms of obsessive-compulsive disorder, and except for the co-occurrence of social and language deficits, many autistic individuals might warrant the diagnosis of an obsessive-compulsive or another anxiety-related disorder. The complexity of the autism phenotype is further supported by the evidence that autism is not the result of a unitary brain abnormality but instead appears to be the result of a range of neural abnormalities, as suggested by the neuroimaging and neuropathological studies showing abnormalities in a number of brain structures and regions (caudate, corpus callosum, amygdaloid-hippocampal complex, cerebellum, anterior cingulate, fusiform gyrus, thalamus, and prefrontal, temporal, occipital, and parietal cortex) (reviewed by Bauman and Kemper 1994; Chugani et al. 1997; Haznedar et al. 1997; Piven et al. 1997a; Schultz et al. 2000; Sears et al.

1999). At yet a more complex level of analysis, the evidence for specific brain-behavior relationships suggests that although related at the syndromic level (defined on the basis of clinical impairment observed when the components of autism occur within a single individual), components of the autism phenotype may, in fact, have distinct and independent pathophysiologies. A recent study by Sears et al. (1999), for example, showed evidence of abnormalities in caudate size in autism that were significantly correlated to stereotyped-repetitive but not social or communication behaviors (paralleling findings of abnormalities in the striatum in obsessive-compulsive disorder and Tourette syndrome [reviewed by Leckman et al. 1997]), suggesting the existence of more specific brain-behavior relationships underlying this complex phenotype.

Disaggregating the Autism Phenotype: Importance of the BAP

Both the quantitative and qualitative characteristics seen in autism (e.g., the wide range of IQ, and the rich and varied behavioral and cognitive deficits, respectively) suggest that the underlying genetic mechanisms in autism are likely to be complex. Based on inheritance patterns for autism observed in family and twin studies, autism has been thought to be the result of at least three to five interacting genes. Although there have been some encouraging overlapping findings from the few genome scan studies published to date (Barrett et al. 1999; IMGSAC 2001), other studies have been strikingly negative (Risch et al. 1999), suggesting the need for complementary strategies for detecting genes in autism. One approach to this enlists our knowledge of the varied components of autism and the BAP to search for independent genetic effects that may underlie these components.

If the oligogenic hypothesis is correct, individuals with autism have most if not all of the genes for this disorder, whereas family members, demonstrating only milder components of the full phenotype, are likely to have a smaller portion of the genes responsible for causing autism. Examination of the components of the BAP[1] in relatives may allow us to

---

[1] *The BAP more appropriately refers to the concept of a milder syndrome of autism in nonautistic relatives who carry genetic liability for autism. Components of the BAP, however, might perhaps be more accurately be referred to as constituting a narrow autism phenotype, because they represent the narrower expression of the underlying genetic liability for autism.*

dissaggregate the genetically meaningful but distinct aspects of the autistic phenotype that segregate independently but together may combine to produce autism. Current efforts at detecting genes for dyslexia, where separate linkages have been demonstrated to distinct reading tasks (e.g., single-word naming and phonological awareness), suggest that this may be a useful approach for detecting genes of moderate effect in genetically heterogeneous, oligogenic disorders (Grigorenko et al. 1997). Given the likelihood that at least some qualitatively distinct aspects of the autism phenotype may be associated with distinct brain abnormalities and distinct genetic effects, it seems as though a similar approach to disaggregating the genetics of autism, exploring for linkage to components of the phenotype in individuals with autism and the BAP, is warranted.

BAP as a Model for Elucidating the Molecular Genetic Basis of Personality

Systematic studies using reliable and standardized measures have now confirmed Kanner's original observation of particular behavioral characteristics aggregating in parents of autistic individuals. These studies suggest that there exists a milder, partial phenotype in the nonautistic relatives of autistic individuals that is genetically related to the full syndrome of autism. This milder, partial phenotype, referred to as the broad autism phenotype, provides a potentially important model for elucidating the genetic basis of personality.

Studies of the genetic basis of personality are limited by the same factors that limit the studies of all complex disorders, but perhaps more so given the difficulties in characterizing the phenotype, etiologic heterogeneity, and the likelihood of multifactorial/polygenic inheritance. The study of the personality characteristics in nonautistic relatives of autistic probands, who themselves have features of the BAP, offers several potential advantages. First, subsetting the range of subjects being studied by first conditioning on their having a relative with autism is likely to minimize the substantial heterogeneity of genes underlying personality in the general population. Second, by focusing on those characteristics of the BAP that parallel the phenotypic characteristics present in the fully affected index case (i.e., in individuals with autism) and by focusing on those aspects of the phenotype that appear to be most heritable (i.e., are highly correlated in two related autistic individuals or related individuals, one of whom is autistic and one of whom demonstrates some features of the BAP), the likelihood of detecting discrete genetic effects should be increased. Third, observations made about psychological phenomena in autistic individuals, such as deficits in executive function or the recognition of complex socioemotional phenomena (e.g., recent research suggesting deficits in theory of mind and ability to detect trustworthiness) (Adolphs et al. 2001; Baron-Cohen et al. 1999) or particular brain-behavior relationships in autism (e.g., the relationship between rigid-stereotyped-repetitive be

haviors and caudate volume in autistic individuals) (Sears et al. 1999) may provide clues to more biologically meaningful phenotypes. Finally, the convergence of abnormalities from multiple domains (e.g., personality, language, and cognition), within individuals and families segregating for autism and the BAP, adds validity to our notions about the constructs we are measuring and may contribute to our understanding of underlying mechanisms, leading to the identification of endophenotypes for studying the genetics of autism, the BAP, and related aspects of personality.

In summary, the cognitive and behavioral features of autism and the BAP provide a useful model for examining the biological and, more specifically, the genetic basis of personality. Ultimately though, the personality characteristics making up the BAP will require validation once genes for autism are found. Given the high heritability of autism and the extreme nature of the phenotype, it seems possible that genes for autism (and genes for components of the BAP) will be found before those for the broader dimensions of personality and may, in turn, lead the way to identifying susceptibility genes underlying personality.

References

Adolphs R, Sears L, Piven J: Abnormal processing of social information from faces in autism. J Cogn Neurosci 13:232–240, 2001

American Psychiatric Association: Diagnostic and Statistical Manual of Mental Disorders, 3rd Edition, Revised. Washington, DC, American Psychiatric Association, 1987

American Psychiatric Association: Diagnostic and Statistical Manual of Mental Disorders, 4th Edition, Text Revision. Washington, DC, American Psychiatric Association, 2000

Bailey A, LeCouteur A, Gottesman I, et al: Autism is a strongly genetic disorder: evidence from a British twin study. Psychol Med 25:63–77, 1995

Baker P, Piven J, Schwartz S, et al: Duplication of chromosomes 15q11–13 in two individuals with autistic disorder. J Autism Dev Disord 24:529–535, 1994

Baker P, Piven J, Sato Y: Autism and tuberous sclerosis complex: prevalence and clinical features. J Autism Dev Disord 28:335–341, 1998

Baron-Cohen S, Ring HA, Wheelwright S, et al: Social intelligence in the normal and autistic brain: an fMRI study. Eur J Neurosci 6:1891–1898, 1999

Barrett S, Beck JC, Bernier R, et al: An autosomal genetic screen for autism. Collaborative Linkage Study of Autism. Am J Med Genet 88:609–615, 1999

Bauman ML, Kemper TL: Neuroanatomic observations of the brain in autism, in The Neurobiology of Autism. Edited by Bauman ML, Kemper TL. Baltimore, MD, Johns Hopkins University, 1994, pp 119–145

Bolton P, Macdonald H, Pickles A, et al: A case-control family study of autism. J Child Psychol Psychiatry 35:877–900, 1994

Bolton PF, Pickles A, Murphy M, et al: Autism, affective and other psychiatric disorders: patterns of familial aggregation. Psychol Med 28:385–395, 1998

Cantwell DP, Baker L, Rutter M: Family factors, in Autism: A Reappraisal of Concepts and Treatment. Edited by Rutter M, Schopler E. New York, Plenum Press, 1976, pp 269–296

Chugani DC, Muzik O, Rothermel R, et al: Altered serotonin synthesis in the dentatothalamocortical pathway in autistic boys. Ann Neurol 42:666–669, 1997

Cook EH Jr, Lindgren V, Leventhal BL, et al: Autism or atypical autism in maternally but not paternally derived proximal 15q duplication. Am J Hum Genet 60:928–934, 1997

Folstein SE, Rutter M: Infantile autism: a genetic study of 21 twin pairs. J Child Psychol Psychiatry 18:297–321, 1977

Fombonne E: The epidemiology of autism: a review. Psychol Rev 29:769–786, 1999

Grigorenko EI, Wood FB, Meyer MS, et al: Susceptibility loci for distinct components of developmental dyslexia on chromosomes 6 and 15. Am J Hum Genet 60:13–16, 1997

Happe F, Frith U: The neuropsychology of autism. Brain 119:1377–400, 1996

Haznedar M, Buchsbaum M, Metzger M, et al: Anterior cingulate gyrus volume and glucose metabolism in autistic disorders. Am J Psychiatry 154:1047–1050, 1997

Hughes C, LeBoyer M, Bouvard M: Executive function in parents of children with autism. Psychol Med 27:209–220, 1997

IMGSAC (International Molecular Genetic Study of Autism Consortium): A genomewide screen for autism: strong evidence for linkage to chromosomes 2q, 7q, and 16p. Am J Hum Genet 69:570–581, 2001

Kanner L: Autistic disturbances of affective contact. Nervous Child 2:217–250, 1943

Landa R, Folstein S, Issacs C: Spontaneous narrative-discourse performance of parents of autistic individuals. J Speech Hear Res 191:1339–1345, 1991

Landa R, Piven J, Wzorek M, et al: Social language use in parents of autistic individuals. Psychol Med 22:245–254, 1992

Leckman F, Peterson BS, Anderson GM, et al: Pathogenesis of Tourette's syndrome. J Child Psychol Psychiatry 38:119–142, 1997

Lotter V: Epidemiology of autistic conditions in young children, I: prevalence. Soc Psychiatry 1:124–137, 1967

Murphy M, Bolton P, Pickles P, et al: Personality traits of the relatives of autistic probands. Psychol Med 30:1411–1424, 2000

Ozonoff S, Rogers S, Farnham J, et al: Can standard measures identify subclinical markers of autism? J Autism Dev Disord 23:429–444, 1993

Ozonoff S, Strayer D, McMahon W, et al: Executive function abilities in autism and Tourette syndrome: an information processing approach. J Child Psychol Psychiatry 35:1015–1032, 1994

Palmer P, Piven J: A comparison of multiple- and single-incidence autism families on perinatal optimality and the broad autism phenotype. J Am Acad Child Adolesc Psychiatry (in press)

Pfohl B, Blum N, Zimmerman M. Structured Interview for DSM-III-R Personality (SIDP-R). Des Moines, University of Iowa, 1989

Piven J, Palmer P: Psychiatric disorder and the broad autism phenotype: evidence from a family study of multiple-incidence autism families. Am J Psychiatry 156:557–563, 1999

Piven J, Gayle J, Landa R, et al: The prevalence of fragile X in a sample of autistic individuals diagnosed using a standardized interview. J Am Acad Child Adolesc Psychiatry 30:825–830, 1991

Piven J, Wzorek M, Landa R, et al: Personality characteristics of parents of autistic individuals. Psychol Med 24:783–795, 1994

Piven J, Harper J, Palmer P, et al: Course of behavioral change in autism: a retrospective study of high-IQ adolescents and adults. J Am Acad Child Adolesc Psychiatry 35:523–529, 1996

Piven J, Bailey J, Ranson BJ, et al: An MRI study of the corpus callosum in autism. Am J Psychiatry 154:1041–1056, 1997a

Piven J, Palmer P, Landa R, et al: Personality and language characteristics in parents from multiple incidence autism families. Am J Med Genet 74:398–411, 1997b

Risch N, Spiker D, Lotspeich L, et al: A genomic screen of autism: evidence for a multilocus etiology. Am J Hum Genet 65:493–507, 1999

Schultz RT, Gauthier I, Klin A, et al: Abnormal ventral temporal cortical activity among individuals with autism and Asperger syndrome during face discrimination. Arch Gen Psychiatry 57:331–340, 2000

Sears LL, Vest C, Mohamed S, et al: An MRI study of the basal ganglia in autism. Prog Neuropsychopharmacol Biol Psychiatry 23:613–624, 1999

Smalley S, Asarnow R, Spence M: Autism and genetics: a decade of research. Arch Gen Psychiatry 45:953–961, 1988

Smalley S, McCracken J, Tanguary P: Autism, affective disorders and social phobia. Am J Med Genet 60:19–26, 1995

Steffenburg S, Gilberg C, Holmgren L: A twin study of autism in Denmark, Iceland, Norway and Sweden. J Child Psychol Psychiatry 30:405–416, 1989

Tyrer P (ed): Personality Assessment Schedule, in Personality Disorders: Diagnosis, Management and Course. London, Butterworth, 1988, pp 140–167

Tyrer P, Alexander J: Classification of personality disorder. Br J Psychiatry 135:163–167, 1979

Tyrer P, Strauss J, Cicchetti D: Temporal reliability of personality in psychiatric patient. Psychol Med 13:393–398, 1983

CHAPTER FOUR

Animal Models of Personality

Jonathan Flint, M.D.

Strictly speaking, there are no animal models of human personality. In fact, although dog breeders have for centuries exploited individual heritable differences in an animal's temperament to create animal breeds with specific behavioral repertoires, it is not at all clear that an animal has a personality. Defining an animal's temperament is also not straightforward. An operational definition would require the animal to show a consistent pattern of responses in a series of behavioral tasks, so that for example, a timid animal would be slow to emerge into a threatening environment but quick to avoid a predator. The difficulty here is whether these tasks measure what they are supposed to measure. How, for instance, do we know that the environment or the predator is threatening to the animal? There may be other cues that determine the response about whose nature we are completely ignorant.

A further problem is that a limited number of behavioral tests are relevant to temperament. The most widely used, and hence those about which we know most, were developed for testing drug efficacy in models of psychiatric disorder. These may not be the best tests for the purposes of understanding personality.

The main justification for the use of animal models is that they allow us to find out things about the neurobiology of temperament and personality. The experimental license animals provide should permit the coupling of behavioral, genetic, cellular, and physiological assays in a way that has been possible in learning and memory experiments. In particular, animal models could identify the biological correlates of personality, thus providing a much needed external validation for personality traits. Most psychologists agree that personality factors can be found from the analysis of trait difference, but an external validation of each factor is lacking: the extraversion factor may emerge from numerous different personality inventories, but the problem is that there is no observable object called extraversion. The large literature on research into the biological basis of human personality has so far turned up very little (Zukerman 1991). Establishing heritability indices for personality factors is not by itself sufficient, first because even if the factor had no heritability it could still have validity in some other domain (for instance as a socially determined set of behaviors) and second because the existence of a heritability coefficient does not by itself guarantee that the trait has a biological basis. For instance the L scale of the Eysenck Personality Questionnaire has a high heritability (Eysenck 1967), but no one has proposed that it constitutes a personality factor. Furthermore, although it is academically interesting to know that there are five personality factors, this observation should be the beginning of further work, for instance, on the biology of personality.

What correlates can we identify? At present the best hope is to find genes that influence personality. There are two ways in which this could happen: either by finding the genes that influence temperament in animals or by looking for the effects of mutations on animal models. Once a gene is identified, then it should be possible to explore the action of that gene and begin to build up a picture of how the gene influences the animal's temperament and, we hope, human personality. Crucial to both expectations is the validity of the animal model. Consequently, I have devoted the first part of this chapter to the available behavioral tests. I argue that the tests relevant to human personality are those developed to study mood disorder. A susceptibility to mood change is a recognized aspect of personality, and both depression and anxiety disorders are known to occur more frequently in those with high neuroticism (or low emotional stability) scores. We know this relationship reflects a common biological mechanism because there is evidence from twin studies that the same genes influence neuroticism, susceptibility to depression, and anxiety (Kendler et al. 1993). Animal models of anxiety and depression may eventually tell us something about human personality (though I accept that the final conclusion may be that the available animal models do not model any aspects of human temperament). Next, we would like to know how best to validate such models.

Two validation methods dominate the literature. First, there is pharmacological validation. A model of depression that does not improve with a serotonin reuptake inhibitor (such as Prozac) does not get a warm reception, but of course this does not mean that the model is wrong. Drugs may work very differently in animals; but because we don't have any other objective standard against which to measure the validity of a test, in general, pharmacological validation remains a major hurdle that any model must overcome.

. The second method of validation is less species specific. A test is validated by correlation with other tests of the same trait and a concomitant lack of correlation with tests of other traits. So a test of depression should correlate with other tests of depression but not with tests of schizophrenia. The use of multiple, correlated tests is central to the development of a valid model. Unfortunately we know that there is considerable comorbidity in psychiatric illnesses and that some of this comorbidity is biologically driven. For instance, as mentioned, depression and one form of anxiety arise from the same genetic predisposition. So we have to be cautious here.

I start this review with a description of the more commonly used behavioral tests. The main interest for the genetic dissection of temperament is that the tests are often used to determine whether genetic mutants show a pattern of behaviors consistent with a change in temperament. I then proceed to discuss a set of experiments on animal strains selectively bred for behavior in such tests. These experiments begin to address more directly the genetic correlates of the measures.

Behavioral Tests of Temperament

Fear-Motivated Behaviors

Both the number of tests and the congruence of results derived from their usage attest to the belief that fear-related behaviors can be successfully modeled in animals. Furthermore at least some of the anatomical and physiological systems responsible for fear-related behaviors are known and are conserved between species.

Table 4–1 lists the most common tests and the measures taken from them. The table is divided into two sections that depend on whether the measures are of conditioned or unconditioned behavior. The motivational basis of unconditioned behaviors is complicated and largely unknown. Conditioned tests have the advantage of allowing the experimenter much more control: they are amenable to experimental manipulation to a degree that is impossible with unconditioned (or ethological) tests. Consequently we know more about the reasons for an animal's behavior in conditioned tests, and the explanations are complex (Gray 1982).

Unconditioned tests typically involve assessing the animal's behavior in a mildly stressful environment. Rats tend to avoid open elevated alleys and prefer closed alleys, a preference that is considered to be driven at least in part by fearfulness. The elevated plus maze, one of the most popular models of anxiety, has four arms, positioned like a cross, two of which are covered and two exposed. The animal is placed in the central platform, and the total number of arm entries is recorded. A fearful animal is expected to show reduced open-arm entries relative to the number of closed-arm entries. The open field exploits the aversive nature of an open space, a plain brightly lit area into which the animal is introduced. Reduced activity, avoidance of the central area, increased defecation and urination, and increased rearing are taken as indices of fearfulness (Rodgers et al. 1997; Willner 1990). The light-dark box (or black-white box) is an emergence test: fearful animals are expected to avoid the brightly lit compartment, preferring to remain in the enclosed dark box. Novelty inhibits eating in rats and other species, so a further measure of fearfulness is the time taken to approach and taste food in a novel environment (hyponeophagia) (Rodgers et al. 1997; Willner 1990). In the hole board apparatus, rodents explore a square board with up to 16 holes into which they tend to put their heads, a behavior that can be encouraged by placing novel objects beneath the holes. Fearful animals are less likely to head-dip (Rodgers et al. 1997; Willner 1990).

The grounds for believing that the unconditioned tests measure fearfulness are twofold. First, there is a large literature on the behavioral effects of anxiolytic and anxiogenic drugs (Rodgers et al. 1997; Willner 1990). The argument for pharmacological validation is that if a test measures fearfulness, then it should be possible to manipulate it specifically with drugs that affect human fearfulness (or anxiety), but not with drugs without such effects. For example, compounds that cause anxiety reduce the percentage of entries into and time spent on the open arms of the elevated plus maze, whereas antidepressants (imipramine, mianserin) and

TABLE 4–1   Animal tests of anxiety and depression

Tests of anxiety

Ethological measures

Elevated plus maze	Ratio of entries to open and closed arms
Light-dark transition	Emergence time
Social interaction	Frequency of social interaction in a novel environment
Hyponeophobia	Latency to start eating
Open field	Activity, defecation, thigmotaxis
Hole board	Head dipping

Conditioned responses

Two-way avoidance conditioning	Rate of acquistion of response
Acoustic startle	Contraction in response to loud noise
Footshock-induced freezing	Contraction in response to conditioned stimulus
Fear-potentiated startle	Contraction in response to loud noise in conjunction with conditioned stimulus
Geller-Seifter	Frequency of conditioned response coincidental to an electrical shock
Vogel conflict	Frequency of conditioned licking coincidental to an electrical shock

Tests of depression

Porsolt swim immobility	Duration of immobility in a forced swim
Learned helplessness	Learning difficulty following exposure to uncontrollable shock
Chronic unpredictable mild stress	Decrease in consumption of weak sucrose solution following mild stress
Separation	Distress calling in isolated chicks

Source. Data from Flint et al. 1995, Gershenfeld and Paul 1997, and Gershenfeld et al. 1997.

antipsychotics (haloperidol) do not. Second, tests can be validated by correlated behaviors. Thus we expect a frightened animal to defecate more and ambulate less in the open field, show a longer latency to emerge in the black-white box, and visit the open arms of the elevated plus maze less often. Factorial-derived constructs should then confirm the observed correlations.

A growing body of evidence indicates the complex motivational structure of the unconditioned tests. Dawson and colleagues provide evidence that the anxiolytic effects of chlordiazepoxide in the elevated plus maze are confounded by increases in motor activity: for instance, psychostimulants such as amphetamine at doses that increase locomotor activity have an anxiolytic profile in the apparatus (Dawson et al. 1995). Factor analysis has also been used to dissect out additional components from fearfulness: in an analysis of five tests of fearfulness, three independent factors were found to account for 85% of the variance (Ramos et al. 1997). Factor 1 loaded primarily on latency measures (time to approach the center of an open field and emerge from a black-white box), whereas factor 2 loaded on activity measures in novel environments. These findings suggest a more complex explanation of unconditioned behavior, though not necessarily one that excludes a fearfulness component (Ramos and Mormède 1998).

Conditioned tests offer more experimental control over potential confounds, and they include the best animal models we have for human emotion and hence for temperament and personality. The term *conditioning* can be misleading here because we are not dealing with classical Pavlovian conditioning. Anxiolytic drugs do not affect classical conditioning, but they do have effects on some forms of instrumental learning, and it is the latter that are involved in the models of fearfulness discussed later.

Not all conditioned tests measure instrumental learning. Many of the studies described next use the following test of conditioned fear: the animal is placed in a conditioning chamber, and a shock, paired with a tone (or light), is administered twice. Animals are returned to the home cage, and on the following day, the amount of time the animal freezes is measured with and without exposure to the tone (or light), the latter now considered to be a conditioned stimulus. Freezing in the chamber without the tone is called freezing to the context (the animal associates the surroundings with the unpleasant experience), and freezing to the tone is called freezing to the conditioned stimulus. The neuronal circuitry of these two responses is different: contextual freezing is mediated by the hippocampus, whereas freezing to the tone is hippocampus independent (Phillips and LeDoux 1992).

In conditioned emotional response, food-deprived animals are trained to press a lever for food. Once the lever pressing is stable (i.e., the animal is unquestionably conditioned) the animal is taught to associate a light with a footshock. The light is then found to suppress bar-pressing. Conditioned emotional response is believed to reflect a central state of fear. However, summarizing a large number of studies, Gray (1982), Davis (1991), and Treit (1985) all point out the variability and inconsistency of drug effects on the conditioned emotional response. This is one of the pieces of evidence that anxiolytics work best when shock depends on the animal's response (i.e., shock is response contingent) and not when the shock is independent of the response. In other words, anxiolytics release punished responding. Consequently, conflict models of fearfulness are preferred to conditioned emotional response models.

The two commonly used conflict models are the Geller-Seifter and the Vogel procedures. In the Geller-Seifter conflict procedure a light or tone introduces footshock in the operant chamber (i.e., where the animal has learned to press a bar for a food reward); in the Vogel water-lick conflict test, thirsty animals are first trained to lick from a tube and then electric shocks are delivered either through the tube or the floor. The suppression of responding in both procedures is attenuated relatively specifically by anxiolytics.

Avoidance learning paradigms are of two sorts. Passive avoidance involves punishing an animal if it makes a response. In active avoidance the animal has to learn to respond to avoid a footshock (Gray 1982). There is an important distinction between one- and two-way active avoidance. Typically both are measured in a box divided into two compartments: in one-way active avoidance the shock is given in one area only, so that the animal learns to associate shock with that compartment; in two-way active avoidance the shock is given in both compartments so that the animal has to shuttle in order to avoid the shock. Two-way active avoidance thus involves more complex learning because the animal has to learn to approach cues that had been associated with shock.

In fear-potentiated startle the animal's fearfulness is measured by how much it jumps in response to a conditioned stimulus to footshock. First light is associated with a footshock. Startle is then elicited by another stimulus, such as a loud noise. Startle is then measured when the conditioned stimulus (the light) is given before the loud noise. Any additional startle (or potentiated startle) is then regarded as a measure of fearfulness. Fear-potentiated startle correlates highly with freezing, but unlike freezing it is open to experimental manipulation. The model has been extensively investigated at the anatomical, cellular, and molecular levels. The brain pathways underlying the startle response have been mapped (Davis 1991), and the amygdala has been implicated in the establishment of conditioned fear.

Overall, the greater degree of experimental manipulation available with conditioned paradigms has resulted in a much more detailed understanding of the mechanisms of fearfulness. As a result, this is one area where animal models have shaped our understanding of human personality (Eysenck 1967; Gray 1987).

Tests of Depression

A well-known model of depression is learned helplessness (Seligman 1974) in which animals are exposed to uncontrollable shock. The hypothesis is that animals learn that their responses no longer have an effect on the environment and consequently become depressed. Although it is true that their impaired learning to escape shock, consequent on the uncontrollable shock, can be improved by antidepressants, there has been extensive debate about the correct interpretation of these findings. Learning impairment is probably secondary to an impairment of attention and not to a change in the animal's emotional state. The same objections can be raised to the other stress models. The forced-swim test consists of leaving the animal to swim in a confined space. Although extensively used in drug development, it is not sensitive to 5-hydroxytryptamine (5-HT) uptake inhibitors (Borsini and Meli 1988).

An alternative to uncontrollable shock is chronic mild stress (Willner et al. 1992). In this procedure the animals are first trained to consume a mild sucrose solution. Half of the animals are then put through a chronic mild stress regime (such as food and water deprivation, overnight illumination, exposure to white noise) during which sucrose consumption is regularly measured and compared with that of the control animals, which are not exposed to stress. A decrease in sucrose consumption is taken as an indication of depressed mood.

Effects of Engineered Mutants on Tests of Temperament

Genetic manipulation of animals has proved to be a very powerful way to explore the neurobiology of learning and memory. More recently the same techniques have been applied to the study of behavior in the tests I described earlier, with the aim of understanding how genes affect mood. Heritable predisposition to a particular mood state is nothing more than a feature of temperament, so the genetically engineered animals should tell us something about the genetics of temperament, and hence of personality. A table of relevant mutants is provided. (Table 4–2). The caveat is of course that the quality of the model determines the value of the information the mutants provide. For the reasons already outlined, we should be particularly wary of trusting too much to data that comes only from unconditioned paradigms, yet in the vast majority of cases it is just

TABLE 4–2 Mice knockout phenotypes relevant to personality

Gene	Contextual fear	Emergence test	Open field	Elevated maze	Novel object	Forced swim	Conditioned fear	References
Adenylate cyclase inhibition								
5-HT$_{1a}$			Reduced activity, less time in center	Less time in open quadrants	Increased latency to approach			Heisler et al. 1998
			Reduced activity, less time in center	Less time in open arms		More active		Ramboz et al. 1998
			Reduced activity, less time in center			More active		Parks et al. 1999
5-HT$_{1b}$			Increased activity	Increased time in open arms		Less active		Malleret et al. 1999; Saudou et al. 1994
Phospholipase C stimulation								
5-HT$_{2c}$	Reduced context-induced freezing	Reduced latency to emerge						Tecott et al. 1998
CRH				Normal			Normal	Weninger et al. 1999
CRH1 receptor		Increased latency to emerge		Less time in open arms				Smith et al. 1998; Timpl et al. 1998
CRH overproduction			Decreased activity	Less time in open arms				Stenzel-Poore et al. 1994

Continued

71

TABLE 4–2 Mice knockout phenotypes relevant to personality (Continued)

Gene	Contextual fear	Emergence test	Open field	Elevated maze	Novel object	Forced swim	Conditioned fear	References
CRH-binding protein		Increased latency to emerge	Reduced center entries	Less time in open arms				Karolyi et al. 1999
Nociceptin/ orphanin FQ		Increased latency to emerge	Decreased activity	Less time in open arms				Koster et al. 1999
GABA$_A$γ2		Increased latency to emerge		Less time in open arms			Increased passive avoidance	Crestani et al. 1999
Puromycin sensitive aminopeptidase								Osada et al. 1999
Dopamine D4 receptor		Increased latency to emerge	Reduced center entries		Increased latency to approach			Dulawa et al. 1999
α-Ca-calmodulin kinase II			Reduced OFD, decreased thigmotaxis					Chen et al. 1994b; Rotenberg et al. 1996; Silva et al. 1992a, 1992b
	Deficient contextual memory	No light-dark preference						Bach et al. 1995; Mayford et al. 1995, 1996

Histamine H1	Decreased open-field avoidance, increased OFD		Normal passive avoidance latency	Inoue et al. 1996
Interleukin 6 overexpression	Normal		Reduced active avoidance	Heyser et al. 1997
PKA RIβ and Cβ 1	Normal	Normal open-field rearing, grooming		Brandon et al. 1995
PKA	Deficient contextual conditioning (at 24 hr)			Abel et al. 1997
PKCγ	Moderate deficit in contextual conditioning			Abeliovich et al. 1993; Chen et al. 1995a

Note. CRH = corticotropin releasing hormone; PKA = protein kinase A; PKC = protein kinase C; OFA = open field activity; OFD = open field defecation.

such tests that are employed to bolster claims for anxiety or depression in knockout mice.

One reason why there are few data from conditioned tests is the difficulty of training mice. Genetic manipulation of the experimental psychologists' preferred organism, the rat, has not yet become a reliable procedure, so we are often faced with interpreting the effect on behavior of a complex biochemical and genetic manipulation with relatively crude behavioral tests.

The power of the genetic engineering technology is impressive, but a number of reservations should be borne in mind (Gerlai 1996, 2000). First, the effects of any knockout experiment are present in all tissues and throughout development. Consequently, effects observed in the adult could be the result of developmental abnormalities. The newer tissue-specific knockouts or those where gene expression is said to be regulated by a tissue-specific promoter are improvements, but they are not perfect models. Second, the genetic background of a mutant can have an effect on the mutant. The choice of the inbred line into which the mutation is bred can be critical because many inbred lines have specific behavioral phenotypes (Crawley et al. 1997). Third, phenotypic effects may derive from compensatory changes, not from the mutant itself. An observer, aware of the compensatory mechanism, could confuse direct and indirect effects.

Mutations in the Serotonin System

The serotoninergic system is implicated in both anxious and depressive mood states and is a contributor to genetic variation in personality differences. Of the 14 known receptor types, one has attracted particular interest: 5-HT$_{1a}$ receptors are autoreceptors, acting to inhibit serotonin release from cells in the raphe nucleus, whose axons project across the whole central nervous system and are the major source of serotonin in the brain. 5-HT$_{1a}$ receptors are good candidates for serotonin regulation. Agonists at the receptor have an anxiolytic effect (DeVry 1996; Lucki 1996), and antagonists may enhance the effectiveness of serotonin reuptake inhibitors (such as Prozac) (Artigas et al. 1996).

Three groups of researchers have made knockouts of the 5-HT$_{1a}$ receptor, and all found that the mutants behave in a way consistent with the receptor's role in modulating fear-related behavior (Heisler et al. 1998; Parks et al. 1999; Ramboz et al. 1998). The knockout mice are less active in the open-field arena, make fewer open-arm entries in the elevated plus maze, and spend less time in the open arms. All groups concluded that the mutants display increased anxiety. If so, we might expect the animals to show abnormalities in other models of mood disorder. Here the picture is not as clear because the knockouts show no increase in duration of immobility in the forced-swim test (in this test of depression, depressed animals are expected to become immobile before controls do). As discussed earlier, the swim test may not measure mood at all, so we cannot draw any conclusions from the test result.

Do the data overall support the view that the mutants are more anxious than wild-type mice? On the behavioral data alone such a conclusion is premature. As discussed earlier, we would need a larger set of unconditioned tests to rule out other motivational states and, preferably, data from conditioned tests with a set baseline. Furthermore, it is not clear that the changes are due to a disruption of the $5\text{-}HT_{1a}$ receptor: Ramboz et al. found no significant changes in total 5-HT or its metabolites in any region of the central nervous system they examined (Ramboz et al. 1998). They suggested that compensation may explain the finding, raising the possibility, mentioned earlier, that the behavioral phenotype is a consequence of the compensatory mechanism.

$5\text{-}HT_{1b}$ receptors also inhibit serotonin release, in this case acting at axon terminals (Boschert et al. 1994); but agonists do not have effects on mood, and there are no available specific antagonists. $5\text{-}HT_{1b}$ knockout mice did not show significant differences with wild-type mice in the elevated plus maze and in fear-conditioning tests (Malleret et al. 1999), though there was a trend in the data toward a reduction in anxiety: knockout mice defecated less and head-dipped more (Brunner et al. 1999).

A GABA$_A$ Receptor Mutation

Benzodiazepines bind to the alpha subunit of the GABA$_A$ receptor, with a consequent increase in inhibition. The importance of benzodiazepines for the treatment of anxiety disorders is only one reason to suspect that the target of these drugs might be important in determining individual differences in anxiety. Patents with anxiety disorders show reduced sensitivity to benzodiazepine agonists and increased sensitivity to antagonists, and a GABA$_A$ receptor deficit has been identified in several brain regions of patients with anxiety disorders (Bell et al. 1999; Nutt et al. 1998). Altogether, these data make altered GABA$_A$ receptor function a prime suspect in the search for a cause of variation in anxiety.

Crestani and colleagues generated mice with a deletion of the GABA$_A\gamma2$ receptor (Crestani et al. 1999). The behavior of the heterozygous mutant animals was consistent with increased anxiety: they spent less time in the open arms of an elevated plus maze, made fewer transitions in the light-dark box, and showed increased passive avoidance. Furthermore, the animals' behavior improved with benzodiazepine treatment, as would be expected if they were more anxious.

Mutations Involving the HPA Axis

Variation in reactivity of the hypothalamic-pituitary-adrenal (HPA) axis has long been known to be involved in emotional states and to be partly under genetic control (Gray 1982, 1987). There has been particular interest in the role of corticotropin releasing hormone or factor (CRH), a 41–amino acid hypothalamic peptide that is the prime mediator of stress-induced HPA axis activation. Administration of CRH produces many of the behavioral responses associated with fear: it enhances the acoustic startle response (Swerdlow et al. 1986) and decreases the amount of time spent in the open arms of an elevated plus maze (Baldwin et al. 1991). Furthermore, CRH antagonists reverse these effects (Heinrichs et al. 1992).

Transgenic mice that overexpress CRH show the expected reduction in exploratory behavior and increased anxiety (Stenzel-Poore et al. 1994). CRH receptor type 1 knockout mice show reduced anxiety: they were more likely to explore a novel environment and lower latencies for emerging from a dark box (Timpl et al. 1998). Mice with mutations of the CRH binding protein are more anxious, as assessed in the elevated plus maze, presumably because of increased levels of free CRH (Karolyi et al. 1999).

Genes Suspected of Regulating Mood

A number of genes have now been implicated in human personality differences, and we would like to know the phenotype of the relevant mouse knockout. One such gene is the dopamine D4 receptor (DRD4): a functional polymorphism has been described and the variant observed to occur more frequently in extraversion or novelty seeking behavior (Benjamin et al. 1996; Ebstein et al. 1996). What is the phenotype of the knockout?

The DRD4 knockout has been tested in the open field, in an emergence test, and by presenting a novel object to the animals (Dulawa et al. 1999). Mutants explored the center of the open field less, took longer to emerge from and spent more time in the dark box, and took longer to approach the novel object. The authors concluded that the knockout reflects a decrease in novelty-related exploration. However, a brief perusal of Table 4–1 or of the foregoing descriptions of the HPA and serotonin system knockouts reveals that an equally valid conclusion would be that the DRD4 mutant animal is more anxious. Here of course the trouble lies with the poor quality of the tests. Without either a better behavioral battery for extraversion (novelty seeking) or ways of ruling out anxiety, there are not sufficient grounds to say that DRD4 knockouts are less extraverted.

Mice with genetic deficits in hippocampal long-term potentiation (LTP) have abnormal fear conditioning, so the genes determining LTP, an activity-dependent form of synaptic strengthening (Bliss and Collingridge 1993), have become candidates for emotionality loci. Most behavioral data are available for mice with mutations in the α-calcium calmodulin kinase II gene (αCaMKII). LTP involves activation of N-methyl-D-aspartate (NMDA) receptors and Ca^{2+} influx, which in turn activates second messenger systems such as protein kinases. Deletion of αCaMKII produces deficits in LTP and impairs spatial learning (Silva et al. 1992a, 1992b) but not contextual fear conditioning. Mutation of the gene to a constitutionally active form (calcium independent) confirmed that dissociation of contextual fear conditioning and spatial memory could be achieved. It suggested that different synaptic mechanisms might be responsible for the two forms of learning (Mayford et al. 1995).

The availability of mutants with regulated expression of Ca^{2+} independent αCaMKII has permitted even more detailed investigation of the genetic control of fear-related behaviors. Mayford et al. (1996) found that mice with high levels of expression of the constitutively active αCaMKII in the lateral amygdala and striatum had severe impairments of cued and contextual fear conditioning that could be reversed by suppressing transgene expression. These results indicate that the genetic effect on fear conditioning is through effects on synaptic plasticity and memory formation, not via alterations of developmental processes.

Finally, there is an intriguing result for the nociceptin/orphanin FQ gene, whose product is an endogenous opioid-like peptide. Nociceptin/orphanin FQ enhances pain perception (nociception) due to a reversal of stress-induced analgesia (Mogil et al. 1996; Reinscheid et al. 1995), suggesting that it may operate on the stress response rather than directly on pain. Further work indicated numerous roles for the peptide, including as an anxiolytic (Jenck et al. 1997). Pharmacological investigation would require the development of specific antagonists, but gene knockouts provide an alternative approach. Koster et al. reported the behavioral phenotype of a nociceptin/orphanin FQ knockout (Koster et al. 1999). The animal displayed anxiety-like behavior in the open field, elevated plus maze, and light-dark box. They argued that nociceptin/orphanin FQ is an important regulator of the neurobiological processing of stress responses, opposing the stress-promoting HPA system.

Testing Whether Genes Are Involved in Mood

In a number of cases genes are implicated in mood solely on the basis of a mutant's behavior in the tests of anxiety and depression. The problem here is that the test battery is open to question, particularly when it consists entirely of ethological tests, which so far has always been the case. For example, transgenic mice expressing the interleukin 6 gene were given an active avoidance learning procedure in which the first arm of a Y maze they entered was deemed the preferred arm and subsequent entries into the wrong arm were punished by footshock (Heyser et al. 1997). At 12 months both heterozygous and homozygous mice showed significantly more errors than did controls. Are we to conclude that interleukin 6 is a gene involved in anxiety? Similarly, problems beset results from knockout studies on preproenkephalin (Konig et al. 1996), histamine H1 receptors (Inoue et al. 1996), puromycin-sensitive aminopeptidase (Osada et al. 1999), and the nicotine receptor (Picciotto et al. 1995).

Genetic Models of Temperament

Potentially the most convincing models of personality traits are those derived from genetic selection experiments. If we have a model that can be defined by a number of correlated tests then genetic selection can be used to test the biological validity of the model. We expect that by selecting for one measure, the correlated measures will also change in the selected animals; if they do not, then we question the validity of the model. If they do, then we can look further at the selected strains to see what other measures have been selected because we strongly suspect that these too tap into the biological basis of the trait. However, we must be careful of assuming that correlated measures in the selected strains have not arisen by chance. The only way to distinguish between a chance association and a true genetic correlation is to perform a segregation test. Segregation tests are not easy to carry out, and they are rare in the literature; by contrast there are many reports of correlated traits in selected strains, and even more from studies of inbred strains, where there is even less expectation that the traits are genetically correlated.

Selected Strains
Animals Selected for Measures of Anxiety

The most convincing case for selectively produced temperamental differences comes from experiments where selection for different tests of the same temperament have equivalent results, so animals selected on test A show the expected difference on test B, and animals selected for test B behave as predicted on test A. The literature contains few examples of this type, no doubt because of the cost and length of time involved in establishing selected strains.

The best example is the production of strains selected for tests of emotionality. Broadhurst performed a genetic selection experiment in the open-field arena in which he selected rats with high and low rates of defecation, eventually producing two strains that consistently differed in their defecation in the open-field (Broadhurst 1960). Rats with high defecation rates were called the Maudsley reactive (MR) strain, and the animals with low defecation rates were called the Maudsley nonreactive (MNR) strain. DeFries performed a similar experiment in mice, selecting the animals for activity rather than defecation in the open field (DeFries and Hegman 1970; DeFries et al. 1970, 1978). In both experiments during and after selection there was a correlated change in the other measure: selection for high activity in the open field resulted in low defecation scores; selection for low defecation scores resulted in high activity.

Open field defecation and activity measures on their own are of course not a convincing test of emotionality, but the case is strengthened by work on a rat model of learning. Bignami established two strains of rat, known as Roman high-avoidance (RHA) and Roman low-avoidance (RLA), by selecting rats for their speed of acquisition in a two-way active avoidance task (Bignami 1965; Broadhurst and Bignami 1965). After five generations of selection the high-avoidance strain rats were consistently better than the low-avoidance strain rats at escaping when shown the light.

One interpretation of this experiment is that RLA rats were freezing in response to the light; they were responding with passive rather than active avoidance (Driscoll et al. 1980). In other words, the selection experiment had produced animals that differed in emotionality. This hypothesis can be tested by seeing whether the animals behave as predicted in other tests of emotionality. Novelty-induced defecation is higher in RLA than RHA rats (Driscoll and Battig 1982). Conversely, rodents that differ on the open-field measures of emotionality should differ in the predicted fashion in tests of active and passive avoidance. Indeed it has been repeatedly shown that the MR rat is poorer at shuttle-box avoidance (active avoidance) than its nonreactive counterpart (Gray 1982).

These experiments go some way to validating the use of these strains as models of emotional behavior. However, there are also important discrepancies in the literature. For instance, no difference in shuttle-box avoidance was found in one test of the Maudsley rats (Overstreet et al. 1992). Some of the inconsistencies in the literature may be due to the creation of substrains of the Maudsley rats. It is possible that the original selection experiment produced animals differing in emotionality, of which defecation differences were one phenotype. Subsequent to the relaxation of selection and with the introduction of new genes from other strains, emotional differences could have been lost, without this necessarily affecting the defecation scores in the open field.

As discussed earlier, one way to test whether the observed phenotypic correlations in selected strains has a genetic basis is to perform a segregation test. This has been carried out for the Roman strains (Castanon et al. 1995); it confirmed a relationship between two-way active avoidance and one endocrine measure of stress (prolactin reactivity), but corticosterone response was not correlated with the avoidance task. Unfortunately the study did not examine the relationship between the different tests of emotionality carried out on the Roman rats, so we still do not know to what extent the associations between behavioral tests are genetically driven.

Animals Selected for Measures of Depression

Selecting animals for depression has not been as popular as selecting animals for anxiety phenotypes, largely because of the lack of good tests for depression. There is only one model that has been extensively investigated: the Flinders sensitive line (FSL) and the Flinders resistant line (FRL) of rats (Overstreet 1993).

The lines were established through selection for sensitivity to an anticholinesterase, and the FSL is the more depressed: animals show exaggerated immobility in the forced swim test, and this improves with antidepressant treatment. Interestingly, a drug response is seen only with chronic administration. The lines do not differ in the elevated plus maze, either with or without benzodiazepine treatment, suggesting they do not differ in emotionality; however, the results of conditioned tests make this interpretation more difficult to sustain (Overstreet 1993). FSL rats are quicker to learn a passive avoidance task than are FRL rats, and they are slower to acquire an active avoidance. Such results indicate the FSL is more emotional than the FRL. Of course, this may mean we cannot dissociate tests of depression and anxiety. Again it would be instructive to have a genetic test to see if the features can be dissociated.

Mapping Genes for Temperamental Differences in Animals

It is forgivable to read the results from the gene knockout experiments as an indication that single-gene effects on behavior are precise and specific models of behavior. The examples I have given appear to demonstrate that there is a relatively straightforward relationship between mutation and behavioral phenotype, for example that the 5-HT_{1a} mutation gives rise to anxiety. If this is so, we might wonder whether there is any value in undertaking the genetic analysis of individual differences in temperament. The undertaking is clearly very difficult, for which the large number of false starts in psychiatric genetics is a witness. Indeed, the difficulties in identifying the genes are so great that it may be best to take an alternative strategy, such as mutagenesis in which large numbers of randomly distributed mutants are generated and each animal is tested for deficiency in a behavioral test of interest.

However, knockouts are not a good model for the way genes influence complex traits. Personality differences, like many other complex behavioral traits, are measured quantitatively, and the genes that influence personality scores are therefore said to be found at quantitative trait loci (QTLs). We know the genetic architecture of personality, again like other complex traits, is determined by many genes, most of which have a small effect. Although knockouts may teach us about the involvement of a specific gene on a behavior, and therefore mutagenesis experiments could find genes crucial for that phenotype, knockouts do not model the complex pattern of gene interactions that give rise to the phenotype. Therefore molecular dissection of personality differences will probably reveal a very different picture from that we have obtained from gene knockouts. It will certainly be complex, and it seems unlikely that mutations will be found. Instead, the small effects we know to be attributed to each gene are likely to be due to changes in regulatory regions, subtly altering gene expression.

QTL Mapping of Emotionality

Genetic mapping of behavioral traits in humans is difficult, but it has proved possible in animals, and the first lesson to be learned from mapping temperament in animals is that the genetic basis need not be complex. In fact, most studies agree that in inbred strains individual differences in the phenotype can be produced by a small number of genes (Table 4–3). The second lesson has been that most loci are pleiotropic. Genetic mapping is a sophisticated way of performing a segregation test. We can use it as a genetic validation of a phenotype, asking whether phenotypic correlations observed in selected strains really reflect common gene action. The DeFries mice were scored for open-field behavior, defecation, and elevated plus maze activity. Of six loci that were significantly associated with activity, three were also significantly associated with defecation and entry into the open arms of the elevated plus maze. Gershenfeld and Paul (1997) mapped thigmotaxis in the open field and light-dark transitions. Thigmotaxis again mapped to chromosome 1, though it was more proximal to the centromere than the previously identified locus for open-field avoidance. Using the number of transitions between light and dark boxes as a measure of exploratory behavior, Gershenfeld and Paul mapped a QTL to chromosome 10. One study of hyperactivity in the rat identified a locus on chromosome 8 that contributed substantially to the variation in spontaneous activity, rearing, and activity in the open field (Moisan et al. 1996). However this is not homologous to loci identified in the mouse.

Genetic loci contributing to variation in fear conditioning have also been mapped, providing an opportunity to test the hypothesis that fear conditioning and open-field behaviors have a common genetic basis. Two F2 intercrosses and one study of recombinant inbred strains identified a locus on chromosome 1 that lies within the region identified by the work on open-field behaviors (Caldarone et al. 1997; Owen et al. 1997; Wehner et al. 1997). It appears likely that a locus on chromosome 1 determines variability in a genetic system mediating fear.

TABLE 4–3   Emotionality quantitative trait loci detected in F2 intercrosses

Closest marker	Position	Lod score	% var.	Cross
D1Mit150	84.4	13.4	9.2	BALBc/J × C57BL/6
D1Mit116	80.2	7.08	6.3	A/J × C57BL/6
D10Mit237 + 2 cM	76	8.76	8.3	A/J × C57BL/6
D12Mit47 + 6 cM	31.5	4.3	4.4	BALBc/J × C57BL/6
D15Mit63 + 3 cM	44	11	8.1	BALBc/J × C57BL/6
D19Mit46	24	3.15	3.2	A/J × C57BL/6

Source. Data from Flint et al. 1995, Gershenfeld and Paul 1997, and Gershenfeld et al. 1997.

However, all these results have been obtained using crosses between inbred animal strains. The strategy has great power (it can detect genes that contribute to as little as 5% of the phenotypic variance of the trait), but it also samples only a fraction of the total variability of a population. Each time a cross is set up, we can look at only two alleles at any locus, and many loci may not be polymorphic in the strain pair that we pick. This explains why results of mapping experiments differ: for example, a locus on chromosome 10 that influences open-field activity was found in a cross between A/J and C57Bl/6J (Gershenfeld and Paul 1997) but not in a cross between BALBcJ and C57Bl/6J (Flint et al. 1995). Thus we cannot yet say if there are any loci that are polymorphic in all strain crosses. Obviously, finding such a locus would tempt us to look in humans at the syntenic region.

Inbred strain analyses have another disadvantage: they do not allow us to fine-map QTLs, a necessary first step toward the molecular identification of the variant. The reason for this is simple: they analyze chromosomes that have been through just one meiosis where recombination is detectable. In other words, the average chromosome will have undergone only a number of recombination events. Thus markers distant from the QTL will still be linked (hence the power of the method); but without many recombinants to divide up the chromosome, we cannot precisely identify where the QTL is on the chromosome (Darvasi 1998). However, it has recently been shown that outbred animals can be used for QTL mapping. Using this new approach one QTL has been mapped to a subcentimorgan level of resolution (within an interval of about 2 Mb of DNA), to the point where positional cloning strategies become feasible (Talbot, et al. 1999).

Thus it may be possible to use gene mapping and cloning in rodents as a way of isolating homologous human genes. The task of finding genes for susceptibility to emotions in humans may not be as daunting as has appeared to be the case from the attempts to map genes for behavioral disorders.

References

Abel T, Nguyen PV, Barad M, et al: Genetic demonstration of a role for PKA in the late phase of LTP and in hippocampus-based long-term memory. Cell 88:615–626, 1997

Abeliovich A, Paylor R, Chen C, et al: PKC gamma mutant mice exhibit mild deficits in spatial and contextual learning. Cell 75:1263–1271, 1993

Artigas F, Romero L, deMontigny C, et al: Acceleration of the effect of selected antidepressant drugs in major depression by 5-HT$_{1A}$ antagonists. Trends Neurosci 19:378–383, 1996

Bach ME, Hawkins RD, Osman M, et al: Impairment of spatial but not contextual memory in CaMKII mutant mice with a selective loss of hippocampal LTP in the range of the theta frequency. Cell 81:905–915, 1995

Baldwin HA, Rassnick S, Rivier J, et al: CRF antagonist reverses the anxiogenic response to ethanol withdrawal in the rat. Psychopharmacology 103:227–232, 1991

Bell CJ, Malizia AL, Nutt DJ: The neurobiology of social phobia. Eur Arch Psychiatry Clin Neurosci 249:S11–S18, 1999

Benjamin J, Li L, Patterson C, et al: Population and familial association between the D4 dopamine receptor gene and measures of Novelty Seeking. Nat Genet 12:81–84, 1996

Bignami G: Selection for high rates and low rates of avoidance conditioning in the rat. Behavioral Research Therapeutics 2:273–280, 1965

Bliss TV, Collingridge GL: A synaptic model of memory: long-term potentiation in the hippocampus. Nature 361:31–39, 1993

Borsini F, Meli A: Is the forced swimming test a suitable model for revealing antidepressant activity? Psychopharmacology 94:147–160, 1988

Boschert U, Amara DA, Segu L, et al: The mouse 5-hydroxytryptamine (1b) receptor is localized predominantly on axon terminals. Neuroscience 58:167–182, 1994

Brandon EP, Zhuo M, Huang Y.-Y, et al: Hippocampal long-term depression and depotentiation are defective in mice carrying a targeted disruption of the gene encoding the RIβ subunit of cAMP-dependent protein kinase. Proc Natl Acad Sci U S A 92:8851–8855, 1995

Broadhurst PL: Application of biometrical genetics to the inheritance of behaviour in Experiments in Personality. London, Routledge and Kegan Paul, 1960, pp. 3–102

Broadhurst PL, Bignami G: Correlative effect of psychogenetic selection: a study of the Roman high and low avoidance strains of rats. Behav Res Ther 2:273–280, 1965

Brunner D, Buhot MC, Hen R, et al: Anxiety, motor activation, and maternal-infant interactions in 5-HT$_{1B}$ knockout mice. Behav Neurosci 113:587–601, 1999

Caldarone B, Saavedra C, Tartaglia K, et al: Quantitative trait loci analysis affecting contextual conditioning in mice. Nat Genet 17:335–337, 1997

Castanon N, Perezdiaz F, Mormede P: Genetic analysis of the relationships between behavioral and neuroendocrine traits in Roman high-avoidance and low-avoidance rat lines. Behav Genet 25:371–384, 1995

Chen C, Kano M, Abelivochi A, et al: Impaired motor coordination correlates with persistent multiple climbing fiber innervation in PKCγ mutant mice. Cell 83:1233–1242, 1995a

Chen C, Rainnie DG, Greene RW, et al: Abnormal fear response and aggressive behavior in mutant mice deficient for alpha-calcium-calmodulin kinase II. Science 267:437, 1995b

Crawley JN, Belknap JK, Collins A, et al: Behavioral phenotypes of inbred mouse strains: implications and recommendations for molecular studies. Psychopharmacology 132:107–124, 1997

Crestani F, Lorez M, Baer K, et al: Decreased GABA-A receptor clustering results in enhanced anxiety and a bias for threat cues. Nat Neurosci 2:833–839, 1999

Darvasi A: Experimental strategies for the genetic dissection of complex traits in animal models. Nat Genet 18:19–24, 1998

Davis M: Animal models of anxiety based on classical conditioning: the conditioned emotional response and fear-potentiated startle effect, in Psychopharmacology of Anxiolytics and Antidepressants. Oxford, UK, Pergamon Press, 1991, pp 187–212

Dawson GR, Crawford SP, Collinson N, et al: Evidence that the anxiolytic-like effects of chlordiazepoxide on the elevated plus-maze are confounded by increases in locomotor activity. Psychopharmacology 118:316–323, 1995

DeFries JC, Hegman JP: Genetic analysis of open-field behavior, in Contributions to Behavior Genetic Analysis: The Mouse As a Prototype. New York, Appleton-Century-Crofts, 1970, pp 23–56

DeFries JC, Wilson JR, McClearn GE: Open-field behavior in mice: selection response and situational generality. Behav Genet 1:195–211, 1970

DeFries JC, Gervais MC, Thomas EA: Response to 30 generations of selection for open field activity in laboratory mice. Behav Genet 8:3–213, 1978

DeVry J: 5-HT$_{1A}$ receptors in psychopathology and the mechanism of action of clinically effective therapeutic agents. Drug News and Perspectives 9:270–280, 1996

Driscoll P, Battig K: Behavioral, emotional and neurochemical profiles of rats selected for extreme differences in active two way avoidance, in Genetics of the Brain. Amsterdam, Elsevier, 1982, pp 95–123

Driscoll P, Woodson P, Fuem H, et al: Selection for two-way avoidance deficit inhibits shock-induced fighting in the rat. Physiol and Behav 24:793–795, 1980

Dulawa SC, Grandy DK, Low, MJ, et al: Dopamine D4 receptor knock-out mice exhibit reduced exploration of novel stimuli. J Neurosci 19:9550–9556, 1999

Ebstein RP, Novick O, Umansky R, et al: Dopamine D4 receptor *(D4DR)* exon III polymorphism associated with the human personality trait of novelty seeking. Nat Genet 12:78–84, 1996

Eysenck HJ: The biological basis of personality. Springfield, IL, Charles C Thomas, 1967

Flint J, Corley R, DeFries JC, et al: A simple genetic basis for a complex psychological trait in laboratory mice. Science 269:1432–1435, 1995

Gerlai R: Gene-targeting studies of mammalian behavior: is it the mutation or the background genotype? Trends Neurosci 19:177–181, 1996

Gerlai R: Targeting genes and proteins in the analysis of learning and memory: caveats and future directions. Rev Neurosci 11:15–26, 2000

Gershenfeld HK, Paul SM: Mapping quantitative trait loci for fear-like behaviors in mice. Genomics 46:1–8, 1997

Gershenfeld HK, Neumann PE, Mathis C, et al: Mapping quantitative trait loci for open-field behavior in mice. Behav Genet 27:201–210, 1997

Gray JA: The Neuropsychology of Anxiety: An Enquiry into the Function of the Septo-Hippocampal System. Oxford, UK, Oxford University Press, 1982

Gray JA: The Psychology of Fear and Stress. Cambridge, UK, Cambridge University Press, 1987

Heinrichs SC, Pich EM, Miczek KA, et al: Corticotropin-releasing factor antagonist reduces emotionality in socially defeated rats via direct neurotropic action. Brain Res 581:190–197, 1992

Heisler LK, Chu H-M, Brennan TJ, et al: Elevated anxiety and antidepressant-like responses in serotonin 5-HT$_{1A}$ receptor mutant mice. Proc Natl Acad Sci U S A 95:15049–15054, 1998

Heyser CJ, Masliah E, Samini A, et al: Progressive decline in avoidance learning paralleled by inflammatory neurodegeneration in transgenic mice expressing interleukin 6 in the brain. Proc Natl Acad Sci U S A 94:1500–1505, 1997

Inoue I, Yanai K, Kitamura D, et al: Impaired locomotor activity and exploratory behavior in mice lacking histamine H$_1$ receptors. Proc Natl Acad Sci U S A 93:13316–13320, 1996

Jenck F, Moreau JL, Martin JR, et al: Orphanin FQ acts as an anxiolytic to attenuate behavioral responses to stress. Proc Natl Acad Sci U S A 94:14854–14858, 1997

Karolyi IJ, Burrows HL, Ramesh TM, et al: Altered anxiety and weight gain in corticotropin-releasing hormone-binding protein-deficient mice. Proc Natl Acad Sci U S A 96:11595–11600, 1999

Kendler KS, Neale MC, Kessler RC, et al: Major depression and phobias: the genetic and environmental sources of comorbidity. Psychol Med 23:361–371, 1993

Konig M, Zimmer AM, Steiner H, et al: Pain responses, anxiety and aggression in mice deficient in pre-proenkephalin. Nature 383:535–538, 1996

Koster A, Montkowski A, Schulz S, et al: Targeted disruption of the orphanin FQ/nociceptin gene increases stress susceptibility and impairs stress adaptation in mice. Neurobiology 96:10444–10449, 1999

Lucki I: Serotonin receptor specificity in anxiety disorders. J Clin Psychiatry 57:5–10, 1996

Malleret G, Hen R, Guillou JL, et al: 5-HT$_{1B}$ receptor knock-out mice exhibit increased exploratory activity and enhanced spatial memory performance in the Morris water maze. J Neurosci 19:6157–6168, 1999

Mayford M, Wang J, Kandel ER, et al: CaMKII regulates the frequency-response function of hippocampal synapses for the production of both LTD and LTP. Cell 81:891–904, 1995

Mayford M, Bach ME, Huang YY, et al: Control of memory formation through regulated expression of α CaMKII transgene. Science 274:1678–1683, 1996

Mogil JS, Grisel JE, Reinscheid KK, et al: Orphanin FQ is a functional anti-opioid peptide. Neuroscience 75:333–337, 1996

Moisan MP, Courvoisier H, Bihoreau MT, et al: A major quantitative trait locus influences hyperactivity in the Wkha rat. Nat Genet 14:471–473, 1996

Nutt DJ, Bell CJ, Malizia AL: Brain mechanisms of social anxiety disorder. J Clin Psychiatry 59:4–11, 1998

Osada T, Ikegami S, Takiguchi-Hayashi K: Increased anxiety and impaired pain response in puromycin-sensitive aminopeptidase gene-deficient mice obtained by a mouse gene-trap method. J Neurosci 19:6068–6078, 1999

Overstreet DH: The Flinders sensitive line rats: a genetic animal-model of depression. Neurosci Biobehav Rev 17:51–68, 1993

Overstreet DH, Rezvani AH, Janowsky DS: Maudsley reactive and nonreactive rats differ only in some tasks reflecting emotionality. Physiol Behav 52:149–152, 1992

Owen EH, Christensen SC, Paylor R, et al: Identification of quantitative trait loci involved in contextual and auditory-cued fear conditioning in BXD recombinant inbred strains. Behav Neurosci 111:1–9, 1997

Parks CL, Robinson PS, Sibille E, et al: Increased anxiety of mice lacking the serotonin 1a receptor. Proc Natl Acad Sci U S A 95:10734–10739, 1999

Phillips RG, LeDoux JE: Differential contribution of amygdala and hippocampus to cued and contextual fear conditioning. Behav Neurosci 106:274–285, 1992

Picciotto MR, Zoli M, Léna C, et al: Abnormal avoidance learning in mice lacking functional high-affinity nicotine receptor in the brain. Nature 374:65–67, 1995

Ramboz S, Oosting R, Amara DA, et al: Serotonin receptor 1A knockout: an animal model of anxiety-related disorder. Proc Natl Acad Sci U S A 95:14476–14481, 1998

Ramos A, Mormède P: Stress and emotionality: a multidimensional and genetic approach. Neurosci Biobehav Rev 22:33–57, 1998

Ramos A, Berton O, Mormede P, et al: A multiple-test study of anxiety-related behaviours in six inbred rat strains. Behav Brain Res 85:57–69, 1997

Reinscheid RK, Nothacker HP, Bourson A, et al: Orphanin-FQ: a neuropeptide that activates an opioid-like G-protein-coupled receptor. Science 270:792–794, 1995

Rodgers RJ, Cao BJ, Dalvi A, et al: Animal models of anxiety: an ethological perspective. Braz J Med Biol Res 30:289–304, 1997

Rotenberg A, Mayford M, Hawkins RD, et al: Mice expressing activated CaMKII lack low frequency LTP and do not form stable place cells in the CA1 region of the hippocampus. Cell 87:1351–1361, 1996

Saudou F, Amara DA, Dierich A, et al: Enhanced aggressive behavior in mice lacking 5-HT1B receptor. Science 265:1875–1878, 1994

Seligman MEP: Depression and learned helplessness, in The Psychology of Depression: Contemporary Theory and Research. Washington, DC, Winston-Wiley, 1974, pp 83–111

Silva AJ, Paylor R, Wehner JM, et al: Impaired spatial learning in α-calcium-calmodulin kinase II mutant mice. Science 257:206–211, 1992a

Silva AJ, Stevens CF, Tonegawa S, et al: Deficient hippocampal long-term potentiation in α-calcium-calmodulin kinase II mutant mice. Science 257:201–206, 1992b

Smith GW, Aubry JM, Dellu F, et al: Corticotropin releasing factor receptor 1–deficient mice display decreased anxiety, impaired stress response, and aberrant neuroendocrine development. Neuron 20:1093–1102, 1998

Stenzel-Poore MP, Heinrichs SC, Rivest S, et al: Overproduction of corticotropin-releasing factor in transgenic mice: a genetic model of anxiogenic behavior. J Neurosci 14:2579–2584, 1994

Swerdlow NR, Geyer MA, Vale W, et al: Corticotropin releasing factor potentiates acoustic startle in rats: blocked by chlordiazepoxide. Psychopharmacology 88:147–152, 1986

Talbot CJ, Nicod A, Cherny SS, et al: High-resolution mapping of quantitative trait loci in outbred mice. Nat Genet 21:305–308, 1999

Tecott LH, Logue SF, Wehner JM, et al: Perturbed dentate gyrus function in serotonin 5-HT$_{2C}$ receptor mutant mice. Proc Natl Acad Sci U S A 95:15026–15031, 1998

Timpl P, Spanagel RS, Kresse A, et al: Impaired stress response and reduced anxiety in mice lacking a functional corticotropin-releasing hormone receptor 1. Nat Genet 19:162–166, 1998

Treit D: Animal models for the study of anti-anxiety agents: a review. Neurosci Biobehav Rev 9:203–222, 1985

Wehner JM, Radcliffe RA, Rosmann ST, et al: Quantitative trait locus analysis of contextual fear conditioning in mice. Nat Genet 17:331–334, 1997

Weninger SC, Dunn AJ, Muglia LJ, et al: Stress-induced behaviors require the corticotropin-releasing hormone (CRH) receptor, but not CRH. Proc Natl Acad Sci U S A 96:8283–8288, 1999

Willner P: Animal models for clinical psychopharmacology: depression, anxiety, schizophrenia. International Review of Psychiatry 2:253–276, 1990

Willner P, Muscat R, Papp M: Chronic mild stress-induced anhedonia: a realistic animal model of depression. Neurosci Biobehav Rev 16:525–534, 1992

Zuckerman M: Psychobiology of Personality. Cambridge, UK, Cambridge University Press, 1991

CHAPTER FIVE

DRD4 and Novelty Seeking

Paolo Prolo, M.D.
Julio Licinio, M.D.

Following the cloning of the dopamine D4 receptor gene *(DRD4)* in 1991 (Van Tol et al. 1991) various attempts have been made to identify a disorder associated with this gene (Asghari et al. 1994; Van Tol et al. 1992). Following the discovery of several sets of variance in the coding region of *DRD4*, a large effort has been made to assess the possible role of these polymorphisms in the pathophysiology of schizophrenia and bipolar disorder (Paterson et al. 1999). Linkage and association studies have failed to demonstrate *DRD4* involvement in either disease. Other reports have already proposed a link between some normal personality traits and variability in dopamine transmission (Cloninger 1987; Zuckerman 1985), without a specific genetic basis. Two independent groups at the 1995 World Congress on Psychiatric Genetics in Cardiff presented work demonstrating an association between the personality trait of novelty seeking in normal human volunteers and the seven-repeat allele of *DRD4*. Those results were published in 1996 (Benjamin et al. 1996; Ebstein et al. 1996).

Paolo Prolo was supported by a grant from Sanofi-Synthélabo Italy S.p.A.

The importance of genetic contribution to personality was proposed long before the genotyping era. It has been known for decades that normal human personality traits show a heritable component (Plomin et al. 1994). The development of reliable measures of personality provided a replicable assessment tool for the study of both normal and pathological personality traits. Several different rating instruments available today are the result of efforts to validate the assessment of personality using replicable measures. They include Cloninger's Tridimensional Personality Questionnaire (TPQ) (Cloninger et al. 1991) and Temperament and Character Inventory (TCI) (Cloninger 1994), the NEO Personality Inventory, Revised (NEO-PI-R) (Kurtz et al. 1999), and the Karolinska Scales of Personality (KSP) (Schalling et al. 1987). The TPQ as well as the TCI have been designed to assess four different types of temperament (novelty seeking, harm avoidance, reward dependence, and persistence) that are supposed to be genetically determined and that are based on specific psychobiological correlates. According to Cloninger's biobehavioral observations on both humans and animals, novelty seeking would be related to dopamine, harm avoidance to serotonin, and reward dependence to norepinephrine (Cloninger 1987). The NEO-PI-R and the KSP are more detailed scales that have been demonstrated to have high reliability and longitudinal stability. TPQ scores can be estimated from the NEO-PI-R through a weighted equation (Ebstein and Belmaker 1997), whereas no such agreement can be reached with the KSP (Jonsson et al. 1997). Overall reliability between TQP and NEO-PI-R is in the range of 70% (Ebstein and Belmaker 1997). Zuckerman's Sensation Seeking Scale (Zuckerman and Link 1968) is rarely used; sensation seeking can be considered phenotypically similar to Cloninger's novelty seeking.

Studies of *DRD4* and Novelty Seeking

Novelty seeking is characterized by impulsiveness, exploration, changeability, excitability, hotheadedness, and extravagance (Cloninger 1987). Subjects with above-average scores on the TPQ Novelty Seeking scale are extravagant, exploratory, excitable, and impulsive. Individuals with TPQ Novelty Seeking scores that are below average are reflexive, stoic, loyal, and frugal. Two earlier studies (Adamson et al. 1995; George et al. 1993) found no connection between *DRD4* and novelty seeking. In 1995 Ebstein and colleagues (published in 1996) and Benjamin and colleagues (published in 1996) were able to simultaneously demonstrate a significant association between above-average TPQ Novelty Seeking scores in normal individuals and the seven-repeat allele in the locus for the D4 gene. That particular polymorphism was chosen because *DRD4* is expressed in limbic regions and the importance of dopamine in the brain's reward system. The convergence of these reports is particularly striking if we consider that Ebstein et al. in Israel analyzed data from 69 males and 55 females with a mean age ($\pm$SD) of 29.8 $\pm$ 8.9 years that were mostly of Jewish background, whereas Benjamin et al. in the United States studied 315 subjects (95% males and 5% females) with a mean age ($\pm$SD) of 32.4 $\pm$ 10.8 years that were predominantly non-Jewish Caucasians. Those findings were later replicated in China and Japan on individuals with substance abuse disorder (Lietal 1997; Muramatsu et al. 1996; Ono et al. 1997), whereas further studies conducted in Europe, in the United States, and in New Zealand (Jonsson et al. 1997) failed to replicate that association, until the reports of Strobel et al. and Ekelund et al. were published in 1999 (Table 5–1). Strobel et al.'s and Ekelund et al.'s careful study designs and findings on normal subjects now lend considerable additional support to the original findings of Benjamin et al. and Ebstein et al. In particular, Strobel et al. (1999) were able to demonstrate an association between long *DRD4* alleles and significantly high scores on the TPQ Novelty Seeking Total scale as well as on the Exploratory Excitability and Extravagance subscales in a young Caucasian population of 48 males and 88 females with an age mean ($\pm$SD) of 23.6 $\pm$ 3.9. Ekelund et al. (1999) administered the TCI to 4,773 individuals from the 1996 birth cohort of northern Finland (Jones et al. 1998). They then selected 200 normal subjects with extreme scores on the Novelty Seeking subscale. They found that the two- and five-repeat alleles were more significantly represented in the high scorers versus the low scorers. This finding suggests that the two-repeat allele might be in linkage disequilibrium with the seven-repeat allele originally studied by Ebstein and colleagues (1996). Given this confluence of results in large independent studies conducted in various populations, it appears that the D4 gene may indeed contribute to the trait of novelty seeking.

Because temperament is the earliest manifestation of personality in children, it is conceivable that temperament in newborns is influenced minimally by the environment and maximally by genes. Brazelton's Neonatal Behavioral Assessment Scale (NBAS) (Brazelton 1989) evaluates neonatal behavior and includes items related to temperament. Only two articles to our knowledge to date have assessed neonatal behavior and its association with *DRD4* (Auerbach et al. 1999; Ebstein et al. 1998). The study by Ebstein et al. shows a significant association between *DRD4* and

TABLE 5–1   Association among DRD4 polymorphisms and novelty-seeking personality and/or substance abuse

Authors	Population	Ethnicity	Mean age (years ± SD)
George et al. 1993	72 alcoholic subjects	Canadian Caucasian	40.5
Adamson et al. 1995	113 alcoholic subjects 113 normal volunteers	Finnish	Unknown
Benjamin et al. 1996	315 normal volunteers	$n = 290$ white non-Hispanic $n = 13$ Asian $n = 9$ Hispanic $n = 2$ African American $n = 1$ Native American	32.4 ± 10.8
Ebstein et al. 1996	114 normal volunteers	$n = 90$ Ashkenazi Jews $n = 25$ Sephardic Jews $n = 5$ mixed Ashkenazi/Sephardic $n = 1$ Arab $n = 1$ Druze $n = 2$ Jews of unknown background	29.8 ± 8.9
Muramatsu et al. 1996	655 alcoholic subjects 144 normal volunteers	Japanese	50.0
Malhotra et al. 1996	193 normal males 138 alcoholic offenders	Finnish	31.1 ± 0.7 33.5 ± 0.8
Ebstein et al. 1997	114 normal volunteers	$n = 90$ Ashkenazi Jews $n = 25$ Sephardic Jews $n = 5$ mixed Ashkenazi/Sephardic $n = 1$ Arab $n = 1$ Druze $n = 2$ Jews of unknown background	29.8 + 8.9
Chang et al. 1997	62 alcoholic subjects 65 normal volunteers	Chinese: Han (21 ± 24) Atayal (21 ± 21) Ami (20 ± 20)	Unknown
Garpenstrand et al. 1997	14 schizophrenic subjects 6 anorexic subjects 3 depressed subjects 2 bipolar subjects 1 obese subject 2 bulimic subjects 21 normal volunteers	Caucasian	Unknown
Geijer et al. 1997	72 alcoholic subjects 67 normal volunteers	Swedish	Unknown
Kotler et al. 1997	110 Israeli normal males 141 male heroin addicts	$n = 54$ Sephardic Jews $n = 56$ Israeli Arabs $n = 107$ Sephardic Jews $n = 34$ Israeli Arabs	45.8 ± 2.28 32.4 ± 0.54
Jonsson et al. 1997	126 normal subjects	Swedish	41 ± 8

Gender	Assessment	Polymorphism	Significance
M = 62 F = 14	Clinical interview	DRD4 exon III repeats	Unclear
M = 113 M = 113	Clinical interview	DRD4 exon III repeats	NS
M = 300 F = 15	NEO-PI-R	Short vs. long DRD4 exon III	$P = 0.002$ (long allele)
M = 69 F = 55	TPQ	7-repeat allele absent 7-repeat allele present 4/4 genotype 4/7 genotype	$P = 0.013$ $P = 0.026$
M = 597 F = 58 M = 70 F = 74	Clinical interview	DRD4 exon III repeats	$P < 0.001$ (in patients)
M = 193 M = 138	TPQ	7-repeat allele	NS NS
M = 69 F = 55	TPQ	Long-repeat DRD4 + 5-HT$_{2Cser}$	Too small cohort expressing both alleles ($n = 6$)
Unknown	Clinical interview	DRD4 exon III repeats	NS
Patients: M = 12 F = 19 Normal subjects: M = 12 F = 9	SSST	DRD4 exon III repeats and trbc MAO	NS
Unknown	Clinical interview	DRD4 exon III repeats	NS
M = 110 M = 141	TPQ	DRD4 exon III 7-repeat allele	$P = 0.02$ (Sephardic heroin dependent) $P = 0.02$ (Arab heroin dependent)
M = 76 F = 50	Karolinska Scales of Personality	Exon III 48 bp Exon I 12-bp repeats Exon I 13-bp deletion	NS NS NS

Continued

TABLE 5–1   Association among DRD4 polymorphisms and novelty-seeking personality and/or substance abuse (Continued)

Authors	Population	Ethnicity	Mean age (years ± SD)
Sander et al. 1997	252 alcoholic subjects	Caucasian	41.9 ± 9.4
Vandenbergh et al. 1997	200 elderly subjects	Unknown (Caucasian)	61.3
Li et al. 1997	121 heroin addicts	Han Chinese	26.97 ± 4.95
Ebstein et al. 1997	94 normal volunteers	Jewish	Unknown
Ono et al. 1997	153 normal volunteers	Japanese	18.7 ± 1.0
Sullivan et al. 1998	86 subjects with major depression	Caucasian (New Zealand)	32.0 ± 11.0
	181 alcoholic subjects		39.7 ± 14.1
Benjamin et al. 1998	124 normal volunteers	n = 91 Ashkenazi Jews n = 33 non-Ashkenazi Jews, Arabs, or others	29.7 ± 9
Pogue-Geile et al. 1998	Same-sex twins (Pennsylvania)	Unknown	18–27
Ebstein et al. 1998	81 newborns	n = 21 Ashkenazi Jews; n = 60 non-Ashkenazi Jews	2 weeks old
Ricketts et al. 1998	95 patients with Parkinson's disease	Caucasian	Patients: 68.9
	47 controls		Controls: 67.5
Mel et al. 1998	143 normal subjects	Israeli	32 ± 0.5
	57 Israeli heroin addicts		
Auerbach et al. 1999	76 infants	Israeli	2 months old
Strobel et al. 1999	136 normal subjects	Caucasian (German)	23.6 ± 3.9
Ekelund et al. 1999	200 normal subjects[b]	Finnish	All born in 1966

Gender	Assessment	Polymorphism	Significance
M = 252	Clinical interview	Exon III 48 bp	NS
M = 116 F = 88	NEO-PI-R	Exon III 7-repeat alleles	NS
M = 88 F = 33	Clinical interview	Long form of exon III vs. short form	$P = 0.02$
Unknown	TPQ	DRD4 exon III 7-repeat allele	$P = 0.01$[a]
F = 153	TPI	DRD4 exon III 48 bp	$P = 0.045$
M = 34 F = 52 M = 90 F = 91	TCI	DRD4 7-repeat allele and 4-repeat allele	NS
M = 69 F = 55	TPQ	DRD4 exon I 12 bp	NS
MZ pairs: M = 43 F = 49 DZ pairs: M = 29 F = 32	TPQ; NST; NEO; Eysenck's extraversion scale; SSST	DRD4 exon I 12 bp DRD4 exon III 48 bp	NS NS
M = 40 F = 41	NBAS	DRD4 exon III 7-repeat allele	$P = 0.02$
M = 60 F = 35 M = 17 F = 30	TPQ	DRD4 exon III 7-repeat allele	$P = 0.039$ (Parkinson's vs. controls) NS (novelty seeking)
M = 143 M = 57	TPQ (38 heroin addicts)	DRD4 exon III 7-repeat allele	$P = 0.04$ (heroin addicts vs. exon III) $P = 0.001$ (novelty seeking)
M = 39 F = 37	IBQ	DRD4 exon III 7-repeat allele	$P = 0.005$ (negative emotionality)
M = 48 F = 88	TPQ	DRD4 exon III 7-repeat allele	$P = 0.001$
M = 100 F = 100	TCI	DRD4 exon III 2-, 3-, 4-, 5-, 6-, 7-, 8-repeat alleles	$P = 0.01$ (2-repeat) $P = 0.03$ (5-repeat)

Note. IBQ = Rothbart's Infant Behavior Questionnaire; NBAS = Brazelton Neonatal Behavioral Assessment Scale; NST = Novelty-Seeking Total Scale; NEO = NEO Personality Inventory; NS = nonsignificant; SSST = Zuckerman's Sensation Seeking Scale; TCI = Temperament and Character Inventory; TPI = Tridimensional Personality Inventory; TPQ = Tridimensional Personality Questionnaire; trbc MAO = thrombocyte monoamine oxidase activity.
[a]In the entire cohort of 218 individuals (including previous papers by Ebstein et al.) and in both ethnic groups (Ashkenazi and Sephardic), the effect of the seven alleles is significant in females (ANOVA, $P = 0.03$) but not in males.
[b]The authors selected 100 individuals with extremely high scores and 100 individuals with extremely low scores on the Novelty Seeking subscale of the TCI within a cohort of 4,773 individuals belonging to the 1966 northern Finland birth cohort study.

four behavioral clusters included in the NBAS: orientation, motor organization, range of state, and regulation of state. These results were confirmed when the same infants were studied at the age of 2 months (Auerbach et al. 1999) using Rothbart's Infant Behavior Questionnaire (Rothbart 1981). Ebstein et al. suggested that the NBAS orientation cluster might precede adult novelty seeking, as implied by longitudinal studies (Korner et al. 1985). In fact, several reports show that early childhood antecedents persist in adult personality traits (Kagan 1997; MacEvoy et al. 1988). A chapter on the dopamine D4 receptor and neonatal temperament is presented in this book (Chapter 7, Dopamine D4 Receptor and Serotonin Transporter Promoter Polymorphisms and Temperament in Early Childhood).

Table 5–1 shows that further confirmation of the first studies published in 1996 has been achieved in those studies that considered exon III alleles in relatively homogeneous populations. In fact, Benjamin and colleagues did not find any significant association with the exon I polymorphism of DRD4 in a group of 124 predominantly Jewish normal volunteers (Benjamin et al. 1998). However, other earlier studies on Finnish subjects from a homogeneous population, with far different ethnic backgrounds from other Europeans, failed to find an association between DRD4 exon III repeats and novelty seeking (Malhotra et al. 1996). The same can be found in Swedish studies, but the Swedish population is undoubtedly more heterogeneous than the Finnish one (Geijer et al. 1997; Jonsson et al. 1997). On the other hand, a positive correlation has been found in a Japanese group, where the long allele polymorphism is rare (Muramatsu et al. 1996; Ono et al. 1997). However, if we look at subjects who participated in certain studies (Muramatsu et al. 1996; Ono et al. 1997), we can see that relationships are based on few individuals, with a predominant prevalence of males and no data on children and adolescents. It has also been suggested that women are more prone to the novelty seeking trait than men (Ebstein and Belmaker 1997). In addition, many other studies were carried out on subjects with substance abuse disorder, most of whom were males (Kotler et al. 1997; Sander et al. 1997). For example, Mel and colleagues analyzed 143 normal volunteers and 57 heroin addicts, all Jewish males, but the TPQ was administered to only 38 of the addicted subjects (Mel et al. 1998). Ebstein and colleagues found a significant association in women, but not in males in a greater cohort (Ebstein and Belmaker 1997; Ebstein et al. 1997b). It is remarkable that Strobel et al. (1999) and Ekelund et al. (1999) found no significant gender effect on Novelty Seeking scores.

Twin studies have not been particularly informative. To our knowledge, only one study on twins and *DRD4* and personality has been published to date, and it failed to find any association between the short or the long allele polymorphisms and same-sex dizygotic and monozygotic twins (Pogue-Geile et al. 1998).

Novelty Seeking scores on the TPQ are inversely correlated with age, with the highest scores found in young individuals. That is further evidenced by the fact that Vandenbergh and colleagues (1997) failed to detect any association in 200 elderly, healthy, Caucasian subjects. Although no studies are available on adolescents, the reports showing a stronger association between *DRD4* and Novelty Seeking were performed on subjects between ages 18 and 32 (Ebstein and Belmaker 1997). Interestingly, the study by Strobel et al. (1999) was performed on subjects with a mean age of 23.6 ± 3.9 years, and the one by Ekelund et al. (1999) was performed on subjects who were all born in 1966 and were age 28 at that time. Thus, it is possible that as individuals age, genetic factors contribute less to personality traits, and that environmental factors have an increasingly greater effect during the course of life. However, a study using the Psychopathic Deviate Scale of the Minnesota Multiphasic Personality Inventory to assess biological and adoptive parents of teenage adoptees (Graham 1977) showed a strong effect of the biological mother's Psychopathic Deviate scores, but no significant effect of the adoptive mother's scores (Willerman et al. 1992).

It appears clear from our review of the literature that all articles on the topic can be divided into two broad categories: association studies on normal volunteers and association studies on subjects with substance abuse disorder (alcoholism or opioid abuse). Only one article to our knowledge refers to another pathology (Parkinson's disease) (Ricketts et al. 1998). Interestingly, Ricketts and colleagues found an association between the *DRD4* exon III polymorphism and Parkinson's disease, but not with the novelty seeking trait. Moreover, the fact that all subjects were more than age 60 may account for the lack of association with novelty seeking.

Dopamine, Personality, and Behavioral Disorders

Early studies have shown that cerebrospinal serotonin and dopamine metabolite levels are reduced in highly aggressive individuals (Limson et al. 1991); however, no correlation between personality inventory scores and monoamine levels has been demonstrated. Eating disorders, particularly bulimia nervosa, have also been shown to be related to personality traits. Brewerton et al. (1993) administered the TPQ to 110 patients with bulimia nervosa, 27 with anorexia nervosa, and age- and sex-matched normal controls. All subjects with eating disorders showed higher scores than did controls on Harm Avoidance ($P < 0.001$). Patients with bulimia also had higher scores on the Novelty Seeking and Impulsivity subscales ($P < 0.001$). Impulsiveness is therefore increasingly seen as a key characteristic of substance abuse, eating disorders, and attention-deficit/hyperactivity disorder, as suggested by Lahoste et al. and Sagvolden et al. (LaHoste et al. 1996; Sagvolden and Sergeant 1998). All of these disorders have been connected with either a hypo- or hyperefficient dopamine system. Data on monoamine transporters obtained from SPECT imaging in subjects with violent behavior (Tiihonen et al. 1997) showed a clear association of impulsivity and serotonin transporter density, whereas data on the dopamine transporter were less conclusive. Animal models can be of use to investigate the underlying biology of specific traits, but they do not fully mimic human personality. For example, a study on the alcohol-preferring P rat strain failed to show that that particular strain could serve as a model for human impulsiveness (McMillen et al. 1998). Another study associated monoamine oxidase B inhibition and L-deprenyl with a reduction in impulsiveness in spontaneously hypertensive rats and Wistar-Kyoto rats (Boix et al. 1998).

Background noise in human genetic studies is usually considerable, and very detailed cohorts need to be studied in order to avoid false positives (Paterson et al. 1999). For that reason, some scientists have researched substance abuse disorder for a possible relation to extremes of temperament. It has long been suggested that descendents of alcoholics show a higher tendency to alcohol-related disorders than do those from families without such a history (Enoch and Goldman 1999; Holden 1991; Sander et al. 1997). Therefore, alcoholics have been targets of intensive investigation on extreme personality traits and alterations in monoamine function. Linkage studies have found an association between an increased frequency of the A1 allele of the *Taq*I restriction fragment length polymorphism of the D2 dopamine receptor gene and alcoholism (Cook and Gurling 1994), but no conclusive data are to date available about the involvement of *DRD4*. Additionally, family studies on heroin addiction are particularly difficult to carry out (Li et al. 1997). Thus, results from different studies in this area are not directly comparable.

It is of note that besides the D4 gene, the dopamine D3 receptor gene *(DRD3)* with the *Bal*I (Gly-Ser) restriction site polymorphism is thought to be involved in personality traits. In fact, a recent article showed that opiate-dependent patients with a Zuckerman's Sensation Seeking score above 24 were more frequently homozygous for both alleles of the D3 gene than were patients with a score of less than 24 ($P = 0.04$) or controls ($P = 0.03$) (Duaux et al. 1998). However, recently, Kotler and colleagues (1999) found no association between *Bal*I *DRD3* and heroin addiction in a group of 193 Israeli heroin addicts. It is likely that for major mental disorders, the combination of a complex genetic makeup involving many genes of weak effect underlies normal personality. As an example, Lesch and colleagues (1996) reported an association between harm avoidance, which can be considered an anxiety-related personality trait, and a polymorphism in the serotonin transporter (5-HTTLPR) gene. However, Ebstein and colleagues (1997a) were unable to find any association between harm avoidance and 5-HTTLPR in their cohort.

Conclusions

Issues of statistical power are crucial to studies where the gene effect might be weak and the risk of false positives is high. If Bonferroni's correction for multiple tests is performed, very few results from the studies summarized in Table 5–1 are still significant. In fact, some studies have used many statistical tests to compare different polymorphisms, genotype sequences, and rating scales. For example, of the 22 tests Benjamin et al. (1996) performed, after Bonferroni's correction, only the overall Novelty Seeking score is significant ($P < 0.02$). That finding has recently been strongly confirmed by Strobel and colleagues (1999), and their association between the *DRD4* seven-allele repeat and Novelty Seeking remains significant at the conservatively Bonferroni's adjusted level of 0.0016. Ekelund's (1999) findings are also very robust.

In conclusion, the effect of *DRD4* on novelty seeking might be so small that some studies may have lacked the necessary power of detection. It is encouraging that an article by Costa and McCrae suggested that NEO validity is universal (Costa and McCrae 1997). It is also possible that the effect may be stronger in younger individuals. The inclusion of cohort effects, stratification, and diverse ethnic groups in the same demographic class may be another reason for a lack of association in some studies. Moreover, another polymorphism may be in linkage disequilibrium with the studied polymorphism in some but not in all populations. The latter possibility needs further investigation and may explain why several studies did not find an association between DRD4 polymorphisms and personality traits. On the other hand, the two original reports conducted in the United States and in Israel and the two recent studies conducted in Finland and in Germany consistently support the hypothesis that the D4 gene contributes to the trait of novelty seeking.

References

Adamson MD, Kennedy J, Petronis A, et al: DRD4 dopamine receptor genotype and CSF monoamine metabolites in Finnish alcoholics and controls. Am J Med Genet 60:199–205, 1995

Asghari V, Schoots O, van Kats S, et al: Dopamine D4 receptor repeat: analysis of different native and mutant forms of the human and rat genes. Mol Pharmacol 46:364–373, 1994

Auerbach J, Geller V, Lezer S, et al: Dopamine D4 receptor (*D4DR*) and serotonin transporter promoter (5-HTTLPR) polymorphisms in the determination of temperament in 2-month-old infants. Mol Psychiatry 4:369–373, 1999

Benjamin J, Li L, Patterson C, et al: Population and familial association between the D4 dopamine receptor gene and measures of Novelty Seeking. Nat Genet 12:81–84, 1996

Benjamin J, Osher Y, Belmaker RH, et al: No significant associations between two dopamine receptor polymorphisms and normal temperament. Human Psychopharmacology: Clinical and Experimental 13:11–15, 1998

Boix F, Qiao SW, Kolpus T, et al: Chronic l-deprenyl treatment alters brain monoamine levels and reduces impulsiveness in an animal model of Attention Deficit/Hyperactivity Disorder. Behav Brain Res 94:153–162, 1998

Brazelton TB: The infant at risk. J Perinatol 9:307–310, 1989

Brewerton TD, Hand LD, Bishop ER Jr: The Tridimensional Personality Questionnaire in eating disorder patients. Int J Eat Disord 14:213–218, 1993

Chang FM, Ko HC, Lu RB, et al: The dopamine D4 receptor gene (DRD4) is not associated with alcoholism in three Taiwanese populations: six polymorphisms tested separately and as haplotypes. Biol Psychiatry 41:394–405, 1997

Cloninger CR: A systematic method for clinical description and classification of personality variants: a proposal. Arch Gen Psychiatry 44:573–588, 1987

Cloninger CR: Temperament and personality. Curr Opin Neurobiol 4:266–273, 1994

Cloninger CR, Przybeck TR, Svrakic DM: The Tridimensional Personality Questionnaire: U.S. normative data. Psychol Rep 69:1047–1057, 1991

Cook CC, Gurling HM: The D2 dopamine receptor gene and alcoholism: a genetic effect in the liability for alcoholism. J R Soc Med 87:400–402, 1994

Costa PT Jr, McCrae RR: Stability and change in personality assessment: the revised NEO Personality Inventory in the year 2000. J Pers Assess 68:86–94, 1997

Duaux E, Gorwood P, Griffon N, et al: Homozygosity at the dopamine D3 receptor gene is associated with opiate dependence. Mol Psychiatry 3:333–336, 1998

Ebstein RP, Belmaker RH: Saga of an adventure gene: novelty seeking, substance abuse and the dopamine D4 receptor (*D4DR*) exon III repeat polymorphism. Mol Psychiatry 2:381–384, 1997

Ebstein RP, Novick O, Umansky R, et al: Dopamine D4 receptor (*D4DR*) exon III polymorphism associated with the human personality trait of Novelty Seeking. Nat Genet 12:78–80, 1996

Ebstein RP, Gritsenko I, Nemanov L, et al: No association between the serotonin transporter gene regulatory region polymorphism and the Tridimensional Personality Questionnaire (TPQ) temperament of harm avoidance. Mol Psychiatry 2:224–226, 1997a

Ebstein RP, Nemanov L, Klotz I, et al: Additional evidence for an association between the dopamine D4 receptor (*D4DR*) exon III repeat polymorphism and the human personality trait of Novelty Seeking. Mol Psychiatry 2:472–477, 1997b

Ebstein RP, Levine J, Geller V, et al: Dopamine D4 receptor and serotonin transporter promoter in the determination of neonatal temperament. Mol Psychiatry 3:238–246, 1998

Ekelund J, Lichtermann D, Jarvelin MR, et al: Association between novelty seeking and the type 4 dopamine receptor gene in a large Finnish cohort sample. Am J Psychiatry 156:1453–1455, 1999

Enoch MA, Goldman D: Genetics of alcoholism and substance abuse. Psychiatr Clin North Am 22:289–299, 1999

Garpenstrand H, Ekblom J, Hallman J, et al: Platelet monoamine oxidase activity in relation to alleles of dopamine D4 receptor and tyrosine hydroxylase genes. Acta Psychiatr Scand 96:295–300, 1997

Geijer T, Jonsson E, Neiman J, et al: Tyrosine hydroxylase and dopamine D4 receptor allelic distribution in Scandinavian chronic alcoholics. Alcohol Clin Exp Res 21:35–39, 1997

George SR, Cheng R, Nguyen T, et al: Polymorphisms of the D4 dopamine receptor alleles in chronic alcoholism. Biochem Biophys Res Commun 196:107–114, 1993

Graham JR: The MMPI: A Practical Guide. New York, Oxford University Press, 1977

Holden C: Alcoholism gene: coming or going? Science 254:200, 1991

Jones PB, Rantakallio P, Hartikainen AL, et al: Schizophrenia as a long-term outcome of pregnancy, delivery, and perinatal complications: a 28-year follow-up of the 1966 north Finland general population birth cohort. Am J Psychiatry 155:355–364, 1998

Jonsson EG, Nothen MM, Gustavsson JP, et al: Lack of evidence for allelic association between personality traits and the dopamine D4 receptor gene polymorphisms. Am J Psychiatry 154:697–699, 1997

Kagan J: Temperament and the reactions to unfamiliarity. Child Dev 68:139–143, 1997

Korner AF, Zeanah CH, Linden J, et al: The relation between neonatal and later activity and temperament. Child Dev 56:38–42, 1985

Kotler M, Cohen H, Segman R, et al: Excess dopamine D4 receptor (D4DR) exon III seven repeat allele in opioid-dependent subjects. Mol Psychiatry 2:251–254, 1997

Kotler M, Cohen H, Kremer I, et al: No association between the serotonin transporter promoter region (5-HTTLPR) and the dopamine

D3 receptor (BalI D3DR) polymorphisms and heroin addiction. Mol Psychiatry 4:313–314, 1999

Kurtz JE, Lee PA, Sherker JL: Internal and temporal reliability estimates for informant ratings of personality using the NEO PI-R and IAS. Assessment 6:103–114, 1999

LaHoste GJ, Swanson JM, Wigal SB, et al: Dopamine D4 receptor gene polymorphism is associated with attention deficit hyperactivity disorder. Mol Psychiatry 1:121–124, 1996

Lesch KP, Bengel D, Heils A, et al: Association of anxiety-related traits with a polymorphism in the serotonin transporter gene regulatory region. Science 274:1527–1531, 1996

Li T, Xu K, Deng H, et al: Association analysis of the dopamine D4 gene exon III VNTR and heroin abuse in Chinese subjects. Mol Psychiatry 2:413–416, 1997

Limson R, Goldman D, Roy A, et al: Personality and cerebrospinal fluid monoamine metabolites in alcoholics and controls. Arch Gen Psychiatry 48:437–441, 1991

MacEvoy B, Lambert WW, Karlberg P, et al: Early affective antecedents of adult type A behavior. J Pers Soc Psychol 54:108–116, 1988

Malhotra AK, Virkkunen M, Rooney W, et al: The association between the dopamine D4 receptor (*D4DR*) 16 amino acid repeat polymorphism and novelty seeking. Mol Psychiatry 1:388–391, 1996

McMillen BA, Means LW, Matthews JN: Comparison of the alcohol-preferring P rat to the Wistar rat in behavioral tests of impulsivity and anxiety. Physiol Behav 63:371–375, 1998

Mel H, Horowitz R, Ohel N, et al: Additional evidence for an association between the dopamine D4 receptor (*D4DR*) exon III seven-repeat allele and substance abuse in opioid dependent subjects: relationship of treatment retention to genotype and personality. Addiction Biology 3:473–481, 1998

Muramatsu T, Higuchi S, Murayama M, et al: Association between alcoholism and the dopamine D4 receptor gene. J Med Genet 33:113–115, 1996

Ono Y, Manki H, Yoshimura K, et al: Association between dopamine D4 receptor (*D4DR*) exon III polymorphism and novelty seeking in Japanese subjects. Am J Med Genet 74:501–503, 1997

Paterson AD, Sunohara GA, Kennedy JL: Dopamine D4 receptor gene: novelty or nonsense? Neuropsychopharmacology 21:3–16, 1999

Plomin R, Owen MJ, McGuffin P: The genetic basis of complex human behaviors. Science 264:1733–1739, 1994

Pogue-Geile M, Ferrell R, Deka R, et al: Human novelty-seeking personality traits and dopamine D4 receptor polymorphisms: a twin and genetic association study. Am J Med Genet 81:44–48, 1998

Ricketts MH, Hamer RM, Manowitz P, et al: Association of long variants of the dopamine D4 receptor exon 3 repeat polymorphism with Parkinson's disease. Clin Genet 54:33–38, 1998

Rothbart M: Measurement of temperament in infancy. Child Dev 52:569–578, 1981

Sagvolden T, Sergeant JA: Attention deficit/hyperactivity disorder: from brain dysfunctions to behaviour. Behav Brain Res 94:1–10, 1998

Sander T, Harms H, Dufeu P, et al: Dopamine D4 receptor exon III alleles and variation of novelty seeking in alcoholics. Am J Med Genet 74:483–487, 1997

Schalling D, Asberg M, Edman G, et al: Markers for vulnerability to psychopathology: temperament traits associated with platelet MAO activity. Acta Psychiatr Scand 76:172–182, 1987

Strobel A, Wehr A, Michel A, et al: Association between the dopamine D4 receptor (DRD4) exon III polymorphisms and measures of novelty seeking in a German population. Mol Psychiatry 4:378–384, 1999

Sullivan PF, Fifield WJ, Kennedy MA, et al: No association between novelty seeking and the type 4 dopamine receptor gene (DRD4) in two New Zealand samples. Am J Psychiatry 155:98–101, 1998

Tiihonen J, Kuikka JT, Bergstrom KA, et al: Single-photon emission tomography imaging of monoamine transporters in impulsive violent behaviour. Eur J Nucl Med 24:1253–1260, 1997

Van Tol HH, Bunzow JR, Guan HC, et al: Cloning of the gene for a human dopamine D4 receptor with high affinity for the antipsychotic clozapine. Nature 350:610–614, 1991

Van Tol HH, Wu CM, Guan HC, et al: Multiple dopamine D4 receptor variants in the human population. Nature 358:149–152, 1992

Vandenbergh DJ, Zonderman AB, Wang J, et al: No association between novelty seeking and dopamine D4 receptor (*D4DR*) exon III seven repeat alleles in Baltimore Longitudinal Study of Aging participants. Mol Psychiatry 2:417–419, 1997

Willerman L, Loehlin JC, Horn JM: An adoption and a cross-fostering study of the Minnesota Multiphasic Personality Inventory (MMPI) Psychopathic Deviate Scale. Behav Genet 22:515–529, 1992

Zuckerman M: Sensation seeking, mania, and monoamines. Neuropsychobiology 13:121–128, 1985

Zuckerman M, Link K: Construct validity for the sensation-seeking scale. J Consult Clin Psychol 32:420–426, 1968

CHAPTER SIX

Serotonin Transporter, Personality, and Behavior

Toward a Dissection of Gene-Gene and Gene-Environment Interaction

K. P. Lesch, M.D., B. D. Greenberg, M.D., Ph.D.
J. D. Higley, Ph.D., A. Bennett, Ph.D., D. L. Murphy, M.D.

The relative influence of genetic and environmental factors on human temperamental and behavioral differences is among the most prolonged and contentious controversies in intellectual history (Degler 1991). Although current views emphasize the joint influence of genes and environment, the complexities of gene-gene and gene-environment interactions (genotypes may *respond* differentially to different environments) as well as gene-environment correlations (genotypes may be *exposed* differentially to environments) represent research areas in their infancy (Bouchard 1994; Loehlin 1992; McGue and Bouchard 1998). Individual differences in behavioral predispositions, referred to as personality traits, are relatively enduring, continuously distributed, and substantially heritable and therefore likely result from the interplay of genetic variations with environmental influences. This perspective has increasingly encouraged the pursuit of dimensional approaches to behavioral genetics, in addition to the traditional strategy of studying individuals with categorically defined psychiatric disorders (Plomin et al. 1994). Genomic variants with a significant impact on

K. P. Lesch is supported by the Hermann and Lilly Schilling Foundation.

the functionality of components of brain monoamine neurotransmitter systems are a rational starting point for this research.

The brain-stem raphe serotonin (5-hydroxytryptamine [5-HT]) system is the most widely distributed neurotransmitter system in the brain; serotonergic raphe neurons diffusely project to a variety of brain regions (e.g., cortex, amygdala, hippocampus) (Hensler et al. 1994). In addition to its neurotransmitter role, 5-HT is an important regulator of morphogenetic activities during early brain development, as well as during adult neurogenesis and plasticity, including cell proliferation, migration, differentiation, and synaptogenesis (Azmitia and Whitaker-Azmitia 1997; Gould 1999; Lauder 1990, 1993). In the brain of adult humans, nonhuman primates, and other mammals, 5-HT neurotransmission is a major modulator of emotional behavior (Westenberg et al. 1996) and integrates cognition, sensory processing, motor activity, and circadian rhythms including food intake, sleep, and reproductive activity. This diversity of physiological functions is due to the fact that 5-HT orchestrates the activity and interaction of several other neurotransmitter systems. Although 5-HT may be viewed as a master control neurotransmitter within this highly complex system of neural communication mediated by more than 14 pre- and postsynaptic receptor subtypes with a multitude of isoforms and subunits, 5-HT's action as a chemical messenger is primarily terminated by reuptake via the 5-HT transporter (5-HTT). The 5-HTT thus plays a critical role in regulating serotonergic neurotransmission in numerous projection fields throughout the brain, including regions crucial to emotional behavior, such as motor behavior, emotional experience, and memory (Lesch 1997). Consistent with this view, brain 5-HTT is the initial site of action of widely used 5-HT reuptake inhibitor antidepressant and antianxiety drugs. Based on converging lines of evidence that the 5-HTT, as the prime modulator of central 5-HT activity, plays an important role in brain development, genetically driven variability of 5-HTT function is likely to influence behavioral predispositions (i.e., personality traits) as well as phenotypic expression of behavior via complementary mechanisms (Lesch and Mossner 1998).

5-HT Transporter Gene Variations: Why This Complexity?

The human 5-HTT is encoded by a single gene on chromosome 17q11.2. It is composed of 14–15 exons spanning approximately 35 kb (Lesch et al. 1994) (Figure 6–1). Comparison of the human and murine 5-HTT genes revealed a striking conservation of both the exon/intron organization and the 5'-flanking transcriptional control region (Bengel et al. 1997), whereas in rats exon 1B is not alternatively spliced. A single mRNA species occurs in rats and mice; however, in the human gene the most proximal signal for polyadenylation deviates from the consensus motif present in the rat and mouse. Although this variant of the consensus polyadenylation signal– like motif leads to alternate usage of additional polyadenylation sites, the functional implications of the resulting multiple mRNA species remain obscure (Austin et al. 1994).

In humans, transcriptional activity of the 5-HTT gene is modulated by a polymorphic repetitive element (5-HTT gene–linked polymorphic region [5-HTTLPR]) located upstream of the transcription start site. Addi-

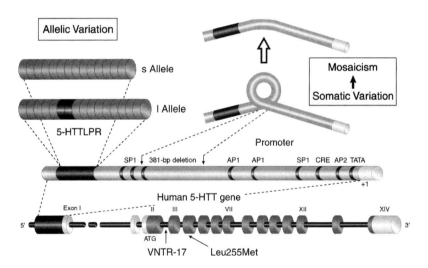

Figure 6–1   Structure of the human 5-HT transporter (5-HTT) gene and its 5'-flanking transcriptional control region. The 5-HTT gene promoter is defined by a TATA-like motif, and several potential binding sites for transcription factors including AP1, AP2, SP1, and a CRE-like motif are present in the 5'-flanking region. The figure depicts the positions of the 5-HTT gene–linked polymorphic region (5-HTTLPR) and a 381-bp somatic deletion [del(17)(q11.2)] resulting in tissue-specific mosaicism of the 5-HTT gene promoter. The localization of the deletion breakpoints adjacent to identical putative signal sequences (CAGCC) suggests a recombinase-like rearrangement event. The locations of a 16/17-bp variable tandem repeat (VNTR-17) located in intron 2 with two common alleles (with 10 or 12 repeats) and one rare allele (with 9 repeats), and a rare structural variant of the 5-HTT protein (Leu255Met) are also indicated.

tional variations have been described in the 5' untranslated region due to alternative splicing of exon 1B (Bradley and Blakely 1997), in intron 2 (variable number of a 16/17-bp tandem repeat) (Lesch et al. 1994), and in the 3' untranslated region (Battersby et al. 1999). Comparison of different mammalian species confirmed the presence of the 5-HTTLPR in platyrrhini and catarrhini (hominoids, cercopithecoids) but not in prosimian primates and other mammals (Lesch et al. 1997). The 5-HTTLPR is unique to humans and simian primates. In humans, the majority of alleles are composed of either 14- or 16-repeat elements (short and long allele, respectively), whereas alleles with 15, 18, 19, 20, or 22 repeat elements, and variants with single-base insertions/deletions or substitutions within individual repeat elements are rare. Great apes, including the orangutan, gorilla, and chimpanzee, display a high prevalence of 18- and 20-repeat alleles. A predominantly Caucasian population displayed allele frequencies of 57% for the long (l) allele and 43% for the short (s) allele, with a 5-HTTLPR genotype distribution of 32% l/l, 49% l/s, and 19% s/s (Lesch et al. 1996); different allele and genotype distributions are found in other populations (Gelernter et al. 1997; Ishiguro et al. 1997; Kunugi et al. 1997).

The unique structure of the 5-HTTLPR gives rise to the formation of a DNA secondary structure (cation-dependent tetrastrands aggregation) that has the potential to regulate the transcriptional activity of the associated 5-HTT gene promoter. The secondary structure of the 5-HTTLPR is also likely to precipitate a 381-bp somatic deletion in the 5-HTT gene's promoter region [del(17)(q11.2)], observed in 20%–60% of genomic DNA isolated from human brain and mononuclear cells (Lesch et al. 1999). The localization of the deletion breakpoints adjacent to identical putative signal sequences (CAGCC) suggests a V(D)J recombinase-like rearrangement event. This suggests that mosaicism of the 5-HTT gene promoter-associated del(17)(q11.2) is likely to be regulated by brain region–selective and possibly 5-HTTLPR-dependent mechanisms. For example, preliminary data from our laboratory indicate a decrease of recombination in recurrent unipolar depression. Moreover, cross-species analysis revealed a similar recombination event in rhesus monkeys *(Macaca mulatta)*. Although this feature is additional evidence for unique 5-HTT gene organization and regulation, it remains to be elucidated whether it is related to reports that the pericentric region of chromosome 17 is highly unstable in humans (Park et al. 1998).

When fused to a luciferase reporter gene and transfected into human 5-HTT expressing cell lines, the short (s) and long (l) 5-HTTLPR variants differentially modulate transcriptional activity of the 5-HTT gene promoter (Lesch et al. 1996). The effect of 5-HTTLPR length variability on 5-HTT function was determined by studying the relationship between 5-HTTLPR genotype, 5-HTT gene transcription, and 5-HT uptake activity in human lymphoblastoid cell lines. Cells homozygous for the l variant of the 5-HTTLPR produced higher concentrations of 5-HTT mRNA than cells containing one or two copies of the s form. Membrane preparations from l/l lymphoblasts showed higher inhibitor binding than did s/s cells. Furthermore, the rate of specific 5-HT uptake was more than twofold higher in cells homozygous for the l form of the 5-HTTLPR than in cells carrying one or two copies of the s variant of the promoter. Further evidence from studies of 5-HTT promoter activity in other cell lines (Mortensen et al. 1999), mRNA concentrations in the raphe complex of human postmortem brain (Little et al. 1998), platelet 5-HT uptake and content (Greenberg et al. 1999; Hanna et al. 1998; Nobile et al. 1999), and in vivo single photon emission computed tomography imaging of human brain 5-HTT (Heinz et al. 1999) confirmed that the s form is associated with lower 5-HTT gene expression and function.

5-HTT and Personality: Searching for Genotype-Phenotype Correlations

Virtually all work in the area of personality supports the idea that there is a substantial heritable component to temperament and personality, typically accounting for between 30% and 60% of the observed variances (for overview see Loehlin 1992). This is convincingly illustrated by the striking similarity of identical twins adopted out and reared apart (Minnesota Twin Study [Bouchard et al. 1990]), some of whom had not known each other prior to the study. On measures of interests, skills, and personality traits, these twins had correlations between 34% and 78%, whereas fraternal twins showed correlations between 7% and 39%.

Anxiety-related traits are a fundamental, enduring, and continuously distributed dimension of normal human personality, with a substantial heritability of 40%–60%, and therefore very likely result from the interplay of genetic variations with environmental influences (Loehlin 1992). This possibility has encouraged many investigators to pursue dimensional approaches to neurobehavioral genetics (Plomin et al. 1994). Functional genetic variants affecting components of brain monoamine neurotransmitter systems are a logical starting point for this research. The contribution of 5-HTTLPR variability to individual phenotypic differences in personality traits was explored in two independent population/family genetics studies. Anxiety-related and other personality traits were assessed by the NEO Personality Inventory, Revised (NEO-PI-R), a self-report inventory based on the five-factor model of personality (Big Five) (Costa and McCrae 1988, 1992), and by the 16PF Personality Inventory (Cattell 1989). The five factors assessed by the NEO-PI-R are Neuroticism (emotional instability), Extraversion, Agreeableness (cooperation, reciprocal alliance formation), Openness (intellect, problem solving), and Conscientiousness (will to achieve).

In our initial study, we found population and within-family associations between the low-expressing s allele and Neuroticism, a trait related to anxiety, hostility, and depression, on the NEO-PI-R in a primarily male population ($n = 505$), and that the s allele was dominant (Lesch et al. 1996). Individuals with either one or two copies of the short 5-HTTLPR variant (group S) had significantly greater levels of neuroticism, defined as proneness to negative emotionality, including anxiety, hostility, and depression, than those homozygous for the long genotype (group L) in the sample as a whole and also within sibships. Individuals with 5-HTTLPR S genotypes also had significantly decreased Agreeableness as measured by the NEO-PI-R. In addition, the group S subjects had increased scores for Anxiety on the separate 16PF Personality Inventory, a trait related to NEO-PI-R Neuroticism. Recently, we reassessed this association in a new sample ($n = 397$, 84% female, primarily sib pairs). The findings robustly replicated the 5-HTTLPR-Neuroticism association and the dominance of the s allele. Combined data from the two studies ($n = 902$) gave a highly significant association between the s allele and higher NEO-PI-R Neuroticism both across individuals and within families (Tables 6–1 through 6–3), reflecting a genuine genetic influence rather than an artifact of ethnic admixture.

Another association encountered in the original study between the s allele and lower scores of NEO-PI-R Agreeableness was also replicated and was stronger in the primarily female replication sample (Tables 6–1 and 6–3). Gender-related differences in 5-HTTLPR–personality trait associations are possible because several lines of evidence demonstrate gender-related differences in 5-HT system functioning in humans and in animals (Fink et al. 1999; McQueen et al. 1997). These findings show that the 5-HTTLPR influences a constellation of neuroticism- and agreeableness-related traits; the associations were strongest for traits de-

TABLE 6–1   Population association between 5-HTTLPR and NEO Personality Inventory, Revised, personality traits: *t* scores by genotype (mean ± SD)

	1/1 **L** ($n = 277$)	1/s + s/s **S** ($n = 625$)	**F**	**S−L**	**P**	**P***
N Neuroticism	54.4 ± 11.7	58.0 ± 11.8	17.8	3.6	**0.0000**	**0.0008**
E Extraversion	55.0 ± 10.6	53.9 ± 11.3	1.8	NS	0.180	0.054
O Openness	57.7 ± 11.7	58.0 ± 11.4	0.2	NS	0.696	0.860
A Agreeableness	49.2 ± 10.5	46.1 ± 11.7	13.2	−3.0	**0.0003**	**0.0007**
C Conscientiousness	45.6 ± 10.3	43.5 ± 12.3	5.6	−2.1	**0.018**	0.077
Neuroticism facets						
N1 Anxiety	54.2 ± 12.0	56.1 ± 11.6	4.9	2.9	**0.028**	0.137
N2 Angry Hostility	51.7 ± 11.0	55.3 ± 11.8	19.4	3.7	**0.0000**	**0.0005**
N3 Depression	53.1 ± 11.0	56.7 ± 11.6	18.9	3.6	**0.0000**	**0.0002**
N4 Self-Consciousness	53.0 ± 11.1	54.5 ± 11.7	3.3	NS	0.070	0.127
N5 Impulsiveness	54.6 ± 11.1	57.0 ± 11.1	8.9	NS	**0.003**	**0.009**
N6 Vulnerability	53.0 ± 10.3	54.9 ± 11.9	5.0	1.9	**0.025**	0.178

Note. Mean scores for the five major traits in the combined populations ($n = 902$) reported by Lesch et al. (1996) and Greenberg et al. (1999), stratified by genotype and genotype group. *F* is the one-way ANOVA statistic, S − L is the mean score for the S genotypes (s/s and l/s) minus the mean score for L genotypes (l/l), *P* is the two-tailed significance, *P** is the two-tailed significance level after including sex, age, and ethnic group as covariates in ANCOVA. Significant *P* values are in bold typeface; *t* scores are raw scores adjusted to a mean of 50 and a standard deviation of 10. NS = not significant.

TABLE 6–2   Population association between 5-HTTLPR and 16 Personality Factor Inventory: *t* scores by genotype (mean ± SD)

	1/1 **L** ($n = 269$)	1/s + s/s **S** ($n = 616$)	**F**	**S − L**	**P**	**P***
Extraversion	5.3 ± 2.1	5.3 ± 2.3	0.3	NS	0.557	0.202
Anxiety	6.1 ± 1.8	6.5 ± 1.7	9.7	0.40	**0.002**	**0.002**
Tough-Mindedness	5.1 ± 1.9	5.2 ± 2.0	0.3	NS	0.599	0.399
Independence	6.5 ± 2.1	6.9 ± 2.3	4.2	0.33	**0.041**	0.090
Self-Control	4.8 ± 1.9	4.6 ± 1.9	2.3	NS	0.137	0.177

Note. Mean scores for the five second-order personality factors measured in the combined populations ($n = 902$) reported by Lesch et al. (1996) and Greenberg et al. (2000), stratified by genotype and genotype group. For symbols see Table 6–1.

fined by the NEO-PI-R. Analysis of the NEO-PI-R subscales helps to define the specific aspects of personality that are reproducibly associated with 5-HTTLPR genotype. For the NEO-PI-R Neuroticism subscales, the com-

TABLE 6–3 Within-family association between 5-HTTLPR and personality traits: standardized scores in genotype-discordant sib pairs (n = 125, mean ± SD)

	L sibling	S sibling	S − L	t^{*a}	P
NEO-PI-R Neuroticism	54.8 ± 11.8	58.5 ± 12.2	3.7	2.3	**0.012**
NEO-PI-R Agreeableness	49.7 ± 9.8	48.1 ± 10.5	−1.6	1.2	0.115
16PF Anxiety	6.3 ± 1.8	6.7 ± 1.8	0.4	1.7	**0.045**

Note. For symbols see Table 6–1.
[a]t score conservatively corrected for nonindependence of sib pairs from a single family.

bined samples from Lesch et al. (1996) and Greenberg et al. (2000) demonstrated significant associations between 5-HTTLPR S genotypes and the facets of increased Depression and Angry Hostility, two of the three facets that showed the most significant associations in the initial sample (Lesch et al. 1996). In contrast, the NEO-PI-R Neuroticism Anxiety facet, which was associated with genotype in the first study at a weaker significance level, was not significantly associated with 5-HTTLPR genotype in the new cohort. With regard to the NEO-PI-R Agreeableness subscales, the previously observed associations of 5-HTTLPR s genotypes with decreased Straightforwardness and Compliance were robustly replicated. It therefore appears more accurate to state that the 5-HTTLPR is associated with traits of negative emotionality related to interpersonal hostility and depression. The relationship between these two aspects of negative emotionality is not unexpected in view of the previously observed negative correlation between Angry Hostility, a facet of Neuroticism, and Agreeableness ($r = -0.48$) (Costa and McCrae 1992), indicating that both measures assess a behavioral predisposition toward uncooperative interpersonal behavior.

The effect sizes for the 5-HTTLPR-personality associations, which were comparable in the two samples, indicate that this polymorphism has a moderate influence on these behavioral predispositions of approximately 0.30 standard deviation units. This corresponds to 3%–4% of the total variance and 7%–9% of the genetic variance, based on estimates from twin studies using these and related measures. Additive contributions of comparable size or epistatic interaction have been found in studies of other quantitative traits. Thus, the results are consistent with the view that the influence of a single, common polymorphism on continuously distributed traits is likely to be small in humans (Plomin et al. 1994).

At first sight, association between the high-activity 5-HTTLPR l allele and lower Neuroticism and related traits seemed inconsistent with the known antidepressant and antianxiety effects of 5-HTT inhibitors (serotonin reuptake inhibitors). Likewise, Knutson et al. (1998) reported that long-term inhibition of the 5-HTT by the serotonin reuptake inhibitor paroxetine reduced indices of hostility through a more general decrease in negative affect, a personality dimension related to neuroticism. The same individuals also demonstrated an increase in directly measured social cooperation after paroxetine treatment, an interesting finding in view of the replicated association between 5-HTTLPR genotype and agreeableness. However, because both 5-HT and 5-HTT play critical roles in brain development that differ from their functions in regulating neurotransmission and neurogenesis in the adult (Azmitia and Whitaker-Azmitia 1997; Gould 1999), this inconsistency may be more apparent than real.

The conclusion that the 5-HTT may affect personality traits via an influence on brain development is strongly supported by recent findings in rodents and nonhuman primates. Studies in rats confirmed that the 5-HTT gene is expressed in brain regions central to emotional behavior during fetal development but not later in life (Hansson et al. 1998, 1999); hence enduring individual differences in personality could result from 5-HTTLPR-driven differential 5-HTT gene expression during pre- and perinatal life. Mice with a targeted disruption of the 5-HTT displayed enhanced anxiety-related behaviors in two animal models of anxiety, the light-dark box and the elevated zero maze (Wichems et al. 1998). Transient 5-HTT gene expression in thalamocortical neurons is required for barrel pattern formation in neonatal rodents, presumably by maintaining extracellular 5-HT concentrations. The somatosensory cortex of 5-HTT$^{-/-}$ mice displays no 5-HT-stained barrels at P7 and only very few cytochrome oxidase–stained whisker barrels both at P7 and adulthood (Persico et al. 2001). Heterozygous (5-HTT$^{+/-}$) mice develop all cortical barrel fields, but frequently present irregularly shaped barrels and septa. The confirmation that a 50% decrease of 5-HTT availability and subtle changes in the dynamics of 5-HT transport in 5-HTT$^{+/-}$ mice (the model that most closely resembles the impact of the s 5-HTTLPR variant on functional 5-HTT gene expression) exerts long-term effects on cortical development and adult brain plasticity may be an important step forward in establishing a neurobiological groundwork for the neurodevelopmental hypothesis of neuroticism-associated personality and affective spectrum disorders.

Additional pertinent evidence comes from studies of rhesus macaques, a higher nonhuman primate species that like humans has a functional 5-HTTLPR polymorphism (Lesch et al. 1997). When tested early in life at postnatal days 7–30, rhesus monkey infants with the low-expression rh-5-HTTLPR s allele displayed higher behavioral stress-reactivity compared with infants homozygous for the l allele (Champoux et al. 1999) (discussed later). Thus, both animal models are consistent with the finding in humans that it is the low-activity s allele that is associated with increased negative emotionality. The findings are intriguing in light of speculations that the recent appearance of the 5-HTTLPR-associated genetic variation may have helped permit more sophisticated modulation of social behaviors during the evolution of higher-order primates (Lesch et al. 1997). The 5-HTT-personality association data also emphasize the advantage of the five-factor NEO-PI-R and the lexical tradition of personality theory on which it is based. This model of personality is consistent with evolutionary perspectives on personality, and the trait terms in natural language may best reflect individual behavioral differences important to group survival and reproductive success (Buss 1991, 1995).

Among a series of subsequent studies, only two attempts to replicate the original finding have been reported using large populations (Jorm et al. 1998; Mazzanti et al. 1998) (Table 6–4). Two of the three available large studies found evidence congruent with an influence of the 5-HTTLPR on Neuroticism and related traits (Lesch et al. 1996; Mazzanti et al. 1998), whereas a large population study not employing a within-family design (Jorm et al. 1998) did not. Smaller population-based studies have had variable but generally negative results. Interpretation of these studies is complicated by their use of relatively small or unusual samples, and the lack of within-family designs to control for population stratification artifacts. This notion is supported by our recent study, which used rigorous family-based protocols.

An additional issue, which applies to both the large and smaller sample studies, is that the personality trait measures have often differed. For example, the most recent large studies (Jorm et al. 1998; Mazzanti et al. 1998) used the Harm Avoidance scale of the Temperament and Character Inventory and the Neuroticism scale of the Eysenck Personality Questionnaire (EPQ), respectively. Given that the magnitude of 5-HTTLPR-personality association is expected to be small, it appears to be critical that attempts to replicate that finding use the same phenotypic definitions. Although the NEO-PI-R and the EPQ Neuroticism scales are correlated in the range of 0.75 (McCrae and Costa 1985), differences in these measures leave a large proportion of the variance measured by one questionnaire

TABLE 6–4 Overview of published data on the association between 5-HTTLPR and anxiety-related traits in general populations and patient samples

	n	Population and study design	Trait assessment/ inventory[a]	Association of s allele, P	Family-based studies, P
Lesch et al. 1996	505	General, U.S. American, males, two subsamples	NEO-PI-R, 16PF	0.023–0.002	0.03–0.004
Ebstein et al. 1997	120	General, Israeli	TPQ	0.75, NS	—
Ball et al. 1997	106	General, German, 5% of highest vs. lowest Neuroticism scores	NEO-FFI	0.89, NS	—
Nakamura et al. 1997	203	General, Japanese, females	NEO-PI-R, TCI	s increased, l is rare	—
Mazzanti et al. 1998	655	Controls, alcoholic violent offenders, Finnish	TPQ	NS	0.45, but 0.003 for HA1 + HA2
Ebstein et al. 1998	81	General, Israeli, neonates (2 weeks old)	NBAS	Interaction with DRD4	—
Ricketts et al. 1998	84	Controls, Parkinson's disease, U.S. American	TPQ	0.04–0.003	—
Gelernter et al. 1998	185 322	Controls, substance dependence, personality disorder, U.S.	NEO-PI-R TPQ	0.47, NS 0.87, NS	—
Jorm et al. 1998	759	General, European Australian	EPQ-R	NS	—
Seretti et al. 1999	132	Depression, bipolar disorder	HAMD, anxiety	0.01	—

Continued

TABLE 6–4 Overview of published data on the association between 5-HTTLPR and anxiety-related traits in general populations and patient samples (Continued)

	n	Population and study design	Trait assessment/ inventory[a]	Association of s allele, P	Family-based studies, P
Murakami et al. 1999	189	General, Japanese	SRQ-AD	0.05	—
Flory et al. 1999	225	General, U.S. American	NEO-PI-R	0.97, NS	—
Kamakiri et al. 1999	144	General, Japanese	NEO-PI-R, TPQ	NS	—
Katsuragi et al. 1999	101	General, Japanese	TPQ	0.007	—
Auerbach et al. 1999	76	General, Israeli, infants (2 months old), follow-up of Ebstein et al. 1998	IBQ	0.05–0.005, interaction with DRD4	—
Menza et al. 1999	32	Parkinson's disease	HAMD	0.05	—
Dreary et al. 1999	204	General, Scottish, 20% of highest vs. lowest Neuroticism scores	NEO-FFI	NS	—
Gustavsson et al. 1999	305	General, Swedish	KSP	NS	—
Osher et al. 1999	148	General, Israeli	NEO-PI-R, TPQ	—	0.06 0.07
Greenberg et al. 1999	397	General, U.S. American, females	NEO-PI-R, 16PF	0.03—0.01	0.01

Note. NS = not significant; — = not determined.

[a]NEO-PI-R and NEO-FFI = Costa and McCrae's NEO Personality Inventory; TPQ = Cloninger's Tridimensional Personality Questionnaire; TCI = Cloninger's Temperament and Character Inventory; 16PF = Catell's 16 Personality Factor Inventory; EPQ-R = Eysenck Personality Questionnaire; KSP = Karolinska Scales of Personality; SRQ-AD = Self-Rating Questionnaire for Anxiety and Depression; HAMD = Hamilton Depression Rating Scale; IBQ = Rothbart's Infant Behavior Questionnaire; NBAS = Brazelton's Neonatal Behavioral Assessment Scale.

unexplained by the other. This amount of variance, approximately 40%, which is very close to estimates of the entire heritable component of neuroticism (Jang et al. 1996; Loehlin 1992), could be critical in assessing the influence of genetic variants of small effect such as the 5-HTTLPR. An additional difference between the five-factor NEO-PI-R and the three-factor EPQ is that the NEO-PI-R Agreeableness domain, which shows a replicated association to 5-HTTLPR genotype, is not measured separately by the EPQ but is instead a component of the Psychoticism dimension (Goldberg 1993). It is possible that the use of a composite trait such as psychoticism might obviate detection of a small 5-HTTLPR influence on traits related to hostility and social cooperation. A final major concern is the lack of a within-family design in that study, raising the possibility of artifacts due to ethnic admixture.

5-HTT Gene-Gene Interaction: Minimizing Environmental Influences by Studying Neonates

The dissection of epistatic gene-gene interaction in the development of personality and behavioral traits is a pertinent and exciting avenue of research. In the evaluation of complex genetic effects it seems to be essential to control for environmental factors. Recent studies have therefore focused on the neonatal period, a time in early development when environmental influences may be minimal and least likely to confound associations between temperament and genes. In this context the term *temperament* is used to refer to the psychological qualities of infants that display considerable variation and have a relatively, but not indefinitely, stable biological basis in the individual's genotype, even though different phenotypes may emerge as the child grows (Kagan 1989; Kagan et al. 1988).

Ebstein and coworkers (1998) investigated the behavioral effects of the variable number tandem repeat polymorphism in exon 3 of the dopamine D4 receptor (DRD4), which had previously been linked to the personality trait of novelty seeking, and of 5-HTTLPR, which seems to influence NEO-PI-R Neuroticism scores and Tridimensional Personality Questionnaire (TPQ) Harm Avoidance scores, in 2-week-old neonates ($n = 81$). Neonatal temperament and behavior were assessed using the Brazelton Neonatal Behavioral Assessment Scale (NBAS). In addition to a significant association of the DRD4 polymorphism across four behavioral clusters relevant to temperament (orientation, motor organization, range of state, and regulation of state), an interaction was observed between the DRD4 polymorphism and 5-HTTLPR. The presence of the 5-HTTLPR s/s genotype decreased the orientation score for the group of neonates lacking the long variant of DRD4. The DRD4 polymorphism–5-HTTLPR interaction was also assessed in a sample of adult subjects. Interestingly, there was no significant effect of the long DRD4 genotype in those subjects homozygous for 5-HTTLPR s, whereas in the group without the homozygous genotype the effect of a long *DRD4* allele was significant and represented 13% of the variance in novelty seeking scores between groups.

Temperament and behavior of the infants were reexamined at 2 months using Rothbart's Infant Behavior Questionnaire (Auerbach et al. 1999). There were significant negative correlations between neonatal orientation and motor organization as measured by the Brazelton Neonatal Assessment Scale at 2 weeks and negative emotionality, especially distress in daily situations, at 2 months. Furthermore, grouping of the infants by DRD4 and 5-HTTLPR polymorphisms revealed significant main effects for negative emotionality and distress. Infants with long *DRD4* alleles had lower scores on Negative Emotionality and Distress to Limitations than infants with short *DRD4* alleles. In contrast, infants homozygous for the 5-HTTLPR s allele had higher scores on Negative Emotionality and Distress than infants with the l/s or l/l genotypes. Infants with the s/s genotype who also were lacking the novelty seeking–associated long *DRD4* alleles showed most negative emotionality and distress, temperament traits that possibly contribute to the predisposition for adult neuroticism.

In addition, an interaction between the 5-HTT gene and the catechol O-methyltransferase gene has been shown to influence the trait of Persistence (RD2), a subscale of TPQ major personality factor Reward Dependence. Persistence is considered to be highly adaptive in the presence of stable intermittent reward patterns. Persistent individuals are eager, ambitious, and determined overachievers (Cloninger 1994). In the presence of catechol O-methyltransferase Val/Val or Met/Met homozygosity, the low-activity 5-HTTLPR s allele significantly raises TPQ RD2 scores, including perfectionism, in a sample of 577 healthy subjects (Benjamin et al. 2000). Because a large number of epistatic interactions could be anticipated with a considerable potential of false positive findings that may lead to meaningless conclusions, gene-gene interaction analyses should at this stage be limited to polymorphisms known to be functional, preferentially within a single neuronal system, or demonstrated to be associated with behavioral phenotypes of interest.

Gene-Environment Interaction:
A Nonhuman Primate Model

Influenced by the sociobiological hypothesis of Edward O. Wilson (Wilson 1975, 1978), there has also been an increasing interest in human personality, particularly the Big Five personality dimensions, from the evolutionary perspective (Buss 1991, 1995). These five dimensions may define the framework for adapting to other people, a crucial task in long-term reproductive success. Extraversion and agreeableness are important to the formation of social structures ranging from pair bonds to coalitions of groups; emotional stability and conscientiousness are critical to the endurance of these structures; and openness may reflect the capacity for innovation. Because the genetic basis of present-day personality dimensions may reflect selective forces among our remote ancestors (Loehlin 1992), we have recently focused our research efforts on rhesus macaques. In this nonhuman primate model, environmental influences are probably less complex, can be more easily controlled, and are thus less likely to confound associations between temperament and genes.

Human and nonhuman primate behavior are similarly affected by deficits in 5-HT function. In rhesus monkeys, 5-HT turnover, as measured by 5-hydroxyindoleacetic acid (5-HIAA) concentrations in cerebrospinal fluid (CSF), has a strong heritable component and is traitlike, with demonstrated stability over an individual's life span (Higley et al. 1991, 1992b, 1993; Kraemer et al. 1989). Moreover, CSF 5-HIAA concentrations are subject to the long-lasting influence of deleterious events early in life as well as by situational stressors. Monkeys separated from their mother and reared in absence of conspecific adults (peer-reared) have altered serotonergic function and exhibit behavioral deficits throughout their lifetimes when compared with their mother-reared counterparts.

Comparison of different mammalian species indicates that the 5-HTTLPR is unique to humans and simian primates. In hominoids, all alleles originate from variation at a single locus (polymorphic locus 1 [PL1]), whereas an alternative locus for a 21-bp length variation (PL2) was found in the 5-HTTLPR of rhesus monkeys (rh-5-HTTLPR) (Lesch et al. 1997). The fact that the 5-HTTLPR is encountered in hominoids and the cercopithecoids, represented by the macaques, indicates remarkable conservation of this part of the 5-HT gene promoter throughout the different lineages of these two superfamilies and suggests that a progenitor 5-HTTLPR sequence possibly representing viral DNA may have been introduced into the genome some 40 million years ago. Appearance of the 5-HTTLPR is therefore an example of a one-time event in the evolutionary history of a species. Although the intervening 5-HTTLPR sequence displays intraspecies and interspecies variability, the 5-HTTLPR-associated insertion/deletion event has been detected at identical positions in humans [del(17)(q11.2)] and rhesus monkeys. The 5-HTTLPR sequence may be informative in the comparison of closely related species and reflects the phylogeny of the old world monkeys, great apes, and humans. The presence of an analogous rh-5-HTTLPR and resulting allelic variation of 5-HTT activity in rhesus monkeys provides a unique model to dissect the relative contribution of genes and environmental sources to central serotonergic function and related behavioral outcomes.

In order to study this genotype-environment interaction, association between central 5-HT turnover and rh-5-HTTLPR genotype was tested in rhesus monkeys with well-characterized environmental histories (Higley et al. 1998). This sample of rhesus monkeys ($n = 177$) showed allele frequencies of 83% for the 24-repeat allele (long [l]) and 16% for the 23-repeat (short [s]) rh-5-HTTLPR variant with a genotype distribution of 68% l/l, 31% l/s, and 1% s/s; one individual was heterozygous for a rare allele with an additional repeat unit (xl) similar to longer alleles found occasionally in humans (Lesch et al. 1997). The monkeys' rearing fell into one of the following categories: mother-reared, either reared with the biological mother or cross-fostered; or peer-reared, either with a peer group of 3–4 monkeys or with an inanimate surrogate and daily contact with a playgroup of peers. Peer-reared monkeys were separated from their mothers, placed in the nursery at birth, and given access to peers at 30 days of age either continuously or during daily play sessions. Mother-reared and cross-fostered monkeys remained with the mother, typically within a social group. At roughly 7 months of age, mother-reared monkeys were weaned and placed together with their peer-reared cohort in large, mixed-gender social groups. The frequency of the l/l genotype was 70% for mother-reared ($n = 79$) and 68% for peer-reared monkeys ($n = 95$); subjects with the rare genotypes s/s and l/xl were excluded from subsequent analyses.

Because the monkey population comprised two groups that received dramatically different social and rearing experience early in life, the interactive effects of environmental experience and the rh-5-HTTLPR on cisternal CSF 5-HIAA levels and 5-HT-related behavior were assessed. CSF 5-HIAA concentrations were significantly influenced by genotype for peer-reared, but not for mother-reared subjects (Bennett et al. 2001). Peer-reared rhesus monkeys with the low-activity rh-5-HTTLPR s allele had significantly lower concentrations of CSF 5-HIAA than their homozygous l/l counterparts. Low 5-HT turnover in monkeys with the s allele is congruent with in vitro studies that show reduced binding and transcriptional efficiency of the 5-HTT gene associated with the 5-HTTLPR s allele (Heils et al. 1996; Lesch et al. 1996). This suggests that the rh-5-HTTLPR genotype is predictive of CSF 5-HIAA concentrations, but that early experiences make unique contributions to variation in later 5-HT functioning. This finding is the first to provide evidence of an environment-dependent association between a polymorphism in the 5′ regulatory region of the 5-HTT gene and a direct measure of 5-HT functioning, and cisternal CSF 5-HIAA concentration, thus revealing an interaction between rearing environment and rh-5-HTTLPR genotype. Similar to the 5-HTTLPR's influence on NEO-PI-R Neuroticism in humans, however, the effect size is small, with 4.7% of variance in CSF 5-HIAA accounted for by the rh-5-HTTLPR–rearing environment interaction.

Intriguingly, the biobehavioral results of deleterious early experiences of social separation are consistent with the notion that the 5-HTTLPR may influence the risk for affective spectrum disorders. Evolutionary preservation of two prevalent 5-HTTLPR variants and the resulting allelic variation in 5-HTT gene expression may be part of the genetic mechanism resulting in the emergence of temperamental traits that facilitate adaptive functioning in the complex social worlds most primates inhabit. Accumulating evidence demonstrates the complex interplay between individual differences in the central 5-HT system and social success. In monkeys, lowered 5-HT functioning, as indicated by decreased CSF 5-HIAA levels, is associated with lower rank within a social group, less competent social behavior, and greater impulsive aggression (Higley et al. 1992a, 1996; Mehlman et al. 1994, 1995). It is well established that although subjects with low CSF 5-HIAA concentrations are no more likely to engage in competitive aggression than other monkeys, when they do engage in aggression it frequently escalates to violent and hazardous levels.

Association between the rh-5-HTTLPR genotype and aggressive behavior was studied by analyzing the joint effects of genotype and early rearing environment on competition-elicited aggression. Socially dominant mother-reared monkeys were more likely than their peer-reared counterparts to engage in competitive aggression. Moreover, under both rearing conditions, monkeys with the low-activity s allele exhibited more aggressive behaviors than their l/l counterparts. The lack of a genotype by rearing interaction for competitive aggression indicates that subjects with the s allele, although unlikely to win in a competitive encounter, are more inclined to persist in aggression once it begins. A role of s allele–dependent low 5-HTT function in nonhuman primate aggressive behavior is in remarkable agreement with the association in humans between NEO-PI-R subscales Neuroticism (increased Angry Hostility) and Agreeableness (decreased Compliance equals increased aggressiveness and hostility) and 5-HTTLPR s genotypes.

As the scope of human studies has been extended to the neonatal period, a time in early development when environmental influences are modest and least likely to confound gene-temperament associations, complementary approaches have recently been applied to nonhuman primates. Rhesus macaque infants heterozygous for the s and l variants of the rh-5-HTTLPR (l/s) displayed higher behavioral stress-reactivity compared with infants homozygous for the long variant of the allele (l/l) (Champoux et al. 1999). Mother-reared and peer-reared monkeys ($n = 36$ and $n = 83$, respectively) were assessed on days 7, 14, 21, and 30 of life, on a standardized primate neurobehavioral test designed to measure orienting, motor maturity, reflex functioning, and temperament. Main effects of genotype, and, in some cases, interactions between rearing condition and genotype, were demonstrated for items indicative of orienting, attention, and temperament. In general, heterozygous animals demonstrated diminished orientation, lower attentional capabilities, and increased affective responding relative to l/l homozygotes. However, the genotype effects were more pronounced for animals raised in the neonatal nursery than for animals reared by their mothers. These results demonstrate the contributions of rearing environment and genetic background, and their interaction, in a nonhuman primate model of behavioral development.

Taken together, these findings provide evidence of an environment-dependent association between allelic variation of 5-HTT gene expression and central 5-HT function (Figure 6–2) and illustrate the possibility that specific genetic factors play a role in 5-HT-mediated social competence in primates. The objective of further studies will be the elucidation of the relationship between the rh-5-HTTLPR genotype and sociability in monkeys, because this behavior is expressed with characteristic individual differences both in daily life and in response to challenge. Because rhesus monkeys exhibit temperamental and behavioral traits that parallel anxiety, depression, and aggression-related personality dimensions associated in humans with the low-activity 5-HTTLPR variant, it may be possible to search for evolutionary continuity in this genetic mechanism for individual

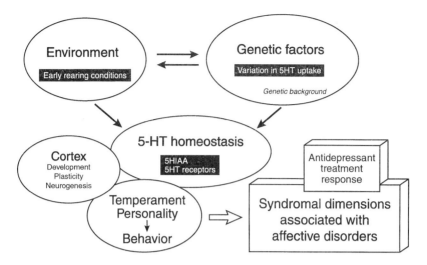

Figure 6–2 The influence of 5-HTT gene–environment interaction on central 5-HT homeostasis in humans and nonhuman primates and its consequences for cortical plasticity, personality, behavior, and the development of affective disorders.

differences. Nonhuman primate studies may also be useful to help identify environmental factors that either compound the vulnerability conferred by a particular genetic makeup or, conversely, act to improve the behavioral outcome associated with that genotype.

In line with this notion our findings encouraged ongoing research exploring possible associations between the 5-HTTLPR or 16/17 variable number tandem repeat variants and categorically defined neuropsychiatric disorders, including depressive syndromes and bipolar affective illness, panic disorder, obsessive-compulsive disorder, autism, schizophrenia, Alzheimer's disease, and substance abuse including alcoholism (for review see Lesch 2000).

Conclusion and Perspective

Converging lines of evidence suggest that allelic variation in functional 5-HTT gene expression plays a critical role in synaptic plasticity, thus setting the stage for expression of complex traits and their associated behavior throughout adult life. Moreover, genetically driven variation of 5-HTT function, in conjunction with other predisposing genetic factors and with inadequate adaptive responses to environmental stressors, is also likely to contribute to the etiopathogenesis and treatment response of affective spectrum disorders emerging from compromised brain development and from neuroadaptive processes.

Several lessons can be learned from past misconceptions in personality and behavioral genetics. First, to detect a small genetic influence, one needs standardized personality behavioral trait assessment with inventories that are characterized by high retest reliability, longitudinal stability, a factor structure that is valid in different populations and cultures, and reasonable correlation between self report and observer ratings. Second, more functionally relevant polymorphisms in genes within a single neurotransmitter system, or in genes that comprise a functional unit in their concerted actions, need to be identified and assessed in both large-population and family-based association studies to avoid stratification artifacts and to elucidate complex epigenetic interactions of multiple loci. Third, genetic influences are not the only pathway that leads to individual differences in personality dimensions, behavior, and psychopathology. Complex traits are most likely to be generated by a complex interaction of environmental and experiential factors with a number of genes and their products. Even pivotal regulatory proteins of neurotransmission, such as the 5-HTT, will have a modest impact, although "noise" from nongenetic mechanisms may seriously hinder identification of relevant genes. Although current methods for the detection of gene-environment interaction in behavioral genetics are largely indirect, the most relevant consequence of identifying genes for personality and behavioral traits may be that it will provide the tools required to systematically clarify the effects of gene-environment interaction (McGue and Bouchard 1998).

The current state of the art of this field illustrates how progress in neuropsychiatric genetics might be accelerated by closer integration of neuroscience and genetic approaches and a dimensional, semiquantitative approach to behavioral phenotypes drawn from a large body of psychometric research. Further studies of the genetics of human behavioral traits using association techniques, linkage strategies, and newer methods in development, such as single nucleotide polymorphism analysis, may be especially useful in refining concepts of the heritable components of personality. Finally, investigating possible genetic differences associated with variation along behavioral dimensions within neuropsychiatric diagnoses may be a useful complement to the traditional strategy of looking for genetic differences between categorically defined neuropsychiatric diagnostic entities.

References

Auerbach J, Geller V, Lezer S, et al: Dopamine D4 receptor (D4DR) and serotonin transporter promoter (5-HTTLPR) polymorphisms in the determination of temperament in 2-month-old infants. Mol Psychiatry 4:369–373, 1999

Austin MC, Bradley CC, Mann JJ, et al: Expression of serotonin transporter messenger RNA in the human brain. J Neurochem 62:2362–2367, 1994

Azmitia EC, Whitaker-Azmitia PM: Development and adult plasticity of serotonergic neurons and their target cells, in Serotonergic Neurons and 5-HT Receptors in the CNS. Edited by Baumgarten HG, Guthert M. Berlin, Springer, 1997, pp 1–39

Battersby S, Ogilvie AD, Blackwood DH, et al: Presence of multiple functional polyadenylation signals and a single nucleotide polymorphism in the 3' untranslated region of the human serotonin transporter gene. J Neurochem 72:1384–1388, 1999

Bengel D, Heils A, Petri S, et al: Gene structure and 5'-flanking regulatory region of the murine serotonin transporter. Brain Res 44:286–292, 1997

Benjamin J, Osher Y, Lichtenberg P, et al: An interaction between the catechol O-Methyltransferase (COMT) and serotonin promoter region (5-HTTLPR) polymorphisms contributes to Tridimensional Personality Questionnaire (TPQ) persistence scores in normal subjects. Neuropsychobiology 41:48–53, 2000

Bouchard TJ: Genes, environment and personality. Science 264:1700–1701, 1994

Bouchard TJ Jr, Lykken DT, McGue M, et al: Sources of human psychological differences: the Minnesota study of twins reared apart. Science 250:223–228, 1990

Bradley CC, Blakely RD: Alternative splicing of the human serotonin transporter gene. J Neurochem 69:1356–1367, 1997

Buss DM: Evolutionary personality psychology. Annu Rev Psychol 42:459–491, 1991

Buss D: Evolutionary psychology: a new paradigm for psychological science. Psychological Inquiry 6:1–30, 1995

Cattell HB: The 16PF: Personality in Depth. Champaign, IL, Institute for Personality Assessment and Testing, 1989

Champoux M, Bennett A, Lesch KP, et al: Serotonin transporter gene polymorphism and neurobehavioral development in rhesus monkey neonates. Society for Neuroscience Abstracts 25:69, 1999

Cloninger C: Temperament and personality. Curr Opin Neurobiol 4:266–273, 1994

Costa P, McCrae R: Personality in adulthood: a six-year longitudinal study of self-reports and spouse ratings on the NEO Personality Inventory. J Pers Soc Psychol 5:853–863, 1988

Costa P, McCrae R: Revised NEO Personality Inventory (NEO PI-R) and NEO Five Inventory (NEO-FFI) Professional Manual. Odessa, FL, Psychological Assessment Resources, 1992

Degler CN: In Search of Human Nature. Oxford, UK, Oxford University Press, 1991

Ebstein RP, Levine J, Geller V, et al: Dopamine D4 receptor and serotonin transporter promoter in the determination of neonatal temperament. Mol Psychiatry 3:238–46, 1998

Fink G, Sumner B, Rosie R, et al: Androgen actions on central serotonin neurotransmission: relevance for mood, mental state and memory. Behav Brain Res 105:53–68, 1999

Gelernter J, Kranzler H, Cubells JF: Serotonin transporter protein (SLC6A4) allele and haplotype frequencies and linkage disequilibria in African- and European-American and Japanese populations and in alcohol-dependent subjects. Hum Genet 101:243–6, 1997

Goldberg L: The structure of phenotypic personality traits. Am Psychol 48:26–34, 1993

Gould E: Serotonin hippocampal neurogenesis. Neuropsychopharmacology 21:46S–51S, 1999

Greenberg BD, Tolliver TJ, Huang SJ, et al: Genetic variation in the serotonin transporter promoter region affects serotonin uptake in human blood platelets. Am J Med Genet 88:83–7, 1999

Greenberg BD, Li Q, Lucas FR, et al: Association between the serotonin transporter promoter polymorphism and personality traits in a primarily female population sample. Am J Med Genetics 96:202–216, 2000

Hanna GL, Himle JA, Curtis GC, et al: Serotonin transporter and seasonal variation in blood serotonin in families with obsessive-compulsive disorder. Neuropsychopharmacology 18:102–111, 1998

Hansson SR, Mezey E, Hoffman BJ: Serotonin transporter messenger RNA in the developing rat brain: early expression in serotonergic neurons and transient expression in non-serotonergic neurons. Neuroscience 83:1185–201, 1998

Hansson SR, Mezey E, Hoffman BJ: Serotonin transporter messenger RNA expression in neural crest–derived structures and sensory pathways of the developing rat embryo. Neuroscience 89:243–265, 1999

Heils A, Teufel A, Petri S, et al: Allelic variation of human serotonin transporter gene expression. J Neurochem 6:2621–2624, 1996

Heinz A, Jones DW, Mazzanti C, et al: A relationship between serotonin transporter genotype and in vivo protein expression and alcohol neurotoxicity. Biol Psychiatry 47:643–649, 1999

Hensler JG, Ferry RC, Labow DM, et al: Quantitative autoradiography of the serotonin transporter to assess the distribution of serotonergic projections from the dorsal raphe nucleus. Synapse 17:1–15, 1994

Higley JD, Suomi SJ, Linnoila M: CSF monoamine metabolite concentrations vary according to age, rearing, and sex, and are influenced by the stressor of social separation in rhesus monkeys. Psychopharmacology 103:551–556, 1991

Higley JD, Mehlman PT, Taub DM, et al: Cerebrospinal fluid monoamine and adrenal correlates of aggression in free-ranging rhesus monkeys. Arch Gen Psychiatry 49:436–441, 1992a

Higley JD, Suomi SJ, Linnoila M: A longitudinal assessment of CSF monoamine metabolite and plasma cortisol concentrations in young rhesus monkeys. Biol Psychiatry 32:127–145, 1992b

Higley JD, Thompson WW, Champoux M, et al: Paternal and maternal genetic and environmental contributions to cerebrospinal fluid monoamine metabolites in rhesus monkeys *(Macaca mulatta)*. Arch Gen Psychiatry 50:615–23, 1993

Higley JD, King ST Jr, Hasert MF, et al: Stability of interindividual differences in serotonin function and its relationship to severe aggression and competent social behavior in rhesus macaque females. Neuropsychopharmacology 14:67–76, 1996

Higley J, Bennett A, Heils A, et al: Serotonin transporter gene variation is associated with CSF 5-HIAA concentrations in rhesus monkeys. Society for Neuroscience Abstracts 24:1113, 1998

Ishiguro H, Arinami T, Yamada K, et al: An association study between a transcriptional polymorphism in the serotonin transporter gene and panic disorder in a Japanese population. Psychiatry Clin Neurosci 51:333–335, 1997

Jang K, Livesley W, Vernon P: Heritability of the big five personality dimensions and their facets: a twin study. J Pers 64:577–591, 1996

Jorm AF, Henderson AS, Jacomb PA, et al: An association study of a functional polymorphism of the serotonin transporter gene with personality and psychiatric symptoms. Mol Psychiatry 3:449–451, 1998

Kagan J: Temperamental contributions to social behavior. Am Psychol 44:664–668, 1989

Kagan J, Reznick JS, Snidman N: Biological bases of childhood shyness. Science 240:167–171, 1988

Knutson B, Wolkowitz OM, Cole SW, et al: Selective alteration of personality and social behavior by serotonergic intervention. Am J Psychiatry 155:373–379, 1998

Kraemer GW, Ebert MH, Schmidt DE, et al; A longitudinal study of the effect of different social rearing conditions on cerebrospinal fluid norepinephrine and biogenic amine metabolites in rhesus monkeys. Neuropsychopharmacology 2:175–189, 1989

Kunugi H, Hattori M, Kato T, et al: Serotonin transporter gene polymorphisms: ethnic difference and possible association with bipolar affective disorder. Mol Psychiatry 2:457–462, 1997

Lauder JM: Ontogeny of the serotonergic system in the rat: serotonin as a developmental signal. Ann N Y Acad Sci 600:297–314, 1990

Lauder JM: Neurotransmitters as growth regulatory signals: role of receptors and second messengers. Trends Neurosci 16:233–240, 1993

Lesch KP: Molecular biology, pharmacology, and genetics of the serotonin transporter: psychobiological and clinical implications, in Serotonergic Neurons and 5-HT Receptors in the CNS. Edited by Baumgarten HG, Guthert M. Berlin, Springer, 1997, pp 671–705

Lesch KP: Serotonin transporter: from genomics and knockouts to behavioral traits and psychiatric disorders, in Molecular Genetics of Mental Disorders. Edited by Briley M, Sulser F. London, Martin Dunitz, 2000

Lesch KP, Mossner R: Genetically driven variation in serotonin uptake: is there a link to affective spectrum, neurodevelopmental, and neurodegenerative disorders? Biol Psychiatry 44:179–192, 1998

Lesch KP, Balling U, Gross J, et al: Organization of the human serotonin transporter gene. J Neural Transm Gen Sect 95:157–162, 1994

Lesch KP, Bengel D, Heils A, et al: Association of anxiety-related traits with a polymorphism in the serotonin transporter gene regulatory region. Science 274:1527–1531, 1996

Lesch KP, Meyer J, Glatz K, et al: The 5-HT transporter gene-linked polymorphic region (5-HTTLPR) in evolutionary perspective: alternative biallelic variation in rhesus monkeys (rapid communication). J Neural Transm 104:1259–1266, 1997

Lesch KP, Jatzke S, Meyer J, et al: Mosaicism for a serotonin transporter gene promoter–associated deletion: decreased recombination in depression. J Neural Transm 106:1223–1230, 1999

Little KY, McLaughlin DP, Zhang L, et al: Cocaine, ethanol, and genotype effects on human midbrain serotonin transporter binding sites and mRNA levels. Am J Psychiatry 155:207–213, 1998

Loehlin JC: Genes and Environment in Personality Development. Newbury Park, CA, Sage Publications, 1992

Mazzanti CM, Lappalainen J, Long JC, et al: Role of the serotonin transporter promoter polymorphism in anxiety-related traits. Arch Gen Psychiatry 55:936–40, 1998

McCrae R, Costa P: Comparison of EPI and psychoticism scales with measures of the five-factor model of personality. Personality and Individual Differences 6:587–597, 1985

McGue M, Bouchard TJ: Genetic and environmental influences on human behavioral differences. Annu Rev Neurosci 21:1–24, 1998

McQueen JK, Wilson H, Fink G: Estradiol-17 beta increases serotonin transporter (SERT) mRNA levels and the density of SERT-binding sites in female rat brain. Brain Res Mol Brain Res 45:13–23, 1997

Mehlman PT, Higley JD, Faucher I, et al: Low CSF 5-HIAA concentrations and severe aggression and impaired impulse control in nonhuman primates. Am J Psychiatry 151:1485–91, 1994

Mehlman PT, Higley JD, Faucher I, et al: Correlation of CSF 5-HIAA concentration with sociality and the timing of emigration in free-ranging primates. Am J Psychiatry 152:907–913, 1995

Mortensen OV, Thomassen M, Larsen MB, et al: Functional analysis of a novel human serotonin transporter gene promoter in immortalized raphe cells. Brain Res Mol Brain Res 68:141–148, 1999

Nobile M, Begni B, Giorda R, et al: Effects of serotonin transporter promoter genotype on platelet serotonin transporter functionality in depressed children and adolescents. J Am Acad Child Adolesc Psychiatry 38:1396–1402, 1999

Park JP, Moeschler JB, Davies W, et al: Smith-Magenis syndrome resulting from a de novo direct insertion of proximal 17q into 17p11.2. Am J Med Genet 77:23–27, 1998

Persico AM, Mengual E, Mossner R, et al: Barrel pattern formation requires serotonin uptake by thalamocortical afferents, and not vesicular monoamine release. J Neurosci 21:6862–6873, 2001

Plomin R, Owen MJ, McGuffin P: The genetic basis of complex human behaviors. Science 264:1733–1739, 1994

Westenberg HG, Murphy DL, Den Boer JA: Advances in the Neurobiology of Anxiety Disorders. New York, Wiley, 1996

Wichems C, Sora I, Andrews AM, et al: Altered responses to psychoactive drugs and spontaneous behavior differences in mice lacking the serotonin transporter. Paper presented at the fourth IUPHAR Satellite Meeting on Serotonin, Rotterdam, 1998

Wilson EO: Sociobiology: The New Synthesis. Cambridge, MA, Belknap Press, 1975

Wilson EO: On Human Nature. Cambridge, MA, Harvard University Press, 1978

CHAPTER SEVEN

Dopamine D4 Receptor and Serotonin Transporter Promoter Polymorphisms and Temperament in Early Childhood

Richard P. Ebstein, Ph.D.
Judith G. Auerbach, Ph.D.

Background

Normal Personality Traits and Their Association With DRD4 and 5-HTTLPR

Only recently has an association between a specific genetic polymorphism and a specific personality trait been reported (Benjamin et al. 1996; Ebstein et al. 1996). Our seminal study catalyzed many investigations by others and ourselves aimed at validating these first reports and identifying other genes contributing to personality factors (see reviews by Baron [1998] and Ebstein and Belmaker [1997]).

The two initial studies (Benjamin et al. 1996; Ebstein et al. 1996) examined the role of the exon III 48-bp repeat polymorphism in the dopamine D4 receptor (DRD4) gene (Lichter et al. 1993; Van Tol 1996, 1998; Van Tol et al. 1992) in personality. This gene has a highly polymorphic

---

This research was partially supported by the Israel Science Foundation founded by the Israel Academy of Sciences and Humanities.

16–amino acid repeat region in the putative third cytoplasmic loop, which varies between 2 and 10 repeats in most populations and changes the length of the receptor protein. Some evidence for a moderate functional significance to the long and short forms of this protein has been shown (Asghari et al. 1994, 1995).

Three recent studies appear to confirm the relevancy of the DRD4 gene to novelty seeking. A Japanese group has characterized several polymorphisms in the upstream promoter region of the DRD4 gene, and one of these was associated with higher novelty seeking scores in a group of Japanese subjects (Okuyama et al. 2000). This particular promoter region polymorphism is functionally significant, and the T variant of the C-521T polymorphism reduces transcriptional efficiency. In a second study, a Finnish group showed an association between the *DRD4* exon III two- and five-repeat alleles and high novelty seeking scores in a very large and homogeneous Finnish birth cohort of more than 4,700 subjects (Ekelund et al. 1999). Both of these studies suggest the possibility that our original observation of an association between the *DRD4* 48-bp repeat region and Tridimensional Personality Questionnaire (Cloninger 1991) Novelty Seeking scores may have been due to linkage disequilibrium between this polymorphism and another polymorphism within the DRD4 gene (perhaps the promoter region?) or in a neighboring gene. Finally, the first genomewide scan in personality genetics in a group of alcoholic families (Cloninger et al. 1998), which reported a linkage between anxiety-related traits and a region on chromosome 8p, also revealed a linkage between novelty seeking and the region on chromosome 11 where the DRD4 gene is located.

Our report of an association between *DRD4* and novelty seeking was followed by Lesch and his colleagues who showed an association between a newly discovered 44-bp deletion in the promoter region of the serotonin transporter promoter region (5-hydroxytryptamine transporter gene–linked polymorphic region [5-HTTLPR]) that affects transcription of the gene (Heils et al. 1996) and neuroticism and harm avoidance (Lesch et al. 1996).

Studies in Neonates and Infants

Assessment of Temperament and Behavior in Neonates

Individual differences in temperament, that is, individual differences in emotional, motor, and attentional reactivity, are apparent from the first days of life. One of the most widely used methods to assess temperament in the first weeks of life is the Neonatal Behavioral Assessment Scale (NBAS) (Brazelton 1990; Brazelton and Nugent 1995).

The NBAS assesses the behavioral repertoire of infants from birth to 1 month. It attempts to capture individual differences in the complexity of behavioral responses to environmental stimuli as the neonate moves from sleep states to alert states to crying states. NBAS scores are a reflection of the baby's capacity to organize his or her autonomic and central nervous system in order to respond to stimuli (both animate and inanimate), and the exam is used to predict the environment's response to the baby as an individual. The NBAS is also related to concurrent and later measures of temperament in infancy and early childhood (Field et al. 1978; Jones and Parks 1983; Tirosh et al. 1992).

Heritability of the NBAS

The heritability of the NBAS-defined clusters has not to our knowledge been directly examined in twin studies. However, the role of genes in determining infant temperament at a somewhat later developmental age has been studied using other testing instruments that measure related behavioral clusters similar to those assessed by the NBAS. For example, in an sample of 604 monozygotic and dizygotic twins ages 3 to 16 months, co-twin similarity in fear and anger and activity level as measured by the Infant Behavior Questionnaire (IBQ) (Rothbart 1981) were best accounted for by additive genetic effects, with genetic and environmental effects best explaining co-twin similarity for interest and persistence (Goldsmith et al. 1999). Similarly, another study of twins (Cyphers et al. 1990) showed high estimates of heritability (0.44–0.65) for eight of the nine temperament scales measured by the New York Longitudinal Study instrument.

More direct evidence for a genetic explanation of the variance in NBAS clusters is provided by a controlled, laboratory study of temperament differences between rhesus monkeys from genetically diverse backgrounds who significantly differed in NBAS cluster scores (Champoux et al. 1994). Temperament characteristics were measured in rhesus monkeys of Indian and Chinese stocks. All infants experienced identical rearing conditions in a neonatal nursery facility. Significant differences were found between Chinese-Indian hybrid and Indian-derived infants on orientation and state control but not on activity and motor maturity clusters.

Similarly, variance in NBAS scores has also been observed between human infants from different cultural and racial backgrounds (Eishima 1992; Nugent et al. 1989; Tronick and Winn 1992). Such differences may be partially determined by diversity in allele frequency of putative temperament genes among these populations. The study by Eishima (1992) is of particular interest because the cross-cultural differences in NBAS scores between British and Japanese neonates were assessed by the same observer. Interestingly, British infants showed better orientation scores, which the current results suggest may be partially determined by the presence of the seven-repeat allele of the DRD4 gene, an allele which is very infrequently encountered in Japanese and Chinese populations (Ono et al. 1997). We believe these studies also suggest that neonatal temperament clusters measured by the NBAS may have some genetic basis. It should be noted, however, that the only twin study of neonates found no evidence for genetic influences (Riese 1990).

Effect of DRD4 and 5-HTTLPR Polymorphisms on Neonatal Temperament Assessed by the NBAS

Experimental Findings

In a first study of its kind (Ebstein et al. 1998), we examined the role of two common polymorphisms on neonatal behavior, evaluated at 2 weeks of age, in 81 neonates (40 males and 41 females) using the NBAS. We note that this initial investigation is the first in a longitudinal study of neonate, infant, and toddler behavior that we have initiated. In the next section of this review we discuss the results obtained at 2 months of age with this same group of children (Auerbach et al. 1999).

The effect of the *DRD4* short (s) versus *DRD4* long (l) (see Chapter 5, DRD4 and Novelty Seeking) and 5-HTTLPR short/short (s/s) versus 5-HTTLPR long/short (l/s) and long/long (l/l) (see Chapter 6, Serotonin Transporter, Personality, and Behavior) alleles on four of the NBAS temperament clusters (Orientation, Range of State, Motor Organization, Regulation of State) was compared by multivariate analysis. A significant association of DRD4 across the NBAS clusters was observed. Univariate F tests showed significant effects of DRD4 on all four of the temperament clusters. Overall, the effect of the presence of the long forms of the *DRD4* exon III repeat region is to raise the mean score for all four of the temperament clusters.

A significant multivariate interaction was observed between DRD4 and 5-HTTLPR, and univariate *F* tests showed a significant interaction between the two polymorphisms on orientation. The interaction between the dopamine and serotonin polymorphisms was further examined as shown in Figure 7–1. The effect size of DRD4 on orientation was much larger in those neonates homozygous for the short (s/s) 5-HTTLPR genotype compared with infants with either the s/l or l/l genotype. Moreover, no significant effect of the *DRD4* long repeat on orientation was observed in neonates grouped by the 5-HTTLPR l/l or l/s alleles, whereas the effect of *DRD4* long repeat alleles was significant in neonates with the s/s 5-HTTLPR genotype. The effect of 5-HTTLPR s/s was to lower the orientation score for the group of neonates lacking the *DRD4* long repeat.

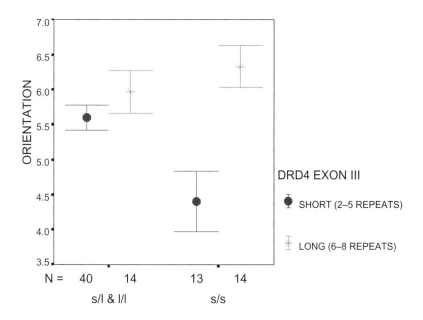

Figure 7–1   NBAS Orientation scores in 2-week-old infants sorted by the dopamine D4 receptor exon III repeat polymorphism and the serotonin transporter promoter region polymorphism. Error bars represent mean values ± SEM.

Source. Reprinted from Benjamin J, Osher Y, Kotler M, et al.: "Association Between Tridimensional Personality Questionnaire Traits and Three Functional Polymorphisms: Dopamine Receptor D4 Serotonin Transporter Promoter Region and Catechol-*O*-Methyltransferase." *Molecular Psychiatry* 5:96–100, 2000. Used with permission.

In summary, the results presented in Figure 7–1 indicate that infants with one or more long alleles of 5-HTTLPR, which is associated with less anxious traits in adults, show no further enhancing effect of the long *DRD4* alleles, which also promote approach-type behaviors in adults. However, in infants with the inhibiting form (at least in adults) of 5-HTTLPR, long *DRD4* alleles, but not short *DRD4* alleles, oppose this inhibition.

Temperament Genes and Developmental Stages: Is NBAS Orientation an Antecedent Behavior of Adult Novelty Seeking?

The longitudinal assessment of temperaments is difficult, especially because the phenotype may subtly and continually change as development evolves. The early antecedents of later novelty seeking behavior that is characterized in adults as impulsive, exploratory, fickle, excitable, quick-tempered and extravagant behavior may not easily be recognizable in earlier stages of development. Our findings on neonates suggest that studies based on examining the genotypic basis of these observed phenotypes may help to unravel the complex temporal expression of temperament.

Only a modest correlation ($r = 0.3$ to 0.4) is generally observed between neonate and infant temperaments across development (reviewed in Ebstein et al. 1998). Such correlations are weak and explain only about 9%–16% of the variance, so that such temperament assessments, although they partially predict group behaviors, may not allow very accurate individual behavioral predictions. Overall, these results suggest, not surprisingly, that much more change than stability is observable from infancy to adulthood. Nevertheless, neonate and infant behavioral assessment instruments apparently tap into some core temperaments that persist, albeit in ever changing expression, into later developmental stages.

Effect of DRD4 and 5-HTTLPR Polymorphisms on Temperament Assessed at 2 Months of Age

We examined the association of DRD4 and 5-HTTLPR and temperament in 76 2-month-old infants (39 boys and 37 girls) who had participated in the neonatal assessment. Mothers completed the IBQ, which is a 94-item, parent questionnaire assessing infant temperament in the first year of life. IBQ scores reflect the ease of elicitation of a given reaction and the intensity of that reaction. Both the stability and validity of the IBQ have been documented (Rothbart 1986; Worobey and Blajda 1989).

Stability of Temperament From 2 Weeks to 2 Months

Temperament stability was examined by calculating bivariate correlation coefficients for the NBAS scales of Orientation, Motor Organization, Regulation of State, and Range of State and the IBQ scales. There were significant negative correlations between Orientation and Negative Emotionality ($r = -0.29$, $P = 0.006$), Orientation and Distress to Limitations ($r = -0.30$, $P = 0.004$), Motor Organization and Negative Emotionality ($r = -0.28$, $P = 0.009$), and Motor Organization and Distress to Limitations ($r = -0.34$, $P = 0.001$).

DRD4 and 5-HTTLPR and 2-Month Temperament

We next considered the effect of the DRD4 and 5-HTTLPR genotypes on the IBQ scales. Two-way ANOVAs (DRD4 and 5-HTTLPR) were computed for each of the IBQ scales. Significant main effects were observed for Negative Emotionality and Distress to Limitations scores when the infants were grouped by the DRD4 (short vs. long alleles) and 5-HTTLPR (s/s vs. l/l and l/s) polymorphisms. Infants with long *DRD4* alleles had significantly lower scores on Negative Emotionality and Distress to Limitations than infants with the short *DRD4* alleles. In contrast, infants with the s/s 5-HTTLPR genotype had higher scores on Negative Emotionality and Distress to Limitations than infants with the l/s or l/l genotypes. A *DRD4* main effect of Distress to Sudden or Novel Stimuli approached significance. Infants with the long *DRD4* alleles were less distressed by sudden or novel stimuli than were infants with the short alleles. Similar results were obtained if the DRD4 genotype was inventoried by either presence or absence of the seven-repeat allele or the two most common genotypes (4/7 and 4/4). In those infants lacking the *DRD4* long-repeat alleles, the effect of the short homozygous form (s/s) of the 5-HTTLPR gene on Negative Emotionality and Distress to Limitations was significant, whereas no effect of this polymorphism was observed in infants possessing the long *DRD4* alleles. In the absence of the long form of the *DRD4* allele, the effect of the s/s form of the 5-HTTLPR gene was to significantly raise the scores for Negative Emotionality and Distress to Limitations.

There was a trend in the same direction for Distress to Sudden or Novel Stimuli. Overall, infants with the s/s form of 5-HTTLPR gene who were lacking the long form of the *DRD4* allele were reported as expressing more negative emotionality, in particular distress to daily situations but also distress when presented with sudden or novel stimuli. No significant effects were found for gender by multivariate or univariate analysis of the temperament scales.

Relationship of NBAS, IBQ, and Genotype

Our findings of significant negative correlations between the NBAS scales of Orientation and Motor Organization and the IBQ scales of Negative Emotionality and Distress to Limitations are in accord with the findings of other studies (Covington et al. 1991; Risholm-Mothander 1989; Worobey and Blajda 1989) that have also examined longitudinally the association of temperament measured neonatally and subsequently through the first year of life. The weak but significant correlation coefficients observed in these studies are similar ($r > 0.3$–0.4) to what we currently report. In particular, it is worth noting that Tirosh and his colleagues (Tirosh et al. 1992) found significant correlations between the NBAS Orientation and Motor clusters and fussy/difficult and unpredictable temperament dimensions at 3 months. In addition, our findings support the suggestion that attention may serve to regulate negative reactivity in various situations (Kochanska et al. 1998).

The findings at 2 months extend our findings on neonates (Ebstein et al. 1998) discussed in the previous section in which we observed a significant multivariate main effect of the DRD4 polymorphism and a significant interaction with 5-HTTLPR across four NBAS temperament clusters. A significant main effect of the DRD4 and 5-HTTLPR genotypes was also observed in our assessment of these infants at 2 months. However, at 2 months the effect of these two polymorphisms was limited to the IBQ scales of Negative Emotionality and Distress to Limitations. Negative emotionality and its components can perhaps be construed as an early precursor of anxiety. Several studies have found a relationship between the temperament dimensions of difficultness and unadaptability, of which negative emotionality is a prime component, and anxiety and inhibition at a later age (Bates and Bayles 1988). The effect of the *DRD4* long alleles was more pervasive on neonatal temperament (and was observed across all four core temperament clusters) than was the effect of this polymorphism on temperament at 2 months of age.

The relationships we are elucidating between the earliest manifestations of temperament in neonates and young infants demonstrate the nonlinear development of these traits. Later temperament dimensions may have little face validity or intuitive relation to the content of earlier manifestation of such temperament. Such relationships, however, are made clearer when it is possible to define the underlying genetic mechanisms. For example, in our longitudinal child study there appears to be a developmentally stable relationship between a gene that is purportedly related to brain activation (DRD4) and a gene that is purported to modulate brain inhibition (the 5-HTTLPR gene). In neonates, orientation, which we suggest is an active exploratory activity, is partially determined by the DRD4 long alleles. In the absence of the long-repeat DRD4 alleles, the short alleles of 5-HTTLPR are inhibitory and reduce Orientation scores. At 2 months, scores for Negative Emotionality and Distress to Limitations, temperament traits perhaps akin to adult neuroticism, are influenced by both the DRD4 and 5-HTTLPR polymorphisms. Similarly, the s/s 5-HTTLPR polymorphism significantly raises Negative Emotionality and Distress to Limitations scores especially in the absence of the long allele of DRD4. Thus, genes contributing to brain activation and brain inhibition may jointly modulate the expression of developmentally dependent behaviors. Our findings are compatible with Cloninger's suggestion (Cloninger 1986) that these systems are functionally interconnected and give rise to integrated patterns of differential responses to punishment, reward, and novelty.

Summary

Using a candidate gene approach, we have been studying the genetic components of temperament spanning human development from neonates to adults. In particular, two common genetic polymorphisms, in DRD4 (a dopaminergic receptor) and 5-HTTLPR (a serotonin transporter), that were initially shown by self-report personality tests to be respectively associated with novelty or sensation seeking traits and harm avoidance or neuroticism, appear to mutually interact from early infancy to adulthood. Our provisional findings are consistent with both human and animal studies that activation of dopaminergic pathways promotes exploratory and impulsive behavior, whereas serotonergic pathways are generally inhibitory and advance avoidance behavior. Similarly, our studies suggest that throughout human development, with temperament as a measure of dopaminergic-serotonergic interactions, the behavioral phenotype conferred by the long DRD4 alleles that furthers exploratory and impulsive behavior is opposed by the 5-HTTLPR polymorphism that acts to constrain this activity.

References

Asghari V, Schoots O, van Kats S, et al: Dopamine D4 receptor repeat: analysis of different native and mutant forms of the human and rat genes. Mol Pharmacol 46:364–373, 1994

Asghari V, Sanyal S, Buchwaldt S, et al: Modulation of intracellular cyclic AMP levels by different human dopamine D4 receptor variants. J Neurochem 65:1157–1165, 1995

Auerbach J, Geller V, Letzer S, et al: Dopamine D4 receptor (D4DR) and serotonin transporter promoter (5-HTTLPR) polymorphisms in the determination of temperament in two month old infants. Mol Psychiatry 4:369–373, 1999

Baron M: Mapping genes for personality: is the saga sagging? Mol Psychiatry 3:106–108, 1998

Bates JE, Bayles K: The role of attachment in the development of behavior problems, in Clinical Implications of Attachment. Edited by Belsky J, Nezworski T. New York, Erlbaum, 1988, pp 253–299

Benjamin J, Li L, Patterson C, et al: Population and familial association between the D4 dopamine receptor gene and measures of novelty seeking. Nat Genet 12:81–84, 1996

Brazelton TB: Saving the bathwater. Child Dev 61:1661–1671, 1990

Brazelton TB, Nugent JK: Neonatal Behavioral Assessment Scale. Cambridge, UK, Cambridge University Press, 1995

Champoux M, Suomi SJ, Schneider ML: Temperament differences between captive Indian and Chinese-Indian hybrid rhesus macaque neonates. Laboratory Animal Science 44:351–357, 1994

Cloninger CR: A unified biosocial theory of personality and its role in the development of anxiety states. Psychiatric Development 4:167–226, 1986

Cloninger CR: The Tridimensional Personality Questionnaire: U.S. normative data. Psychol Rep 69:1047–1057, 1991

Cloninger CR, Van Eerdewegh P, Goate A, et al: Anxiety proneness linked to epistatic loci in genome scan of human personality traits. Am J Med Genet 81:313–317, 1998

Covington C, Cronenwett L, Loveland-Cherry C: Newborn behavioral performance in colic and noncolic infants. Nurs Res 40:292–296, 1991

Cyphers LH, Phillips K, Fulker DW, et al: Twin temperament during the transition from infancy to early childhood. J Am Acad Child Adolesc Psychiatry 29:392–397, 1990

Ebstein RP, Belmaker RH: Saga of an adventure gene: novelty seeking, substance abuse, and the dopamine D4 receptor (D4DR) exon III repeat polymorphism. Mol Psychiatry 2:381–384, 1997

Ebstein RP, Novick O, Umansky R, et al: Dopamine D4 receptor (D4DR) exon III polymorphism associated with the human personality trait of novelty seeking. Nat Genet 12:78–80, 1996

Ebstein RP, Levine J, Geller, V, et al: Dopamine D4 receptor and serotonin transporter promoter in the determination of neonatal temperament. Mol Psychiatry 3:238–246, 1998

Eishima K: A study on neonatal behaviour comparing between two groups from different cultural backgrounds. Early Hum Dev 28:265–277, 1992

Ekelund J, Lichtermann D, Jarvelin MR, et al: Association between novelty seeking and the type 4 dopamine receptor gene in a large Finnish cohort sample. Am J Psychiatry 156:1453–1455, 1999

Field T, Hallock N, Ting G, et al: A first-year follow-up of high-risk infants: formulating a cumulative risk index. Child Dev 49:119–131, 1978

Goldsmith HH, Lemery KS, Buss KA, et al: Genetic analyses of focal aspects of infant temperament. Dev Psychol 35:972–985, 1999

Heils A, Teufel A, Petri S, et al: Allelic variation of human serotonin transporter gene expression. J Neurochem 66:2621–2624, 1996

Jones C, Parks P: Mother–, father–, and examiner-reported temperament across the first year of life. Res Nurs Health 6:183–189, 1983

Kochanska G, Coy KC, Tjebkes TL, et al: Individual differences in emotionality in infancy. Child Dev 64:375–390, 1998

Lesch KP, Bengel D, Heils A, et al: Association of anxiety-related traits with a polymorphism in the serotonin transporter gene regulatory region. Science 274:1527–1531, 1996

Lichter JB, Barr CL, Kennedy JL, et al: A hypervariable segment in the human dopamine receptor D4 (DRD4) gene. Hum Mol Genet 2:767–773, 1993

Nugent JK, Lester EZ, Brazelton TB: The Cultural Context of Infancy. Norwood, NJ, Ablex, 1989

Okuyama Y, Ishiguro H, Nankai M, et al: Identification of a polymorphism in the promoter region of DRD4 associated with the human personality trait of novelty seeking. Mol Psychiatry 5:64–69, 2000

Ono, Y., Manki, H., Yoshimura, K., et al: Association between dopamine D4 receptor (D4DR) exon III polymorphism and novelty seeking in Japanese subjects. Am J Med Genet 74:501–503, 1997

Riese ML: Neonatal temperament in monozygotic and dizygotic twin pairs. Child Dev 61:1230–1237, 1990

Risholm-Mothander P: Predictions of developmental patterns during infancy: assessments of children 0–1 years. Scand J Psychol 30:161–167, 1989

Rothbart MK: Measurement of temperament in infancy. Child Dev 52:569–578 1981

Rothbart MK: Longitudinal observation of infant temperament. Dev Psychol 22:356–365, 1986

Tirosh E, Harel J, Abadi J, et al: Relationship between neonatal behavior and subsequent temperament. Acta Paediatr 81:829–831, 1992

Tronick EZ, Winn SA: The neurobehavioral organization of Efe (pygmy) infants. J Dev Behav Pediatr 13:421–4, 1992

Van Tol HH: The dopamine D4 receptor. NIDA Res Monogr 161:20–38, 1996

Van Tol HH: Structural and functional characteristics of the dopamine D4 receptor. Adv Pharmacol 42:486–90, 1998

Van Tol HH, Wu CM, Guan HC, et al: Multiple dopamine D4 receptor variants in the human population. Nature 358:149–52, 1992

Worobey J, Blajda VM: Temperament ratings at 2 weeks, 2 months, and 1 year: differential stability of activity and emotionality. Dev Psychol 25:257–263, 1989

CHAPTER EIGHT

Personality, Substance Abuse, and Genes

Richard P. Ebstein, Ph.D.
Moshe Kotler, M.D.

Background

Addictive Drugs as Positive Reinforcers in the Brain Dopaminergic Reward System

In the early history of addiction research the predominant concept of addiction was that compulsive drug self-administration was due to the drug's ability to alleviate aversive withdrawal symptoms, the so-called negative reinforcement model. More recently, theories of addiction have underscored the role of drugs in positive reinforcement and euphoria. The mesolimbic dopamine system is strongly implicated in the habit-forming properties of several classes of abused drugs, suggesting a common ground for addictions. Addictive drugs would then appear to mimic aspects of natural reinforcers and interact with identical brain reward

This research was supported in part by the Israel Science Foundation founded by the Israel Academy of Sciences and Humanities (R.P.E. and M.K.) and the Israeli Anti-Drug Authority (Dr. Rachel Bar-Hamberger, Grant Administrator).

mechanisms (Kalivas and Nakamura 1999; Robbins and Everitt 1996; Schultz 1997; Wise 1996a, 1996b).

Reward Mechanisms in Humans: Relationship to Personality Traits and Cognition

The motivational and reinforcement value that people attribute to particular environmental events and stimuli clearly differs among individuals. Such personality traits combine with situational manipulations to produce motivational states that in turn affect cognitive performance (Revelle 1989). The encoding of environmental demands reflects differences in biological sensitivities to cues for rewards and punishment, as well as the prior contents of memory. In the past two decades it has become possible to assess such differences and attribute them to underlying neural mechanisms.

Novelty or Sensation Seeking

Zuckerman, in his book *Behavioral Expressions and Biosocial Bases of Sensation Seeking* (Zuckerman 1994), cogently discusses the notion that sensation seeking (sometimes referred to as novelty seeking) is a primary drive in both animals and humans. Sensation seeking has its expression in human personality and furthermore is closely linked to brain reward mechanisms.

Self-Report Personality Questionnaires Measure Novelty Seeking

Impulsive, unsocialized sensation seeking or novelty seeking is a major factor discovered in factor analyses of scales used in psychobiological research and appears as a higher-order factor in most self-report questionnaires (Zuckerman 1994). As Zuckerman has noted (1994), Zuckerman's Sensation Seeking scale is strongly convergent with Eysenck's P dimension, Conscientiousness in the Big Five model of personality (Costa and McCrae 1997), (Impulsiveness in the Big Five is a subscale of Neuroticism), and Cloninger's Tridimensional Personality Questionnaire (TPQ) (Cloninger 1987) trait of Novelty Seeking. Factor analyses suggest that sensation seeking (or novelty seeking) together with impulsivity and asocial tendencies constitute the dimension of personality that the Eysencks called *psychoticism*. Risk taking for the sake of novel experience is part of the definition of sensation seeking or novelty seeking and includes both physical risk taking and a broader concept of legal, social, and financial risk taking.

Genes and Personality

A large number of twin studies demonstrate firstly that personality traits measured by self-report questionnaires show moderate heritability and secondly that almost all the environmental variance is nonshared, although environmental influence is also important (Loehlin 1992). Heritabilities in the 30%–50% range are typical. Extraversion, a trait akin to novelty seeking or sensation seeking, is one of the most highly heritable categories (~50%), closely followed by neuroticism, akin to Harm Avoidance on the TPQ, or emotional stability (the converse trait name) on some instruments (~40%).

Dopamine D4 Receptor and Novelty Seeking

Only recently has an association between a specific genetic polymorphism and a specific personality trait, novelty seeking, been reported (Benjamin et al. 1996; Ebstein et al. 1996). Our seminal study catalyzed many investigations by others, and we aimed at validating these first reports and identifying other genes that contribute to personality factors. The two initial studies examined the role of the exon III 48-bp repeat polymorphism of the dopamine D4 receptor (DRD4) (Lichter et al. 1993; Van Tol 1996, 1998; Van Tol et al. 1992) in personality. The DRD4 gene codes for a highly polymorphic 16–amino acid repeat region in the putative third cytoplasmic loop that varies between 2 and 10 repeats in most populations and changes the length of the receptor protein. There is some evidence that differences between the long and short forms of this protein have a moderate functional significance (Asghari et al. 1994, 1995).

Novelty Seeking and Psychopathology

Two DSM-IV-TR (American Psychiatric Association 2000) disorders in particular, substance abuse and attention-deficit/hyperactivity disorder (ADHD), show exaggerated elements of impulsive and excitable behavior somewhat akin to TPQ Novelty Seeking. Most interesting is that adult ADHD subjects score higher on Novelty Seeking and are often comorbid for substance abuse, antisocial personality disorder, and depressive disorders (Downey et al. 1996, 1997). Novelty Seeking scores are also higher in substance abusers than in control subjects (Cloninger et al. 1988).

Studies

Substance Abuse and DRD4

The role of dopamine in mediating TPQ Novelty Seeking scores in humans and this neurotransmitter's importance in mediating drug reinforcement and reward mechanisms as discussed earlier prompted us to examine a group of Israeli heroin addicts for prevalence of the DRD4 repeat polymorphism. We demonstrated that the seven-repeat allele is significantly overrepresented in the opioid-dependent cohort (Kotler et al. 1997). To our knowledge this was the first report of an association between a specific genetic polymorphism and opioid addiction. A subsequent study we conducted confirmed an excess of the seven-repeat allele in another group of heroin addicts (Mel et al. 1998).

Similar results showing an excess of the long alleles ($\geq$5) of DRD4 were obtained in a group of Chinese heroin addicts and Japanese alcoholics (Li et al. 1997; Muramatsu et al. 1996). Although the seven-repeat allele is quite rare in Asian populations, the only two seven-repeat alleles observed were among the addicts in the Chinese study. The DRD4 polymorphism has also been examined in a study of alcoholism that illustrated the importance of gene interactions in determining such phenotypes. A point mutation in the aldehyde dehydrogenase 2 (ALDH2) allele is considered a genetic deterrent for alcoholism. Nevertheless, 80 of 655 Japanese alcoholics had the protective ALDH2 allele (Muramatsu et al. 1996). Genotype factors that might increase susceptibility by overriding the deterrent included a higher frequency of a five-repeat allele of the DRD4 polymorphism in alcoholics with ALDH2 than in 100 other alcoholics and 144 controls. Alcoholics with the five-repeat allele also abused other drugs more often than did those without this polymorphism.

Shields and his colleagues found an association between the DRD4 genotype and smoking (Shields et al. 1998). These results are consistent with a study in a DRD4 knockout mouse that was characterized as supersensitive to ethanol, cocaine, and methamphetamine (Rubinstein et al. 1997). However, in three studies with Caucasian populations (Geijer et al. 1997; Sander et al. 1997; Vandenbergh et al. 1997b) and one study in Taiwan (Chang et al. 1997), no evidence for an association between DRD4 and substance abuse was found.

Substance Abuse and the Serotonin Promoter Region and Dopamine D3 Receptor *Bal*I Polymorphisms

We have examined two other polymorphisms, the serotonin transporter promoter region polymorphism (5-HTTLPR) and the dopamine D3 receptor (DRD3) *Bal*I polymorphism (linked to the personality traits of harm avoidance or neuroticism [Lesch et al. 1996] and reward [Ebstein et al. 1997], respectively) in a group of Israeli heroin addicts (Kotler et al. 1999a). DRD3 has also been linked in one study to novelty seeking in a small group of bipolar disorder patients (Duaux et al. 1998) and in two studies to substance abuse in schizophrenia (Duaux et al. 1998; Krebs et al. 1998). We failed to replicate the relationship between DRD3 and substance abuse in our sample of 186 heroin addicts and 217 gender- and ethnically matched controls. DRD3 has also been examined in alcoholism, again with conflicting results (Dobashi et al. 1997; Higuchi et al. 1996; Parsian et al. 1997). Nor did we observe an association between 5-HTTLPR polymorphism and heroin addiction (Kotler et al. 1999a).

DRD4 and Attention-Deficit/Hyperactivity Disorder

Several studies have examined the DRD4 polymorphism in ADHD (Castellanos et al. 1998; Eisenberg et al. 2000; LaHoste et al. 1996; Rowe et al. 1998; Smalley et al. 1998; Swanson et al. 1998). With the exception of a family-based study from our own group (Eisenberg et al. 2000) and a single case-control report (Castellanos et al. 1998), these investigations show an excess of the seven-repeat allele in ADHD. Overall, these results strengthen the notion that DRD4 contributes modestly to impulsive and novelty seeking behaviors presenting in children as ADHD and in adults as substance abuse. The dopamine transporter polymorphism has also been examined in ADHD and a positive association reported (Comings et al. 1996; Cook et al. 1995; Gill et al. 1997). Recently the dopamine transporter has also been shown to be associated with novelty seeking and cigarette addiction (Sabol et al. 1999).

Catechol *O*-Methyltransferase

Another polymorphism we have examined in ADHD (Eisenberg et al. 1999), violent schizophrenia (Kotler et al. 1999b), personality traits (Benjamin et al. 2000; Kotler et al. 1999a), studies of executive function (hypnotizability) (Lichtenberg et al. 2000), and heroin addiction (Horowitz et al. 2000) is catechol *O*-methyltransferase (COMT). A common COMT polymorphism coding for a thermolabile low-activity enzyme has been recognized for two decades (Lotta et al. 1995; Weinshilboum and Dunnette 1981). Lachman and his colleagues (Lachman et al. 1996) found a common biallelic polymorphism (Val/Met) that results in high (Val/Val), low (Met/Met), and intermediate (Val/Met) levels of enzyme activity. COMT contributes to the clearance of dopamine and norepinephrine but not serotonin.

Using the case-control design, Vandenbergh and his colleagues (Vandenbergh et al. 1997a) showed an association between the high-activity COMT polymorphism and polysubstance abuse in a group of North American subjects. We confirmed these results by genotyping 38 Israeli heroin addicts and both parents, using the haplotype relative risk strategy (Horowitz et al. 2000).

COMT and Personality: Multiple Gene Interactions

We examined three functional genetic polymorphisms, in DRD4, 5-HTTLPR, and catechol O-methyltransferase (COMT Val $\rightarrow$ Met), for association with TPQ personality factors in $N = 455$ subjects, and significant interactions were observed (Benjamin et al. 2000).

In the absence of the short 5-HTTLPR allele and in the presence of *COMT* homozygosity especially for the high-enzyme Val/Val genotype, Novelty Seeking scores are higher in the presence of the *DRD4* seven-repeat allele than in its absence (Figure 8–1).

These results are consistent with two earlier reports in which we demonstrated an interaction between the 5-HTTLPR and *DRD4* seven-repeat allele in 2-week-old neonates and in the same children assessed again at 2 months of age (Auerbach et al. 1999; Ebstein et al. 1998). In both infants and adults, short alleles of 5-HTTLPR and long alleles of *DRD4* oppose each other's effects; that is, approach behaviors (orientation to environmental stimuli in infants and novelty seeking in adults) are promoted by long *DRD4* alleles, whereas short alleles of 5-HTTLPR increase avoidance behaviors.

Summary

In our review we discuss the concept of reward, as understood from animal experiments, and extend these concepts to humans. We also examine some recent human genetic studies suggesting that common dopaminergic polymorphisms contribute to individual differences in personality traits and the propensity for substance abuse, kindred phenomena grounded in the mesolimbic motive circuit.

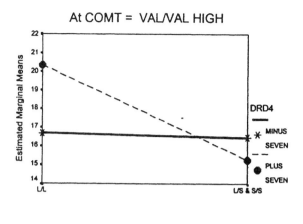

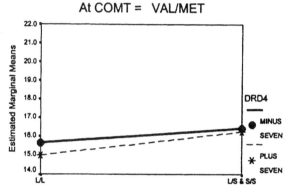

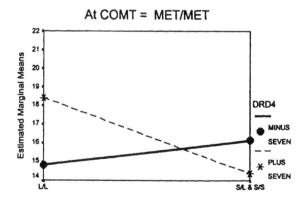

Figure 8–1   Marginal mean value of Tridimensional Personality Questionnaire Novelty Seeking (adjusted for age and sex covariates) scores grouped by three types of polymorphisms: COMT, DRD4, and 5-HTTLPR. The left y axis groups subjects with the long/long 5-HTTLPR and the right y axis with the short genotypes.

We discuss a number of recent genetic studies including many from our own laboratory suggesting that common dopaminergic polymorphisms account for some of the variance in personality traits such as novelty seeking and harm avoidance. Novelty seeking is a personality trait that seems to govern how much stimulation we need from environmental events to reach each individual's optimal level of arousal. Thrill or sensation seekers clearly need more stimulation than the average, and some of these thrill seekers obtain their stimulation by bungee jumping and others in less socially acceptable ways such as substance use and abuse.

References

American Psychiatric Association: Diagnostic and Statistical Manual of Mental Disorders, 4th Edition, Text Revision. Washington, DC, American Psychiatric Association, 2000

Asghari V, Schoots O, van Kats S, et al: Dopamine D4 receptor repeat: analysis of different native and mutant forms of the human and rat genes. Mol Pharmacol 46:364–373, 1994

Asghari V, Sanyal S, Buchwaldt S, et al: Modulation of intracellular cyclic AMP levels by different human dopamine D4 receptor variants. J Neurochem 65:1157–1165, 1995

Auerbach J, Geller V, Letzer S, et al: Dopamine D4 receptor (D4DR) and serotonin transporter promoter (5-HTTLPR) polymorphisms in the determination of temperament in two month old infants. Mol Psychiatry 4:369–373, 1999

Benjamin J, Li L, Patterson C, et al: Population and familial association between the D4 dopamine receptor gene and measures of novelty seeking. Nat Genet 12:81–84, 1996

Benjamin J, Osher Y, Kotler M, et al: Association between Tridimensional Personality Questionnaire (TPQ) traits and three functional polymorphisms: dopamine receptor D4 (DRD4), serotonin transporter promoter region (5-HTTLPR) and catechol O-methyltransferase (COMT). Mol Psychiatry 5:96–100, 2000

Castellanos FX, Lau E, Tayebi N, et al: Lack of an association between a dopamine-4 receptor polymorphism and attention-deficit/

hyperactivity disorder: genetic and brain morphometric analyses. Mol Psychiatry 3:431–434, 1998

Chang FM, Ko HC, Lu RB, et al: The dopamine D4 receptor gene (DRD4) is not associated with alcoholism in three Taiwanese populations: six polymorphisms tested separately and as haplotypes. Biol Psychiatry 41:394–405, 1997

Cloninger CR: A systematic method for clinical description and classification of personality variants: a proposal. Arch Gen Psychiatry 44:573–588, 1987

Cloninger CR, Sigvardsson S, Bohman M: Childhood personality predicts alcohol abuse in young adults. Alcohol Clin Exp Res 12:494–505, 1988

Comings DE, Wu S, Chiu C, et al: Polygenic inheritance of Tourette syndrome, stuttering, attention deficit hyperactivity, conduct, and oppositional defiant disorder: the additive and subtractive effect of the three dopaminergic genes—DRD2, D beta H, and DAT1. Am J Med Genet 67:264–288, 1996

Cook EH Jr, Stein MA, Krasowski MD, et al: Association of attention-deficit disorder and the dopamine transporter gene. Am J Hum Genet 56:993–998, 1995

Costa PT Jr, McCrae RR: Stability and change in personality assessment: the revised NEO personality inventory in the year 2000. J Pers Assess 68:86–94, 1997

Dobashi I, Inada T, Hadano K: Alcoholism and gene polymorphisms related to central dopaminergic transmission in the Japanese population. Psychiatr Genet 7:87–91, 1997

Downey KK, Pomerleau CS, Pomerleau OF: Personality differences related to smoking and adult attention deficit hyperactivity disorder. J Subst Abuse 8:129–35, 1996

Downey KK, Stelson FW, Pomerleau OF, et al: Adult attention deficit hyperactivity disorder: psychological test profiles in a clinical population. J Nerv Ment Dis 185:32–38, 1997

Duaux E, Gorwood P, Griffon N, et al: Homozygosity at the dopamine D3 receptor gene is associated with opiate dependence. Mol Psychiatry 3:333–336, 1998

Ebstein RP, Novick O, Umansky R, et al: Dopamine D4 receptor (D4DR) exon III polymorphism associated with the human personality trait of novelty seeking. Nat Genet 12:78–80, 1996

Ebstein RP, Segman R, Benjamin J, et al: 5-HT2C (HTR2C) serotonin receptor gene polymorphism associated with the human personality trait of reward dependence: interaction with dopamine D4 receptor (D4DR) and dopamine D3 receptor (D3DR) polymorphisms. Am J Med Genet 74:65–72, 1997

Ebstein RP, Levine J, Geller V, et al: Dopamine D4 receptor and serotonin transporter promoter in the determination of neonatal temperament. Mol Psychiatry 3:238–246, 1998

Eisenberg J, Mei-Tal G, Steinberg A, et al: A haplotype relative risk study of catechol-O-methyltransferase (COMT) and attention deficit hyperactivity disorder (ADHD): association of the high-enzyme activity val allele with ADHD impulsive-hyperactive phenotype. Am J Med Genet 88:497–502, 1999

Eisenberg J, Zohar A, Mei-Tal G, et al: A haplotype relative risk study of the dopamine D4 receptor (DRD4) exon III repeat polymorphism and attention deficit hyperactivity disorder (ADHD). Am J Med Genet 96:258–261, 2000

Geijer T, Jonsson E, Neiman J, et al: Tyrosine hydroxylase and dopamine D4 receptor allelic distribution in Scandinavian chronic alcoholics. Alcohol Clin Exp Res 21:35–39, 1997

Gill M, Daly G, Heron S, et al: Confirmation of association between attention deficit hyperactivity disorder and a dopamine transporter polymorphism. Mol Psychiatry 2:311–313, 1997

Higuchi S, Muramatsu T, Matsushita S, et al: No evidence of association between structural polymorphism at the dopamine D3 receptor locus and alcoholism in the Japanese. Am J Med Genet 67:412–414, 1996

Horowitz R, Shufman A, Aharoni S, et al: Confirmation of an excess of the high enzyme activity COMT val allele in heroin addicts in a family based haplotype relative risk study. Am J Med Genet 95:599–603, 2000

Kalivas PW, Nakamura M: Neural systems for behavioral activation and reward. Curr Opin Neurobiol 9:223–227, 1999

Kotler M, Cohen H, Segman R, et al: Excess dopamine D4 receptor (D4DR) exon III seven repeat allele in opioid-dependent subjects. Mol Psychiatry 2:251–4, 1997

Kotler M, Cohen H, Kremer I, et al: No association between the serotonin transporter promoter region (5-HTTLPR) and the dopamine D3 receptor (*Bal*I D3DR) polymorphisms and heroin addiction. Mol Psychiatry 4:313–314, 1999a

Kotler, M., Peretz, B., Cohen, H., et al: Homicidal behavior in schizophrenia associated with a genetic polymorphism determining low catechol *O*-methyltransferase (COMT) activity. Am J Med Genet 88:628–633, 1999b

Krebs MO, Sautel F, Bourdel MC, et al: Dopamine D3 receptor gene variants and substance abuse in schizophrenia. Mol Psychiatry 3:337–341, 1998

Lachman HM, Papolos DF, Saito T, et al: Human catechol-*O*-methyltransferase pharmacogenetics: description of a functional polymorphism and its potential application to neuropsychiatric disorders. Pharmacogenetics 6:243–250, 1996

LaHoste GJ, Swanson JM, Wigal SB, et al: Dopamine D4 receptor gene polymorphism is associated with attention deficit hyperactivity disorder. Mol Psychiatry 1:121–124, 1996

Lesch KP, Bengel D, Heils A, et al: Association of anxiety-related traits with a polymorphism in the serotonin transporter gene regulatory region. Science 274:1527–1531, 1996

Li T, Xu K, Deng H, et al: Association analysis of the dopamine D4 gene exon III VNTR and heroin abuse in Chinese subjects. Mol Psychiatry 2:413–416, 1997

Lichtenberg P, Bachner-Melman R, Gritsenko I, et al: Exploratory association study between catechol *O*-methyltransferase (COMT) high/low enzyme activity polymorphism and hypnotizability. Am J Med Genet 96:771–774, 2000

Lichter JB, Barr CL, Kennedy JL, et al: A hypervariable segment in the human dopamine receptor D4 (DRD4) gene. Hum Mol Genet 2:767–773, 1993

Loehlin JC: Genes and Environment in Personality Development, Newbury Park, CA, Sage, 1992

Lotta, T., Vidgren, J., Tilgmann, C., et al: Kinetics of human soluble and membrane-bound catechol O-methyltransferase: a revised mechanism and description of the thermolabile variant of the enzyme. Biochemistry 34:4202–4210, 1995

Mel H, Horowitz R, Ohel N, et al: Additional evidence for an association between the dopamine D4 receptor (D4DR) exon III seven-repeat allele and substance abuse in opioid dependent subjects: relationship of treatment retention to genotype and personality. Addiction Biology 3:473–481, 1998

Muramatsu T, Higuchi S, Murayama M, et al: Association between alcoholism and the dopamine D4 receptor gene. J Med Genet 33:113–115, 1996

Parsian A, Chakraverty S, Fisher L, et al: No association between polymorphisms in the human dopamine D3 and D4 receptors genes and alcoholism. Am J Med Genet 74:281–285, 1997

Revelle W: Personality, Motivation, and Cognitive Performance, in Learning and Individual Differences: Abilities, Motivation, and Methodology. Edited by Ackerman P, Kanfer R, Cudeck R. Hillsdale, NJ, Erlbaum, 1989, pp 297–341

Robbins TW, Everitt BJ: Neurobehavioural mechanisms of reward and motivation. Curr Opin Neurobiol 6:228–236, 1996

Rowe DC, Stever C, Giedinghagen LN, et al: Dopamine DRD4 receptor polymorphism and attention deficit hyperactivity disorder. Mol Psychiatry 3:419–426, 1998

Rubinstein M, Phillips TJ, Bunzow JR, et al: Mice lacking dopamine D4 receptors are supersensitive to ethanol, cocaine, and methamphetamine. Cell 90:991–1001, 1997

Sabol SZ, Nelson ML, Fisher C, et al: A genetic association for cigarette smoking behavior. Health Psychol 18:7–13, 1999

Sander T, Harms H, Dufeu P, et al: Dopamine D4 receptor exon III alleles and variation of novelty seeking in alcoholics. Am J Med Genet 74:483–487, 1997

Schultz W: Dopamine neurons and their role in reward mechanisms. Curr Opin Neurobiol 7:191–197, 1997

Shields PG, Lerman C, Audrain J, et al: Dopamine D4 receptors and the risk of cigarette smoking in African-Americans and Caucasians. Cancer Epidemiol Biomarkers Prev 7:453–458, 1998

Smalley SL, Bailey JN, Palmer CG, et al: Evidence that the dopamine D4 receptor is a susceptibility gene in attention deficit hyperactivity disorder. Mol Psychiatry 3:427–430, 1998

Swanson JM, Sunohara GA, Kennedy JL, et al: Association of the dopamine receptor D4 (DRD4) gene with a refined phenotype of attention deficit hyperactivity disorder (ADHD): a family based approach. Mol Psychiatry 3:38–41, 1998

Van Tol HH: The dopamine D4 receptor. NIDA Res Monogr 161:20–38, 1996

Van Tol HH: Structural and functional characteristics of the dopamine D4 receptor. Adv Pharmacol 42:486–90, 1998

Van Tol HH, Wu CM, Guan HC, et al: Multiple dopamine D4 receptor variants in the human population. Nature 358:149–152, 1992

Vandenbergh DJ, Rodriguez LA, Miller IT, et al: High-activity catechol-*O*-methyltransferase allele is more prevalent in polysubstance abusers. Am J Med Genet 74:439–442, 1997a

Vandenbergh DJ, Zonderman AB, Wang J, et al: No association between novelty seeking and dopamine D4 receptor (D4DR) exon III seven repeat alleles in Baltimore longitudinal study of aging participants. Mol Psychiatry 2:417–419, 1997b

Weinshilboum R, Dunnette J: Thermal stability and the biochemical genetics of erythrocyte catechol-*O*-methyl-transferase and plasma dopamine-beta-hydroxylase. Clin Genet 19:426–437, 1981

Wise RA: Addictive drugs and brain stimulation reward. Annu Rev Neurosci 19:319–340, 1996a

Wise RA: Neurobiology of addiction. Curr Opin Neurobiol 6:243–251, 1996b

Zuckerman M: Behavioral Expressions and Biosocial Bases of Sensation Seeking. New York, Cambridge University Press, 1994

CHAPTER NINE

Role of *DRD2* and Other Dopamine Genes in Personality Traits

David E. Comings, M.D.
Gerard Saucier, Ph.D.
James P. MacMurray, Ph.D.

Dopaminergic neurons in humans play a major role in a wide range of behaviors including impulsivity, aggression, sexual behavior, appetite, reward, and regulation of pituitary hormones. The dopamine D2 receptor is part of a superfamily of G-protein-coupled receptors having seven membrane-spanning domains (Civelli et al. 1991). The five dopamine receptors can be placed into two subgroups: D1 and D5 stimulate the production of cyclic AMP; and D2, D3, and D4 inhibit the production of cyclic AMP. The interaction between the D1 and D2 receptors has been emphasized in a wide range of behaviors including schizophrenia, cataplexy, cocaine abuse, and others (Spealman et al. 1992; Waddington 1990). The gene for the rat and human dopamine D2 receptor was cloned and sequenced by Civelli and colleagues (Bunzow et al. 1988; Grandy et al. 1989), and a *Taq*I polymorphism located 3' to the gene was described by Grandy et al. (1989).

Supported in part by the Tobacco Related Research Disease Program (Grant 4RT-0110), the Gaming Entertainment Research and Education Foundation, National Center for Responsible Gaming, and the Mary Ellen Gerber Foundation.

DRD2 and Alcoholism

The first molecular genetic association studies in psychiatric genetics were performed with the dopamine receptor D2 (DRD2) gene using the *Taq*I polymorphism and reported in 1990 by Blum and colleagues. Of 22 Caucasian alcoholics studied, 64% carried the A1 allele compared with 17% of 24 controls ($P = 0.003$). This report was widely publicized as having identified a "gene for alcoholism." However, some subsequent reports refuted this finding. The first was by Bolos et al. (1990). They reported that 38% of 40 ambulatory Caucasian alcoholics carried the A1 allele compared with 30% of 127 controls ($P = 0.369$). In addition, there was no evidence for linkage between the *DRD2* A1 allele and alcoholism in two families. The next two reports, published in 1991 in the same issue of the *Journal of the American Medical Association,* were by Comings et al. (1991) and Gelernter et al. (1991). Comings et al. (1991) reported the presence of the A1 allele in 43.4% of 104 alcoholics with and without comorbid drug abuse versus 24.5% of 314 controls ($P < 0.001$). They also reported a significant increase in the prevalence of the A1 allele (45% to 55%) in a range of impulsive behaviors including Tourette syndrome and attention-deficit/hyperactivity disorder (ADHD) (see the section "*DRD2* in Tourette Syndrome and Attention-Deficit/Hyperactivity Disorder"). Gelernter et al. (1991) reported the presence of the A1 allele in 43.2% of 44 ambulatory alcoholics versus 35.3% of 68 random controls. Although the prevalence of the A1 allele in alcoholism was similar to that reported by Comings et al., the frequency in their controls was sufficiently higher such that the difference was not significant ($P = 0.40$). However, this report was complicated by the fact that many of these controls were from Tourette syndrome families.

In the ensuing years many reports of the association of the *DRD2 Taq*I A1 allele with alcoholism were published (Blum et al. 1995; Noble 1993). About half were confirmatory. These early studies of the role of the DRD2 gene in alcoholism took the brunt of the learning curve in our knowledge of how to undertake studies of polygenic disorders and with it came a great deal of skepticism about the DRD2 gene. However, the difficulties in uniform replication of the results for the DRD2 genes were subsequently seen in all association studies of single genes in polygenic disorders. Like alcoholism, personality is a polygenic trait (Plomin et al. 1994). Thus before progressing to examine the potential role of the DRD2 gene in personality and other traits, it is critical to understand the unique nature of polygenic disorders.

Single-Gene Versus Polygenic Inheritance

Because single-gene disorders have been the focus of attention by human geneticists for the past century, much of the thinking about the role of genes in polygenic behavioral disorders has been based on these single-gene concepts. This has led to a number of misperceptions about polygenic disorders and what to expect of association studies of the genes involved in polygenic disorders. Some of these misperceptions are as follows: 1) To provide valid information the polymorphisms studied must be inside the reading frame of the gene, in the promoter, or located where they can directly affect the function of the gene. 2) Polygenic disorders are similar to single-gene disorders except that a few more genes (oligogenic inheritance) are involved. 3) The type of mutations that are associated with single-gene disorders are similar to those involved in polygenic disorders. 4) When a gene is found to be significantly associated with a given polygenic disorder, it is legitimate to claim that a so-called major gene for that disorder has been found. 5) As with single-gene inheritance, lod score linkage and sib-pair analysis are the most accurate ways of identifying the genes for polygenic disorders. 6) If an initial association study is not replicated by most or all of the subsequent studies, the initial claims are probably invalid. 7) If only half or fewer of the replication studies confirm an initial result, all the studies are probably in error. 8) If the frequency of a given allele is higher in the relatives than in the probands, that gene is not associated with the disorder. 9) The variability from study to study in population-based association studies is most likely due to ethnic stratification of the sample, that is, differences in the ethnic composition between the subjects and the controls. 10) Because of the latter, family-based studies such as the haplotype relative risk (Falk and Rubinstein 1987) or transmission disequilibrium test (Spielman and Ewens 1996) are uniformly better than population-based association studies. 11) The genotypes of specific genes that are associated with a given behavior tend to be constant for similar behaviors.

Some of these subjects have been discussed in more detail elsewhere (Comings 1996, 1998a, 1998b, 1999c; Comings et al. 2000, 2001), and it is not our purpose to have this chapter be a dissertation on polygenic inheritance. On the other hand, if some of the unique aspects of polygenic inheritance are not understood, it is impossible to understand the role of the DRD2 gene or other genes in personality traits. Thus, before progressing we will review some basic aspects of polygenic inheritance. Because some of these issues are still not totally resolved, what we are presenting are in part our personal views. Also, instead of individually discussing each of the misperceptions we present a general review of polygenic inheritance.

The key characteristic of polygenic inheritance is that traits and disorders are caused when an individual inherits a critical number of variants of genes that affect a given function. In the case of behavioral disorders, the variants affect genes involved in the synthesis, degradation, transport, and binding of neurotransmitters, neuropeptides, and hormones. One of the most enlightening observations to come out of our studies over the past 10 years on 70 different genes and a range of behavioral phenotypes is that each gene on average accounts for less than 5.0% and usually less than 1.5% of the variance of a trait (Comings 1996, 1998a, 1998b; Comings et al. 2000). Risch and Merikangas (1996) and Risch (2000) have shown that when genes account for such a small percentage of the variance (low λ), lod score and sib-pair linkage analyses lack the power to identify these genes. Thus, when a classical linkage study purports to have ruled out the role of a given gene in a polygenic disorder, such a statement instead means that a major effect of the gene has been ruled out.

A second characteristic of polygenic disorders is that they are genetically heterogeneous. For example, if variants at 100 different genes can contribute to a disorder but only 10 such variants are required to produce the disorder in a given individual, it is very likely that if one group of investigators reports a significant association with a specific gene, that association may not be replicated in a second study. Although the failure of replication of different population-based association studies can be due to hidden ethnic stratification, it is much more likely to be due to the very small percentage of the variance contributed by each gene, and genetic heterogeneity. Variable results have also been reported in series of studies using transmission disequilibrium test analyses.

A third characteristic is that the genetic variants involved in polygenic disorders are likely to be fundamentally different from those involved in single-gene disorders. For example, if common diseases require the additive effect of multiple genes, the variants of those genes must be very common. By contrast, the mutations that cause single-gene disorders are usually present in less than 0.01% of the population, and all the single-gene disorders combined affect less than 2% of the population. We have argued elsewhere (Comings 1998a) that the common microsatellite polymorphisms have a modest effect on gene regulation and may be responsible for a significant proportion of the variation for polygenic disorders.

Because the effect of these polymorphisms extends over the domain of more than one gene (Paquette et al. 1998), and because each gene is often associated with multiple microsatellites, it is likely that each gene is present in a wide range of hypo- and hyperfunctional variants (Comings 1999b). This also makes it likely that any common single-nucleotide polymorphism, whether directly affecting gene function or not, tends to divide the population into groups varying in the function of the gene with which they are associated (Comings 1999b).

A fourth characteristic is that because the key feature in polygenic inheritance is that an individual possesses a certain threshold number of genetic variants to produce a given phenotype, the relatives can actually show a higher frequency for a given allele but still be unaffected because they do not carry the threshold number.

Fifth, in polygenic disorders, similar genes but different alleles or genotypes of those genes may be involved in different traits (Comings et al. 2000).

In conclusion, polygenic inheritance is much more complex than single-gene inheritance, and the rules of single-gene inheritance do not hold. Before reviewing the specific role of *DRD2* and other dopamine genes in personality traits, we review the role of *DRD2* in a range of impulsive, compulsive, and addictive behaviors, using the observations just stated to help interpret the results.

DRD2 in Tourette Syndrome and Attention-Deficit/Hyperactivity Disorder

When we first observed the variability in the results in the studies of *DRD2* and alcoholism, we wondered if part of the problem might have been that only a subset of alcoholics, such as Cloninger's type II alcoholics associated with childhood ADHD (Cloninger et al. 1988; Tarter et al. 1977) and antisocial behavior (Cadoret et al. 1987; Earls et al. 1988), might be associated with the DRD2 gene. Thus, the variable results might have been due to the inclusion of alcoholism resulting from other causes. In 1991 we reported our studies of the association of the *DRD2 Taq*I A1 allele and Tourette syndrome, ADHD, and related disorders. The prevalence of the A1 allele in 314 controls screened to exclude alcoholism and drug abuse was 24.5%. In subjects with Tourette syndrome, ADHD, autism, substance abuse, and posttraumatic stress disorder (PTSD), the prevalence ranged from 42.3% to 54.6%, and *P* values were less than or equal to 0.005. Viewed from the perspective of single-gene disorders these results were unimpressive because in most cases fewer than 50% of the subjects carried the A1 allele. However, viewed from the perspective of a polygenic disorder they suggested the DRD2 gene was one of a set of genes contributing to a range of impulsive, compulsive, and addictive behaviors.

Supportive of a role of the DRD2 gene in behavioral disorders are studies of Noble et al. (1991) showing that the presence of the A1 allele was associated with a lower B_{max} for the dopamine D2 receptors in brain tissue. Using positron emission tomography and ^{18}F-deoxyglucose, Noble et al. (1997) also found that A1 carriers showed a significantly lower relative glucose metabolism in the putamen, nucleus accumbens, frontal and temporal gyri, and medial prefrontal, occipitotemporal, and orbital cortices than those with the A22 genotype. These studies are important because glucose metabolism is a measure of blood flow, and blood flow is a measure of function. Thus, the DRD2 gene was playing a direct role in the function of these portions of the brain.

Heterosis and Physiological Correlates With *DRD2*

Heterosis appears to play a role in the interpretation of *DRD2 Taq*I A1/A2 association studies. Heterosis, or overdominance, refers to a situation in which the heterozygous phenotype is more robust than either homozygous phenotype. Heterosis is termed positive when the value of the phenotype is higher in heterozygotes and is termed negative when the value is lower in heterozygotes. Although heterosis is most often used to described plant or animal hybrids that are more robust than the parental strains (hybrid vigor), it can also apply at the level of individual molecular genetic polymorphisms (Comings 1999a; Comings and MacMurray 1997a, 1997b). We have reviewed the subject of molecular heterosis for many genes, including the DRD2 gene, elsewhere (Comings and MacMurray 2000).

In summary, a number of studies provide evidence that the *Taq*I A1/A2 polymorphism is in linkage disequilibrium with a locus that regulates *DRD2* function (possibly a microsatellite polymorphism), and that half of heterozygotes show significantly lower receptor density in the striatum and lower blood flow in many areas of the brain. Given the importance of the dopamine D2 receptor in a range of central nervous system functions, *DRD2* becomes an important candidate gene in behavioral disorders and personality traits.

DRD2 and Posttraumatic Stress Disorder

Because Tourette syndrome and ADHD are stress-related disorders, and because dopamine is released in the mesolimbic system following stress (Thierry et al. 1976), we postulated the DRD2 gene would be involved in PTSD. To test this we examined "battle-hardened" non-Hispanic Caucasian Vietnam veterans for the presence of DSM-III-R (American Psychiatric Association 1987) criteria of PTSD. There were 32 subjects in the initial study (Comings et al. 1996a). Of the 24 that met criteria for PTSD, 58% carried the *DRD2* A1 allele compared with 12.5% of the 8 without PTSD ($P = 0.041$). In a replication study we examined an additional 24 subjects. Here, of the 13 that met criteria for PTSD, 61.5% carried the *DRD2* A1 allele compared with 0% of the 11 without PTSD ($P = 0.002$). For the combined set, $P = 0.0001$. In this study we also found that the *DRD2* A1 allele was significantly associated with a history of childhood conduct disorder and imprisonment for violent behaviors as an adult. Gelernter et al. (1999) found no increase in the prevalence of the A1 allele in subjects with PTSD compared with controls. However, he did not compare the prevalence in battle-hardened veterans with or without PTSD as was done in our study.

DRD2 in Pathological Gambling

Pathological gambling has often been referred to as the perfect addiction to study for research purposes because it is not confounded by the problems of ingestion of an addicting drug. We found that 50.9% of 171 pathological gamblers carried the *DRD2* A1 allele compared with 25.9% of the 714 known non-Hispanic Caucasian controls screened to exclude drug and alcohol abuse ($P < 0.000001$, odds ratio $= 2.96$). The DRD2 gene was associated with severity in that the *DRD2* A1 allele was present in 63.8% of those in the upper half of severity (odds ratio vs. controls $= 5.03$) compared with 40.9% in the lower half of severity. Of those who had no comorbid substance abuse, 44.1% carried the *DRD2* A1 allele, compared with 60.5% of those who had comorbid substance abuse. These results suggest that genetic variants of *DRD2* play a role in pathological gambling and support the concept that variants of this gene are a risk factor for impulsive and addictive behaviors.

DRD2 in Smoking

We also examined the role of the *DRD2* A1 allele in smoking. The *DRD2* A1 allele was present in 48.7% of 317 non-Hispanic Caucasians who had attempted to stop smoking and could not, compared with 25.9% in 714 controls ($P < 0.0001$). Studies by Noble et al. (1994b), Spitz et al. (1998), and Lerman et al. (1999) have shown very similar results. Some studies have been negative (Bierut et al. 2000; Singleton et al. 1998).

DRD2 in Obesity

Compulsive eating with obesity can also be considered an addictive behavior. We examined the role of the DRD2 gene in obesity using *DRD2* haplotypes based on two other polymorphisms of the DRD2 gene (Comings et al. 1993). Different alignments of these two polymorphisms produced four different haplotypes. This showed a significant association between body mass index and height with the fourth haplotype. Noble et al. (1994b) and Blum et al. (1996) have independently also observed an association between the *DRD2* A1 allele and obesity.

DRD2 and Personality

Given the number of positive associations between the DRD2 gene and a range of impulsive, compulsive, and addictive behaviors, it would be anticipated that this gene might also be associated with various personality traits, especially those relating to novelty seeking, impulsivity, aggression, and externalizing traits. We divide this section into two parts, prior studies presenting published or in press studies completed prior to this review, and new studies presenting studies we carried out specifically for this chapter.

Prior Studies

Defense Style Questionnaire (DSQ): immature defenses. The first study of the role of the DRD2 gene in personality traits was reported by Comings et al. (1995) using *DRD2* haplotypes. The DSQ was originally developed by Bond et al. (1990) to evaluate a subject's style of dealing with conflict. The final version (Andrews et al. 1993) is a 40-item instrument with two questions to evaluate each of 20 different defense styles. These are divided into Mature Defenses (sublimation, humor, anticipation, and suppression), Neurotic Defenses (undoing, pseudoaltruism, idealization, and reaction formation), and Immature Defenses (projection, passive aggression, acting out, isolation, devaluation, autistic fantasy, denial, displacement, dissociation, splitting, rationalization, and somatization). We observed a significant association of the DRD2 gene with the Immature Defenses scores.

Millon Personality Inventory: schizoid avoidant behavior. In a study of a range of personality traits based on the Millon Personality Inventory, Blum et al. (1997) found the *DRD2* A1 allele to be associated with high scores for Schizoid Avoidant Behavior.

Neuroticism. Eley et al. (1998) examined polymorphisms at a number of dopamine genes *(DRD1, DRD2, DRD3, DRD4,* and *DAT1)* and found no association with either high or low neuroticism scores. They concluded the dopamine genes were more likely to be associated with externalizing than internalizing disorders.

Novelty seeking. In a review of the *DRD2* alcoholism data, Cook and Gurling (1996) suggested the gene was associated with spontaneity and impulsiveness. In a study of the DRD2 gene in cocaine abusers, Compton et al. (1996) reported an association between the *DRD2 Taq*I A1 allele and Novelty Seeking using the Tridimensional Personality Questionnaire (Cloninger 1987b; Cloninger et al. 1991) with 40 cocaine abusers. There was no association with Harm Avoidance, Reward Dependence, or with Extraversion or Introversion scales of the Eysenck Personality Inventory (Eysenck and Eysenck 1996). Noble et al. (1998) examined the association between the DRD2 and DRD4 genes in 119 healthy Caucasian boys who were administered the Tridimensional Personality Questionnaire. They found that the Novelty Seeking scale was significantly associated with boys carrying all three *DRD2* alleles A1, B1, and intron 6 1 compared with boys without any of these alleles. Boys with the seven-repeat allele of *DRD4* also had significantly higher Novelty Seeking scores. The greatest difference was in those carrying both the three *DRD2* alleles and the *DRD4* seven-repeat allele, indicating an additive effect of the two genes. Neither *DRD2* nor *DRD4* differentiated the total Harm Avoidance scale. *DRD2* but not *DRD4* differentiated subjects with high scores on the Persistence subscore of the Reward Dependence scale. In an unpublished study from our group, Saucier et al. (G. Saucier, P. F. Collins, D. E. Comings, et al., personal communication, February 2000) found no association between the *DRD2* A1 allele and the Novelty Seeking scale of the Temperament and Character Inventory (TCI) but did find an association with the Extravagance (vs. Reserve) subcomponent of Novelty Seeking.

New Studies

As part of our ongoing studies of the role of a number of genes in addictive and other behaviors, we collected DNA samples and performed extensive personality testing on a series of students from a local university (California State University of San Bernardino) and subjects from a Veterans Administration hospital addiction treatment unit. Combining the two groups provided a wider range of scores than examining either group alone. Although both genders were represented in the control group, because virtually all of the subjects in the addiction treatment unit were males, to avoid gender as a confounding variable we examined only males in both groups. To avoid the confounding variable of race, we also restricted this study to non-Hispanic Caucasians. This produced a final group of 81 control subjects and 123 addiction treatment unit subjects, 204 in all. Although we genotyped these individuals for polymorphisms associated with 59 different genes, these are part of a subsequent, more complete study (Comings et al. 2001). Because this set of genes included six different dopamine genes *(DRD1, DRD2, DRD3, DRD4, DRD5,* and *DAT1)* including two different polymorphisms for the DRD2 gene, we felt it would provide a more useful report to include all six genes rather than restrict this report to the DRD2 gene.

Since our initial study of the interactive role of three different dopamine genes *(DRD2, DAT1,* and *DBH)* on an ADHD score in our Tourette syndrome probands (Comings et al. 1996b), we have been interested in the role of the interaction of multiple genes in polygenic disorders. The technique we found to be most useful is to assign each of the three major genotypes of each gene a score of 0, 1, or 2 based on results in the prior literature showing which genotypes are most associated with addictive, compulsive, and impulsive behaviors. The genes and the polymorphisms used and the literature on which the scoring was based are given elsewhere (Comings et al. 2000). Each gene is scored on the basis of 1 of 12 different modes of inheritance. The scores for all six dopamine genes were then included in a multivariate linear regression analysis with backward elimination to identify the genes that contributed most to the traits. The *pin* was set at 0.10 and the *pout* at 0.30. This conservative setting is more likely to retain genes that have previously been found to be associated with various personality traits. Those genes that were included in the equation were considered to play a role in the personality trait in question. The final r, r^2, F ratio, and P value for the combined set provided the correlation coefficient, fraction of the variance, F ratio, and significance for the entire set of dopamine genes. The printout also provided the individual r, r^2, and P values for each gene included in the equation. The SPSS statistical package for Macintosh, 1995 was used (SPSS, Inc. 1995).

These subjects were assessed with the following tests: Cloninger's TCI (Cloninger et al. 1993), the NEO Five Factor Personality Inventory, (NEO-FFI) (Costa and McCrae 1992), the Brown Attention-Deficit Disorder Scales (BADDS) (Brown 1996), the Buss-Durkee Hostility Inventory (Buss and Durkee 1957), the IPC Locus of Control Inventory (IPC-LOCI) (Levenson 1981; Sadowski and Wenzel 1982), and the DSQ (Andrews et al. 1993). Because Cloninger et al. (1993) found a significant effect of age on the traits in the TCI, and because substance abuse itself could be a confounding factor, we used residual scores of the different traits after controlling for age and sample group. The results for each of these tests using the literature-based gene scores are given in Tables 9–1 through 9–6. A caveat of these studies is that they were limited to males. The results with females might be different.

For the seven summary TCI traits, the genes were also scored on the basis of examining by ANOVA the magnitude of the different continuous personality traits for the three genotypes of each gene. Because this was done on the same database used to examine the effect of multiple genes, the absolute values of the total r, r^2, and P are optimized. This approach is valid for examining the relative influence of different genes, and the relative importance of different genotypes of those genes, for the traits in question. Table 9–7 illustrates the results obtained when the optimized gene scores were used for the seven variables of the TCI. The gene scores used are also listed. Four dopamine receptor genes, *DRD1, DRD2, DRD4,* and *DAT1,* contributed to 5.25% of the variance of the Novelty Seeking score ($P = 0.032$). *DRD1* contributed the most, 2.95% of the variance. Three genes, *DRD2, DRD3,* and *DRD4,* contributed to 5.14% of the variance of Reward Dependence ($P = 0.015$) with *DRD4* contributing the most, 4.04%. Four genes, *DRD1, DRD2, DRD5,* and *DAT1,* contributed to 8.84% of the variance of Harm Avoidance, with *DRD5* contributing the most, 6.86% ($P = 0.0002$). Three to five genes contributed to 2.45% to 9.64% of the variance of the remaining four traits. Interestingly, the dopamine genes made a greater contribution to Self-Transcendence (9.64%

TABLE 9–1   Temperament and Character Inventory: dopamine genes (*DRD1–DRD5* and *DAT1*) included in the multivariate regression equation using literature-based gene coding and residuals of personality scores after controlling for age and sample

Scale	Genes included	r	r^2	P
Novelty Seeking	*DRD1*	0.131	0.017	0.064
	DRD2 ins/del	−0.092	0.0085	0.190
	Total	0.163	0.0265	0.071
Harm Avoidance	*DRD5*	0.268	0.0718	0.0001
	DRD1	−0.084	0.0071	0.211
	Total	0.280	0.0784	0.0003
Reward Dependence	*DRD4*	−0.213	0.0453	0.0024
	DRD2	0.091	0.0083	0.189
	Total	0.228	0.0522	0.005
Persistence	*DRD2*	0.096	0.0092	0.174
	DRD1	−0.077	0.0059	0.271
	DRD3	−0.076	0.0058	0.276
	Total	0.142	0.0202	0.252
Cooperativeness	*DRD2*	0.098	0.0096	0.16
	DRD4	−0.088	0.0077	0.21
	DRD5	−0.085	0.0072	0.23
	Total	0.152	0.0233	0.19
Self-Directedness	*DRD5*	−0.186	0.0345	0.0091
	DRD4	−0.093	0.0086	0.189
	Total	0.203	0.0411	0.018
Self-Transcendence	*DRD4*	0.167	0.0279	0.018
	DAT1	−0.119	0.0142	0.091
	DRD3	0.102	0.0104	0.15
	DRD5	0.078	0.0061	0.27
	Total	0.233	0.0543	0.028

Note. pin = 0.10, pout = 0.30.

of the variance) than any other trait, with *DRD4* contributing to 5.43% of the variance ($P = 0.0008$).

Rather than comment on the results for each trait, we instead list the conclusions we have reached based on these results.

1. *Each gene accounts for only a small percentage of the variance.* Using literature scoring, the percentage of the variance explained based on r^2 for the included genes ranged from 0.55% to 7.18%, with the majority accounting for less than 2%. The following genes and scores accounted for 2% or more of the variance:

DRD5	7.18% TCI Harm Avoidance
DRD5	6.45% NEO-FFI Neuroticism
DRD5	6.10% DSQ Immature Defenses
DRD2I	5.93% BADDS diagnosis
DRD4	4.53% TCI Reward Dependence
DRD5	3.45% TCI Self-Determination
DRD3	3.15% DSQ Neurotic Defenses.
DRD4	2.79% TCI Self-Transcendence
DRD4	2.49% BADDS diagnosis
DRD3	2.31% DSQ Immature Defenses
DRD5	2.22% NEO-FFI Extraversion
DRD5	2.04% BADDS diagnosis
DRD2	2.02% IPC-LOC Chance

TABLE 9–2   NEO Five Factor Personality Inventory: dopamine genes (*DRD1–DRD5* and *DAT1*) included in multivariate regression equation using literature-based gene coding and residuals of the personality scores after controlling for age and sample

Scale	Genes included	r	r^2	P
Agreeableness	*DRD4*	−0.133	0.0176	0.072
	DRD5	−0.099	0.0098	0.176
	Total	0.157	0.0248	0.100
Conscientiousness	*DRD3*	−0.110	0.0121	0.137
	DRD5	−0.098	0.0096	0.185
	DRD4	−0.094	0.0088	0.205
	Total	0.175	0.0307	0.134
Extraversion	*DRD5*	−0.149	0.0222	0.043
	DRD2	0.089	0.0079	0.223
	DRD1	0.084	0.0070	0.253
	Total	0.199	0.0395	0.063
Neuroticism	*DRD5*	0.255	0.0645	0.0004
	DRD4	0.100	0.0100	0.16
	DRD3	0.097	0.0094	0.17
	DRD2I	0.096	0.0092	0.175
	DRD1	−0.081	0.0066	0.252
	DAT1	0.076	0.0058	0.280
	Total	0.322	0.1034	0.0028
Openness	*DRD2*	0.101	0.0102	0.172
	DRD3	0.077	0.0059	0.294
	Total	0.127	0.0162	0.228

Note. pin = 0.10, pout = 0.30.

TABLE 9–3   Brown Attention-Deficit Disorder Scales: dopamine genes (*DRD1–DRD5* and *DAT1*) multivariate regression equation using literature-based gene coding and residuals of the personality scores after controlling for age and sample

Scale	Genes included	r	r^2	P
Attention	DRD5	0.108	0.0117	0.12
Energy	DRD5	0.099	0.0098	0.16
	DRD4	0.091	0.0083	0.19
	Total	0.129	0.0168	0.18
ADHD Diagnosis	DRD4	−0.158	0.0249	0.021
(yes = 1, no = 2)	DRD5	−0.143	0.0204	0.039
	DRD2I	0.077	0.0593	0.264
	Total	0.219	0.0482	0.019
Irritability	No genes included			
Memory	No genes included			
Organization	DRD3	0.107	0.0114	0.126
	DRD5	0.074	0.0055	0.291
	DRD4	0.073	0.0053	0.300
	Total	0.148	0.0221	0.213
Total	DRD5	0.112	0.0125	0.109
	DRD4	0.096	0.0092	0.171
	Total	0.142	0.0202	0.128

Note. pin = 0.10, pout = 0.30.

The genes that were most often included were *DRD5* (six times), *DRD4* (three times), *DRD2* (two times), and *DRD3* (two times). When optimized gene scoring for the TCI was used (Table 9–7, Figure 9–1), each gene accounted for 0.52% to 6.86% of the variance. The following genes and scores accounted for 2% or more of the variance, listed in descending order:

DRD5	6.86%	Harm Avoidance
DRD4	5.43%	Self-Transcendence
DRD4	4.04%	Reward Dependence
DRD3	3.96%	Self-Transcendence
DRD5	3.34%	Self-Directedness
DRD1	2.95%	Novelty Seeking

The major difference was that when optimized gene scoring was used, the scoring for Self-Transcendence for *DRD4* changed from 002 to 012, indicating that differentiating the four-or-fewer-repeat alleles from the 4/4 genotype increased the percentage of the variance. The scoring also

TABLE 9–4   Buss-Durkee Hostility Inventory: dopamine genes *(DRD1–DRD5* and *DAT1)* included in the multivariate regression equation using literature-based gene coding and residuals of the personality scores after controlling for age and sample

Scale	Genes included	r	r^2	P
Assault	DRD5	0.083	0.0069	0.239
Feelings of Guilt	DRD5	0.128	0.0163	0.069
	DRD2I	0.077	0.0059	0.269
	Total	0.148	0.0220	0.110
Indirect Hostility	No genes included			
Irritability	No genes included			
Negativism	DRD4	0.093	0.0086	0.188
Resentment	DRD2	−0.120	0.0144	0.087
	DRD5	0.093	0.0086	0.188
	Total	0.153	0.023	0.093
Suspicion	DRD5	0.098	0.0096	0.165
	DRD1	−0.095	0.0090	0.179
	DAT1	−0.082	0.0067	0.244
	Total	0.156	0.0244	0.181
Verbal Hostility	DRD4	0.095	0.0090	0.180
Total	No genes included			

Note. pin = 0.10, pout = 0.30.

TABLE 9–5   Locus of Control Scale: dopamine genes *(DRD1–DRD5* and *DAT1)* included in the multivariate regression equation with residual scores for age and sample

Scale	Genes included	r	r^2	P
Chance	DRD2	−0.142	0.0202	0.043
	DAT1	0.099	0.0098	0.154
	DRD2I	0.092	0.0084	0.189
	Total	0.187	0.0352	0.066
Internal	DRD1	0.135	0.0182	0.052
	DRD5	−0.126	0.0158	0.068
	DRD3	−0.113	0.0127	0.102
	DRD2	0.091	0.0083	0.190
	DRD2I	−0.078	0.0061	0.256
	Total	0.253	0.0639	0.022
Powerful Others	DRD1	−0.102	0.0104	0.147
	DRD3	0.074	0.0055	0.294
	Total	0.125	0.0156	0.205

Note. pin = 0.10, pout = 0.30.

TABLE 9–6   Defense Style Questionnaire: dopamine genes *(DRD1–DRD5 and DAT1)* included in the multivariate regression equation

Scale	Genes included	r	r^2	P
Immature Defenses	DRD5	0.247	0.0610	0.0004
	DRD3	0.152	0.0231	0.027
	DRD4	0.119	0.0141	0.083
	DRD1	−0.091	0.0082	0.188
	DRD2	−0.090	0.0081	0.191
	Total	0.339	0.115	0.0003
Neurotic Defenses	DRD3	0.177	0.0315	0.011
Mature Defenses	DRD3	0.122	0.0148	0.084
	DRD5	−0.082	0.0070	0.259
	Total	0.147	0.0218	0.115

Note. pin = 0.10, pout = 0.30.

changed for *DRD4* from 002 to 210 for Self-Directedness, again indicating the potentially important role of the four or fewer repeats. This is consistent with our studies showing that for some traits or disorders, the four-or-fewer-repeat alleles (especially the two-repeat allele) were more important than the seven-repeat allele (Comings et al. 1999).

2. *The inclusion of substance abuse subjects did not alter the results.* Because we used a combination of normal controls and individuals with different types of substance abuse, we were concerned that the results would be driven more by the substance abuse than the personality traits themselves. To correct for this we partialed age and sample group out of the dependent variable to correct for the effects of age and sample group. However, to further determine if substance abuse played a role we compared the results for of the TCI scales using the residual scores instead of the raw scores. The results for the two sets of scores were remarkably similar.

3. *Sets of dopamine genes also account for a small percentage of the variance.* Despite examining the additive effect of several dopamine genes, they still accounted for only 1.56% to 10.34% of the variance of the respective traits. The highest values were 11.5% for five genes for DSQ Immature Defenses and 10.34% for five genes for the NEO-FFI Neuroticism scale. Using optimized gene scoring, three dopamine genes accounted for 9.64% of the TCI Self-Transcendence scale.

TABLE 9–7   Temperament and Character Inventory: dopamine genes
(*DRD1–DRD5* and *DAT1*) included in the multivariate regression equation
using optimized scoring with residual scores from age and sample group

Scale	Genes included	Gene score	*r*	*r²*	*P*
Novelty Seeking	DRD1	200	0.172	0.0295	0.0145
	DAT1	201	0.104	0.0108	0.137
	DRD2	021	0.083	0.0069	0.234
	DRD4	201	0.076	0.0058	0.275
	Total		0.229	0.0525	0.032
Reward Dependence	DRD4	120	0.201	0.0404	0.0042
	DRD2	120	0.090	0.0081	0.198
	DRD3	201	0.081	0.0066	0.228
	Total		0.227	0.0514	0.015
Harm Avoidance	DRD5	210	0.262	0.0686	0.0002
	DRD1	021	0.081	0.0066	0.231
	DAT1	012	0.076	0.0058	0.265
	DRD2	012	0.072	0.0052	0.291
	Total		0.297	0.0884	0.001
Persistence	DAT1	021	0.104	0.0108	0.076
	DRD2	021	0.115	0.0132	0.097
	DRD3	120	0.112	0.0125	0.106
	DRD5	002	0.104	0.0108	0.134
	DRD1	021	0.095	0.0090	0.171
	Total		0.243	0.0592	0.032
Cooperativeness	DRD2	120	0.102	0.0104	0.151
	DRD4	210	0.093	0.0086	0.191
	DRD5	012	0.085	0.0072	0.226
	Total		0.156	0.0245	0.179
Self-Directedness	DRD5	012	0.183	0.0334	0.010
	DRD4	210	0.108	0.0116	0.128
	DAT1	210	0.078	0.0061	0.271
	DRD2	210	0.074	0.0055	0.299
	Total		0.231	0.0534	0.032
Self-Transcendence	DRD4	012	0.233	0.0543	0.0008
	DRD3	210	0.199	0.0396	0.0038
	DAT1	120	0.108	0.0117	0.116
	Total		0.310	0.0964	0.0002

Note. pin = 0.10, pout = 0.30.

4. *Many other genes are involved in personality traits.* The small percentage of the total variance explained by the dopamine genes
means that the dopamine genes represent just a portion of the total
genes involved. Many other genes including those for serotonin,

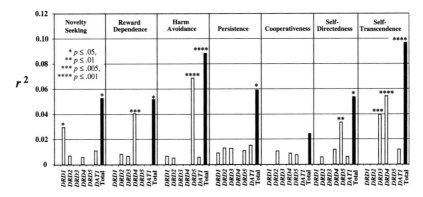

Figure 9–1 Summary of results. Fraction of the variance, r^2, on the ordinate, and the dopamine genes for the seven Temperament and Character Inventory traits on the abscissa.

norepinephrine, GABA, and other neurotransmitters, as well as neuropeptides, hormones, and the genes involved in secondary messengers, are also involved. Our studies examining the role of these other genes in personality traits are now complete (Comings et al. 2001). As described later (p. 184), they modify some of the conclusions based on examining only dopamine genes.

5. *Many personality traits have genes in common.* Even the most cursory glance at Tables 9–1 through 9–7 shows that all of the different personality traits have genes in common. Thus, in marked contrast to single-gene disorders, where each disorder is due to a different gene, in polygenic disorders, many traits and disorders have genes in common. Different combinations of *DRD5, DRD4,* and *DRD2* were especially common, but the other three were also utilized.

6. *Genotype variation is as important as gene variation.* With literature-based gene scoring, many of the genes listed showed negative correlation coefficients, or *r* values. This means that in these cases the optimized gene scoring was different from that based on the literature. Because there are 12 different ways to score each gene, a negative value does not necessarily mean a precise inverse coding was used, but it does indicate a variation from the literature coding. This was especially common for *DRD4.* Although the seven-repeat alleles, or the four-or-more-repeat alleles, have been widely emphasized in the literature, we have previously shown that for some traits the two-repeat allele, or the four-or-fewer-repeat alleles,

are more important (Comings et al. 1999). Because *DRD4* was scored as 002 (<4/<4 = 0, 4/4 = 0, >4/>4 = 2), a negative *r* indicates that for that trait the four-or-more-repeat alleles were not the ones associated with the phenotype. This was the case in 6 of the 13 times (46%) *DRD4* was involved in a trait. The four-or-more-repeat alleles have been especially implicated in novelty seeking and ADHD (Benjamin et al. 1996; Comings et al. 1999; Epstein et al. 1996; Faraone et al. 2001; Grice et al. 1996; Lahoste et al. 1996; Rowe et al. 1998). Our observations of a positive, but not necessarily significant, correlation with the ADHD diagnosis of the BADDS (where a negative score is a positive correlation with the diagnosis because yes = 1 and no = 2), and the Impulsiveness versus Reflection subscore for TCI Novelty Seeking (not shown) for the four-or-more-repeat alleles are consistent with these findings. However, in our series *DRD4* was not one of the genes included in the total TCI Novelty Seeking score. It was of interest that the four-or-more-repeat alleles of *DRD4* were significantly involved in the TCI Self-Transcendence scores. Using 012 scoring it accounted for 5.43% of the variance of the total score ($P = 0.0008$). Of interest, Svrakic et al. (1993) reported a modest positive correlation ($r = 0.20$) between Novelty Seeking and Self-Transcendence. Some of the variability between *DRD4* and Novelty Seeking may be related to variations in different groups in the association of Novelty Seeking with Self-Transcendence.

The same results of a mixture of positive and negative *r* values were seen for the other genes as well. We found that the same principle held for our studies of ADHD, oppositional defiant disorder, and conduct disorder (Comings et al. 2000a, 2000b). We term this phenomenon *genotype variability*. Because it was based on optimal gene scores, Table 9–7 provides the best evidence for genotype variability in that scoring of the same gene was often different for each trait. This is understandable if each gene comes in a wide range of hypo- and hyperfunctional variants (Comings 1999b) and different traits and disorders are due to the critical combination of different hypo- and hyperfunctional alleles.

7. *Personality and behavioral traits are polygenic.* Many of the same conclusions reached above also applied to our studies of ADHD, oppositional defiant disorder, conduct disorder (Comings et al. 2000a, 2000b), pathological gambling, and other behavioral disorders, indicating all are polygenic, each gene contributes to a small

percentage of the total variance, many genes are involved, different traits have genes in common, and the variation in the genotypes is as important as the variation in the genes.

8. *Personality traits are not due to specific functional types of genes.* Cloninger proposed that novelty seeking was predominately regulated by dopaminergic genes, reward dependence by serotonergic genes, and harm avoidance by noradrenergic genes (Cloninger 1987a). The present studies show that for each of these traits, even using optimized gene scores, dopamine genes accounted for only 5.25% of the variance of TCI Novelty Seeking. If more than 25% of the variance of these traits is genetic, genes other than the dopamine genes account for most of the variance. In addition, dopamine genes accounted for even more of the variance for Harm Avoidance (8.84%), Persistence (5.92%), Self-Directedness (5.34%), and Self-Transcendence (9.64%). These results are summarized in Figure 9–1. However, a major caveat is that when many other nondopamine genes were added to the regression equation, the results were somewhat different (Comings et al. 2001). With these additional genes, dopamine genes played a greater role in novelty seeking than in harm avoidance and reward dependence, and as Cloninger predicted, norepinephrine genes were more involved in reward dependence than in novelty seeking or harm avoidance. These studies also showed that the different functional groups of genes were involved in all of the traits, that all traits have these genes in common just as they share dopamine genes, that genotype variability is as important or more important than the utilization of different genes, and that genes other than dopamine genes play a significant role in novelty seeking. Again, these findings are consistent with the earlier discussion of polygenic inheritance, suggesting that each gene comes in a range of hypo- and hyperfunctional variants, and it is the unique combination of a wide range of genes and genotypes of genes involved in neurotransmitter and hormonal function that is crucial, rather than a predominant role of a few specific genes.

References

American Psychiatric Association: Diagnostic and Statistical Manual of Mental Disorders, 3rd Edition, Revised. Washington, DC, American Psychiatric Association, 1987

Andrews G, Singh M, and Bond M: The Defense Style Questionnaire. J Nerv Ment Dis 181:246–256, 1993

Benjamin J, Li L, Patterson C, et al: Population and familial association between the D4 dopamine receptor gene and measures of novelty seeking. Nat Genet 12:81–84, 1996

Bierut LJ, Rice JP, Edenberg HJ, et al: Family based study of the association of the dopamine D2 receptor gene (DRD2) with habitual smoking. Am J Med Genet 90(4):299–302, 2000

Blum K, Noble EP, Sheridan PJ, et al: Allelic association of human dopamine D2 receptor gene in alcoholism. JAMA 263:2055–2059, 1990

Blum K, Wood RC, Sheridan PJ, et al: Dopamine D2 receptor gene variants: association and linkage studies in impulsive, addictive and compulsive disorders. Pharmacogenetics 5:121–141, 1995

Blum K, Braverman ER, Wood RC, et al: Increased prevalence of the *Taq*I A1 allele of the dopamine receptor gene (DRD(2)) in obesity with comorbid substance use disorder: a preliminary report. Pharmacogenetics 6:297–305, 1996

Blum K, Braverman ER, Wu S, et al: Association polymorphisms of dopamine D2 receptor (DRD2), dopamine transporter (DAT1) with schizoid/avoidant behaviors (SAB). Mol Psychiatry 2:239–246, 1997

Bolos A., Dean M, Lucas-Derse S, et al: Population and pedigree studies reveal a lack of association between the dopamine D2 receptor gene and alcoholism. JAMA 26:3156–3160, 1990

Bond M, Gardner ST, Christian J, et al: Empirical study of self-rated defense styles. Arch Gen Psychiatry 40:333–338, 1990

Brown TE: Brown Attention-Deficit Disorder Scales. San Antonio, TX, Psychological Corporation Harcourt Brace, 1996

Bunzow JR, Van Tol HH, Grandy DK, et al: Cloning and expression of a rat D2 dopamine receptor cDNA. Nature 336:783–787, 1988

Buss AH, Durkee A: An inventory for assessing different kinds of hostility. J Consult Clin Psychol 21:343–349, 1957

Cadoret RJ, Troughton E, O'Gorman TW: Genetic and environmental factors in alcohol abuse and antisocial personality. J Stud Alcohol 48:1–8, 1987

Civelli O, Bunzow JR, Grandy DC, et al: Molecular biology of the dopamine receptors. Eur J Pharmacol 207:277–286, 1991

Cloninger CR: Neurogenetic adaptive mechanisms in alcoholism. Science 236:410–416, 1987a

Cloninger CR: A systematic method for clinical description and classification of personality variants: a proposal. Arch Gen Psychiatry 44:573–588, 1987b

Cloninger CR, Sigvardsson S, Bohman M: Childhood personality predicts alcohol abuse in young adults. Alcoholism Clinical and Experimental Research 12:494–505, 1988

Cloninger CR, Przybeck TR, Svrakic DM: The Tridimensional Personality Questionnaire: U.S. normative data. Psychol Rep 69:1047–1057, 1991

Cloninger CR, Svrakic DM, Przybeck TR: A psychobiological model of temperament and character. Arch Gen Psychiatry 50:975–990, 1993

Comings DE: Polygenetic inheritance of psychiatric disorders, in Handbook of Psychiatric Genetics. Edited by Blum K, Noble EP, Sparks RS, et al. Boca Raton, FL, CRC Press, 1996, pp 235–260

Comings DE: Polygenic inheritance and micro/minisatellites. Mol Psychiatry 3:21–31, 1998a

Comings DE: Why different rules are required for polygenic inheritance: lessons from studies of the DRD2 gene. Alcohol 16:61–70, 1998b

Comings DE: Molecular heterosis as the explanation for the controversy about the effect of the DRD2 gene on dopamine D2 receptor density. Mol Psychiatry 4:213–215, 1999a

Comings DE: SNPs and polygenic disorders: a less gloomy view. Mol Psychiatry 4:314–316, 1999b

Comings DE: Tourette syndrome: a polygenic disorder. CNS Spectrums 4:14–15, 1999c

Comings DE, MacMurray JM: Molecular heterosis: implications for complex inheritance. Am J Hum Genet 61:A196, 1997a

Comings DE, MacMurray JM: Molelcular heterosis: implications for psychiatric genetics. Am J Med Genet 74:656, 1997b

Comings DE, MacMurray JM: Molecular heterosis: a review. Mol Genet Metab 71:19–31, 2000

Comings DE, Comings BG, Muhleman D, et al: The dopamine D2 receptor locus as a modifying gene in neuropsychiatric disorders. JAMA 266:1793–1800, 1991

Comings DE, Flanagan SD, Dietz G, et al: The dopamine D2 receptor (DRD2) as a major gene in obesity and height. Biochemical Medicine and Metabolic Biology 50:176–185, 1993

Comings DE, MacMurray J, Johnson P, et al: Dopamine D2 receptor gene (DRD2) haplotypes and the Defense Style Questionnaire in substance abuse, Tourette syndrome, and controls. Biol Psychiatry 37:798–805, 1995

Comings DE, Muhleman D, Gysin R: The dopamine D2 receptor (DRD2) gene in posttraumatic stress disorder: a study and replication. Biol Psychiatry 40:368–372, 1996a

Comings DE, Wu H, Chiu C, et al: Polygenic inheritance of Tourette syndrome, stuttering, ADHD, conduct, and oppositional defiant disorder: the additive and subtractive effect of the three dopaminergic genes DRD2, DβH, and DAT1. Am J Med Genet 67:264–288, 1996b

Comings DE, Gonzalez N, Wu S, et al: Studies of the 48 bp repeat of the *DRD4* gene in impulsive-addictive behaviors: Tourette syndrome, ADHD, pathological gambling, and substance abuse. Am J Med Genet 88:358–368, 1999

Comings DE, Gade-Andavolu R, Gonzalez N, et al: Comparison of the role of dopamine, serotonin, and noradrenergic genes in ADHD, ODD and conduct disorder: multivariate regression analysis of 20 genes. Clin Genet 57:178–196, 2000a

Comings DE, Gade-Andavolu R, Gonzalez N, et al: Multivariate analysis of associations of 42 genes in ADHD, ODD, and conduct disorder. Clin Genet 58:31–40, 2000b

Comings DE, Gade-Andavolu R, Gonzalez N, et al: A multivariate analysis of 59 candidate genes in personality traits: the Temperament Character Inventory. Clin Genet 58:375–385, 2001

Compton PA, Anglin MD, Khalsa-Denison ME, et al: The D2 dopamine receptor gene, addiction, and personality: clinical correlates in cocaine abusers. Biol Psychiatry 39:302–304, 1996

Cook CC, Gurling HM: The D2 dopamine receptor gene and alcoholism: a genetic effect in the liability for alcoholism. J R Soc Med 87:400–402, 1996

Costa PTJ, McCrae RR: Revised NEO Personality Inventory (NEO PI-R) and NEO Five Inventory (NEO-FFI) Professional Manual. Odessa, FL, Psychological Assessment Resources, 1992

Earls F, Reich W, Jung KG, et al: Psychopathology in children of alcoholic and antisocial parents. Alcoholism Clinical and Experimental Research 12:481–487, 1988

Ebstein RP, Novick O, Umansky R, et al: Dopamine D4 receptor (D4DR) exon III polymorphism associated with the human personality trait of novelty seeking. Nat Genet 12:78–80, 1996

Eley TC, Ball D, Hill L, et al: Association study of extreme high and low neuroticism, with genetic markers for the dopaminergic system. Am J Med Genet 81:487, 1998

Eysenck HJ, Eysenck SBG: Manual for Eysenck Personality Inventory. San Diego, CA, Educational and Industrial Testing Service, 1996

Falk CT, Rubinstein P: Haplotype relative risks: an easy reliable way to construct a proper control sample for risk calculations. Ann Hum Genet 51:227–233, 1987

Faraone SV, Doyle AE, Mick E, et al: Meta-analysis of the association between the 7-repeat allele of the dopamine D(4) receptor gene and attention deficit hyperactivity disorder. Am J Psychiatry 158:1052–1057, 2001

Gelernter J, O'Malley SO, Risch N, et al: No association between an allele at the D2 dopamine receptor gene (DRD2) and alcoholism. JAMA 266:1801–1807, 1991

Gelernter J, Southwick S, Goodson S, et al: No association between D-2 dopamine receptor (DRD2) "A" system alleles, or DRD2 haplotypes, and posttraumatic stress disorder. Biol Psychiatry 45:620–625, 1999

Grandy DK, Litt M, Allen L, et al: The human dopamine D2 receptor gene is located on chromosome 11 at q22–q23 and identifies a *Taq*I RFLP. Am J Hum Genet 45:778–785, 1989

Grice DE, Leckman JF. Pauls DL, et al: Linkage disequilibrium of an allele at the dopamine D4 receptor locus with Tourette's syndrome by TDT. Am J Hum Genet 59:644–652, 1996

Lahoste GJ, Swanson JM, Wigal SB, et al: Dopamine D4 receptor gene polymorphism is associated with attention deficit hyperactivity disorder. Mol Psychiatry 1:121–124, 1996

Lerman C, Caporaso NE, Audrain J, et al: Evidence suggesting the role of specific genetic factors in cigarette smoking. Health Psychol 18:14–20, 1999

Levenson H: Differentiating among internality, powerful others and chance, in Research With the Locus of Control Construct, Vol 1. Edited by Lefcourt HM. New York, Academic Press, 1981, pp 15–63

Noble EP, Blum K, Ritchie T, et al: Allelic association of the D2 dopamine receptor gene with receptor-binding characteristics in alcoholism. Arch Gen Psychiatry 48:648–654, 1991

Noble EP: The D_2 dopamine receptor gene: a review of association studies in alcoholism. Behav Genet 73:119–129, 1993

Noble EP, Jeor ST, Ritchie T, et al: D2 dopamine receptor gene and cigarette smoking: a reward gene? Med Hypothesis 42:257–260, 1994a

Noble EP, Noble RE, Ritchie T, et al: D2 receptor gene and obesity. Int J Eat Disord 15:205–217, 1994b

Noble EP, Gottschalk LA, Fallon JH, et al: D2 dopamine receptor polymorphism and brain regional glucose metabolism. Am J Med Genet 74:162–166, 1997

Noble EP, Ozkaragoz TZ, Ritchie TL, et al: D2 and D4 dopamine receptor polymorphisms and personality. Am J Med Genet 81:257–267, 1998

Paquette J, Giannoukakis N, Polychronakos C, et al: The INS 5′ variable number of tandem repeats is associated with IGF2 expression in humans. J Biol Chem 273:14158–14164, 1998

Plomin R., Owen MJ, McGuffin P: The genetic basis of complex human behaviors. Science 264:1733–1739, 1994

Risch N, Merikangas K: The future of genetic studies of complex human diseases. Science 273:1516–1517, 1996

Risch N: Searching for genetic determinants in the new millennium. Nature 405:847–56, 2000

Rowe DC, Stever C, Giedinghagen LN, et al: Dopamine DRD4 receptor polymorphism and attention deficit hyperactivity disorder. Mol Psychiatry 3:419–426, 1998

Sadowski CJ, Wenzel DM: The relationship of locus of control dimensions to reported hostility and aggression. J Psychol 112:227–230, 1982

Singleton AB, Thomson JH, Morris CM, et al: Lack of association between the dopamine D2 receptor gene allele DRD2*A1 and cigarette smoking in a United Kingdom population. Pharmacogenetics 8:125–128, 1998

Spealman RD, Bergman J, Madras BK, et al: Role of D_1 and D_2 dopamine receptors in the behavioral effects of cocaine. Neurochem Int 20:147S–152S, 1992

Spielman RS, Ewens WJ: The TDT and other family based tests for linkage disequilibrium and association. Am J Hum Genet 59:983–989, 1996

Spitz MR, Shi H, Yang F, et al: Case-control study of the D2 dopamine receptor gene and smoking status in lung cancer patients. J Natl Cancer Inst 90:358–363, 1998

SSPS, Inc: SPSS User Manual. Chicago, IL, SPSS, Inc., 1995

Svrakic DM, Whitehead C, Przybeck TR, et al: Differential diagnosis of personality disorders by the seven-factor model of temperament and character. Arch Gen Psychiatry 50:991–999, 1993

Tarter RE, McBride H, Bounpane N, et al: Differentiation of alcoholics: childhood history of minimal brain dysfunction, family history, and drinking pattern. Arch Gen Psychiatry 34:761–768, 1977

Thierry AM, Tassin JP, Blanc G, et al: Effects of stimulation of the mesocortical dopaminergic system by stress. Nature 263:242–244, 1976

Waddington JL: Functional interactions between D-1 and D-2 dopamine receptor systems: their role in the regulation of psychomotor behavior, putative mechanisms and clinical relevance. Am J Hum Genet 47:828–834, 1990

CHAPTER TEN

Genetics of Sensation Seeking

Marvin Zuckerman, Ph.D.

History of the Construct

The first sensation seeking scale (SSS) was developed to predict responses to the experimental situation of sensory deprivation (Zuckerman et al. 1964). The scale was based on an earlier construct called *optimal level of stimulation* (Eysenck 1967; Hebb 1949; Wundt 1893; Yerkes and Dodson 1908). The theory was that too little stimulation or too much stimulation led to inefficient performance and negative affect, whereas at some optimal level people functioned and felt better. Other theories put the emphasis on the arousal or excitement produced by stimulation and suggested *optimal levels of arousal* (Berlyne1960; Breuer and Freud 1895/1937; Hebb 1955). All of these theories, including Freud's, based the construct on the characteristics of the cerebral cortex, and Hebb added the feedback regulation of the cortex by the reticular activating system.

Development of Sensation Seeking Scales

The optimum level of stimulation and optimum level of arousal ideas were incorporated in a theory that attempted to explain individual differences in responses to sensory deprivation (Zuckerman 1969). The first form of the SSS was developed partly from Berlyne and Madsen's (1973) theory of the qualities of stimulation that create their concept of arousal potential, such as novelty, intensity, complexity, incongruity, and change. The items of the SSS translated these qualities into life behaviors, or intentions for future behaviors. The first published form (form II) of the SSS contained only a General scale consisting of items most highly related to the Total score and to the first unrotated factor derived from factor analysis. At first we applied the SSS to the limited goal of predicting responses to sensory deprivation.

Results Using the Sensation Seeking Scale

We were surprised to find that high sensation seekers were overrepresented among those volunteering for sensory deprivation and hypnosis experiments being done at that time in our lab (Zuckerman et al. 1967). Broader studies of volunteering revealed that high sensation seekers are likely to volunteer for any kind of experiment promising some type of novel or arousing experience, even if the experiments are regarded as risky. In the sensory deprivation experiment high sensation seekers (highs) became more restless than low sensation seekers (lows) during 8-hour sensory deprivation or monotonous confinement situations (Zuckerman et al. 1966). Restlessness was measured by recording random movements on the bed to which they were confined. Lows maintained a low level of movement throughout the experiment.

Over the years the SSS has shown concurrent and predictive validity in a broad variety of experiments and life behaviors including various kinds of risky behaviors such as fast and reckless driving, gambling, risky financial activities, smoking, alcohol and drug use, sex with many partners, and risky sports. The trait was also shown to be involved in vocational choices and preferences, job satisfaction, social and sexual premarital and marital relationships, eating habits and food preferences, media and art preferences, humor, fantasy, creativity, and social attitudes. These behavioral expressions of sensation seeking are not described in this chapter except where they are directly relevant to the genetics of the trait by virtue of a common genetic factor involved in both. Interested readers can find descriptions in two major books on sensation seeking (Zuckerman 1979, 1994).

Soon after the appearance of form II of the SSS it was suggested that there might be more than one general factor describing the trait and its different kinds of expression. Additional items were written, and item factor analyses were conducted. Four factors were defined and used as the bases for subscales in forms IV (Zuckerman 1971) and V (Zuckerman et al. 1978). The factor structure has been fairly well replicated in English and translated forms around the world (Zuckerman 1994). Form V has been the one most widely used in genetic research, so a description of its subtests is important for understanding the results of this research.

The four factors in forms IV and V of the SSS are described here in terms of the content of their items, but construct validity requires a study of the research using these forms, and of the results relating specifically to one or two rather than to all of the subscales. Results relating to all or most of the subscales provide construct validity for the broad sensation seeking factor represented by the Total score on form V or the General score in forms II and IV.

- *Thrill and Adventure Seeking.* The items in this subscale describe a desire to engage in various somewhat risky sports or activities involving speed, adventure, defiance of gravity, or unusual sensations in general. None of the items ask about actual experience in these activities.
- *Experience Seeking.* The items in this subscale cover a broad range of experience or desired experience through the mind and the senses, through travel, art, food, dress, and nonconformist friends and groups.
- *Disinhibition.* The items in this subscale describe experiences or attitudes relating to seeking sensation through other exciting people, disinhibited parties, and sexual variety.
- *Boredom Susceptibility.* These items concern boredom and an intolerance for repetition of any kind, monotonous conditions or boring people, and restlessness when alone in familiar surroundings for any length of time.

The SSS form V contains 10 items for each of these four subscales. The Total score is the sum of the sensation seeking choices on all 40 items or all four scales. A new form of the SSS was recently developed based on factor analyses of many personality scales and items in these scales (Zuckerman et al. 1991, 1993). One of the five major factors that consistently emerged from these analyses combined impulsivity and sensation seeking items and therefore was called impulsive sensation seeking (Impulsive Sensation Seeking scale [ImpSS]). One advantage of this new scale over the General or Total score forms of the older SSS is that the items are stated in general form and do not refer to specific activities such as sports, drinking, drugs, or sex. The SSS form V did contain such items, and investigators had to remove them to avoid confounding when using the SSS to predict the specific activities.

Correlations With Other Scales

Personality test constructors have a tendency to give different names to tests measuring the same thing. Scales may be based on different constructs, but correlations with other scales may reveal strong similarities. Examples of scales that are near equivalents of the SSS General or Total scales are the Change Seeker Index, Stimulus Variation Seeking Scales, Need for Change, Venturesomeness, Monotony Avoidance, Reducing-Augmenting, Arousal Seeking, and Arousal Avoidance (reviewed in Zuckerman 1994).

Cloninger (1987) developed a temperament inventory that includes a scale called Novelty Seeking. This scale is of particular interest in this book because the Novelty Seeking scale has been significantly related several times to alleles of the D4 dopamine receptor (DRD4) gene (see Chapter 5, *DRD4* and Novelty Seeking). Zuckerman and Cloninger (1996) correlated their personality questionnaires and found a correlation of 0.68 between Cloninger's Novelty Seeking scale and Zuckerman and Kuhlman's ImpSS. If corrected for attenuation due to unreliability of both scales, this would approach perfect correlation, so that the Novelty Seeking scale may be considered as a near equivalent of the ImpSS. Apart from the phenomenal similarity in the content of the scales, they are related to the same kinds of dysfunctional behavior, such as drug and alcohol abuse, and have a similar postulated biochemical basis, but with some differences as is described later.

Genetics of Sensation Seeking

Animal Models

I initially suggested that the open-field test might be a good animal model for sensation seeking (Zuckerman 1984). The evolutionary theory of sensation seeking points out the adaptive value of exploration in the spread of our species over the entire globe and in willingness to take risks in hunting large animals and seeking mates from outside of the primary band

(Zuckerman 1990, 1994). Simmel (1984) argued that the open-field test is merely a test of exploration of open spaces and does not measure approach reactions to novelty, which lie at the heart of the definition of sensation seeking. However, responses to the open-field test are not entirely situation specific because strains of mice that are most active in the initial trials in the open-field test also show reactivity to novelty in other types of situations (McClearn 1959). Explorativeness, as assessed by the tendency to enter the novel arms of a maze rather than remain in the familiar ones, is related to the readiness of rats to ingest addictive drugs such as cocaine, again suggesting a link with sensation seeking in humans because the latter is predictive of substance use and abuse (Bardo et al. 1996). A strain of rats that shows a link with human sensation seeking through a common psychophysiological marker is also likely to develop a taste for alcohol in tests of tolerance for this substance (Siegel et al. 1993). The C57 strain of mice, notable for their activity in the open-field test, is a strain that readily takes to ingesting alcohol, and the BALB strain, which is inhibited and fearful in the open-field test, rarely gets beyond the first lick of an alcohol solution. We can never be entirely sure of the validity of animal models for human individual differences, but the ones discussed show some promise in this regard and suggest that sensation seeking is an evolved trait with some genetic basis. However, only studies of humans can assess the strength of the genetic basis of this trait in our species.

Human Behavior Genetic Studies of Sensation Seeking

The first study of the genetics of sensation seeking used SSS data from 422 pairs of twins residing in the London area (Fulker et al. 1980). Using the Jinks and Fulker (1970) method of analysis, 58% of the variance in the Total score could be attributed to heredity, and the remainder of the variance was due to the specific or nonshared environmental influence and error of trait measurement. There was no evidence of an influence of shared environment. The heritability was raised to 0.69 if corrected for the unreliability of the trait measure. This is a high heritability for personality traits, where uncorrected heritabilities usually fall between 0.22 and 0.46 and average 0.40 (Bouchard 1994; Loehlin 1992). About 70% of the genetic variation in sensation seeking was due to a general additive genetic factor common to both genders, but the remaining 30% reflected an interaction of gender and the genetic factor suggesting that sex-linked genetic factors might control the specific patterns among the subtests, particularly on the

Thrill and Adventure Seeking and Disinhibition subscales. These are the two subscales that show the largest gender differences in the SSS, men scoring higher than women. The interaction of genotype and gender could indicate that different genes may be operating in men and women, or that the same genes may be operating but with different effects in each gender. The authors concluded that the former possibility is more likely than the latter, although the issue could not be fully resolved with the data.

Eysenck (1983) further analyzed the data from this study for the proportions of common and specific variance of the four subscales due to genetic and environmental factors. His results for the total genetic and nonshared environmental factors are shown in Table 10–1 for men and women separately. The table also shows data from two other studies to be discussed shortly.

The genetic component of the variation in all of the subscales was relatively high, and particularly so for Experience Seeking (57%–58%). Heritability of Disinhibition was higher in men (0.51) than in women (0.41). Nearly all of the genetic effects of Experience Seeking were due to a genetic factor common to all the subscales, but the predominant genetic effects of each of the other subscales came from genetic factors specific to each factor. For Thrill and Adventure Seeking, Experience Seeking, and Boredom Susceptibility, environmental effects were largely due to specific factors, but for Disinhibition the environmental factor was a

Table 10–1   Proportions of genetic (G) and environmental (E) variance in the subscales of the Sensation Seeking Scale

| | Eysenck (1983) | | | | Koopmans et al. (1995) | | | | Hur and Bouchard (1997) | | |
| | Males | | Females | | Males | | Females | | Males and females | | All five[a] |
SSS	G	E	G	E	G	E	G	E	G	E	G
Dis	0.51	0.49	0.41	0.59	0.62	0.38	0.60	0.40	0.46	0.54	0.50
TAS	0.45	0.55	0.44	0.56	0.62	0.38	0.63	0.37	0.54	0.46	0.54
ES	0.58	0.42	0.57	0.43	0.56	0.44	0.58	0.42	0.55	0.45	0.57
BS	0.41	0.59	0.34	0.66	0.48	0.52	0.54	0.46	0.40	0.60	0.43

Note. SSS = Sensation Seeking Scales; Dis = Disinhibition; TAS = Thrill and Adventure Seeking; ES = Experience Seeking; BS = Boredom Susceptibility.
[a]Average of genetic (G) proportions among the five groups in the three studies.

common one. Eysenck applied the same method of analysis to data from impulsivity scales given to the same population. The total genetic effects were less than found for sensation seeking scales, ranging from 15 to 40% compared with 34% to 58% for the sensation seeking scales.

Table 10–1 shows the results of a semireplication study by Koopmans et al. (1995) using a Dutch version of the SSS form IV containing the same four factors but using a Likert-type item format instead of the forced-choice form used in the SSS forms IV and V. The subjects were 1,591 twin pairs from cities throughout the Netherlands. A model with only additive genetic variance and unique environmental factors best described the pattern of variances and covariances in monozygotic and dizygotic twins. The genetic variances for all subscales were higher in this study than in the previously described one: 48%–62% for men and 54%–63% for women. There was no calculation of heritability for the total score, but the heritabilities for the four individual scales lead to an estimate of about the same (0.58) or even higher heritability for the total score than found by Fulker et al. (1980). The highest heritabilities in this study for both men and women were for Disinhibition and Thrill and Adventure Seeking (0.60, 0.63), whereas the heritabilities for Experience Seeking were just about the same as in the previous study (0.56, 0.58). Boredom Susceptibility had the lowest proportions of genetic variance in all studies, probably because of its lower reliability (Zuckerman 1979). Unlike the previous study, this one found no evidence that different genes influence sensation seeking in men and women. The genetic correlations among subscales were substantial, but an attempt to fit a genetic common factor model was not successful, and the authors concluded that they could find no evidence for one genetic common factor underlying all four subfactors. The highest genetic correlations were between Experience Seeking and Thrill and Adventure Seeking (0.51) and Disinhibition and Boredom Susceptibility (0.54) for men, and between Disinhibition and Boredom Susceptibility (0.54) for women. It may be that there are actually two genetic factors among the subscales rather than four discrete ones: one involving Disinhibition and Boredom Susceptibility and the other Thrill and Adventure Seeking and Experience Seeking. The first of these could correspond to what is now called *impulsive sensation seeking* in our new scale.

The third study shown in Table 10–1, by Hur and Bouchard (1997), was conducted on 106 twins of both genders separated at or near birth and raised in different families. The twins took the SSS form V and the Control scale of the Multidimensional Personality Questionnaire, a reverse measure of impulsivity. As in many other studies age was negatively related to all sensation seeking scales, and men scored higher than women on all but the Experience Seeking subscale. All scores were adjusted for gender, age, and their interactions. The analysis was by Cholesky model-fitting, similar to the method in the Koopmans et al. study. The Control scale was negatively correlated with all of the sensation seeking subscales, and the covariance between the SSS and the Control scale was determined largely by shared genetic influences. Although the published study did not provide the results for the Total score, a personal communication (June 1992) by David Lykken gave a separated monozygotic twin correlation of 0.54 and a separated dizygotic twin correlation of 0.32, based on a slightly lower sample size than in the published results. Because the correlation between separated monozygotic twins is a direct measure of the genetic portion of the variance, this gives a heritability of 0.54, which is very close to the 0.58 in the Fulker et al. (1980) study. Doubling the separated dizygotic correlation of 0.32 would give a heritability of 0.64. The mean of these two estimates is 0.59, almost exactly the heritability from the Fulker et al. (1980) study based on twins reared together. Shared family environment does not seem to be important in the sensation seeking trait.

Looking at the results for the subscales, the strongest genetic heritabilities are for the Thrill and Adventure Seeking and Experience Seeking subscales (54%–55%). The Control scale, not shown in the table, had a genetic variance estimate of 49%. Of this variance, 45% was specific to the Control scale and the rest of the variance was attributed to the genetic variance in common with the SSS. This finding is supportive of our new measure of sensation seeking (the ImpSS), which combines impulsivity with sensation seeking items. Although the genetic correlation with Boredom Susceptibility, Disinhibition, and Experience Seeking ranged from 0.46 to 0.53, the genetic correlation of Thrill and Adventure Seeking with the Control scale was only 0.23. It could be that the genetic basis of ImpSS scores is not the same as that for Thrill and Adventure Seeking scores, although the phenomenal correlations between ImpSS and Thrill and Adventure Seeking, Experience Seeking, and Disinhibition are all about the same (Zuckerman et al. 1993).

Looking across the five groups (male and female groups were reported separately in the first two studies) in the studies in Table 10–1, the average heritability is highest for Experience Seeking (0.57) followed closely by Thrill and Adventure Seeking (0.54) and Disinhibition (0.50). Boredom Susceptibility has a lower heritability (0.40), but this is probably because of the larger error variance for this scale, which is added in with the specific environmental component. Except for Boredom Susceptibility, all the sensation seeking subscales have higher heritabilities than the majority of personality traits in the literature.

Specific Genes for Sensation Seeking

The molecular genetics of sensation seeking or novelty seeking is treated in Chapter 5 (DRD4 and Novelty Seeking) in this volume so I only briefly describe the topic in this chapter. Ebstein et al. (1996) first reported the association between the trait of novelty seeking and the *DRD4* exon III genotypes. The longer, seven-repeat form of the allele was associated with high scores on Cloninger's Novelty Seeking scale from his Tridimensional Personality Questionnaire. Because Novelty Seeking scores correlate very highly with ImpSS scores, it is likely that a similar association between DRD4 and ImpSS will be found, although this remains to be demonstrated.

An immediate replication was reported in the same issue of *Nature Genetics* using both the Tridimensional Personality Questionnaire Novelty Seeking scale and the NEO Personal Inventory, Revised scale (Benjamin et al. 1996). Novelty or impulsive sensation seeking are not primary factors in the latter, but they resemble some of the subscales of its major factors. Among the five primary factors, Extraversion and Conscientiousness were associated with DRD4. Among the subscales of the broad Extraversion factor, Warmth, Excitement Seeking, and Positive Emotions were significantly associated with the long allele of *DRD4*. Within the Conscientiousness factor only Deliberation was associated with DRD4. Those with the shorter form of *DRD4* allele were more deliberate and less impulsive.

Within a year Ebstein and Belmaker (1997) summarized the literature, including two more replications and three failures to replicate the original two positive findings. Baron (1998) took a negative view of these outcomes, even though four positive results out of seven studies is quite remarkable given the record of replication in the field of psychiatric disorders.

Other Correlates of DRD4 Relevant to Sensation Seeking
Opiate Abuse

In Chapter 8 (Personality, Substance Abuse and Genes) Ebstein and Kotler discuss the findings of association between DRD4 gene and opiate abuse. Sensation seeking has been shown to be associated with and predictive of drug use and abuse in many studies in many countries (Zuckerman 1994). Delinquents with a history of heroin abuse in a youth detention center scored higher than prisoners who had not used heroin on the General and Experience Seeking scales of the SSS (Platt and Labatte 1976). Sensation seeking is correlated with all types of drugs that are abused, and although there is some indication of higher scores in stimulant users than in opiate users, the major finding is that sensation seeking is related to the number of drugs used (polydrug use) rather than the specific drug of greatest use. Users of any illegal drugs are higher sensation seekers than alcohol-only users, and the latter are higher than abstainers. Nearly all drugs that are used recreationally release dopamine from the reward centers in the medial forebrain bundle (nucleus accumbens, ventral tegmental area, lateral hypothalamus) of the mesolimbic brain, where D4 receptors are most dense.

Pathological Gambling Disorder

Pathological Gambling Disorder has been associated with the long allele of *D4DR* (Castro et al. 1997). Although certain forms of gambling in the community have been associated with sensation seeking, pathological gamblers in treatment do not exhibit high levels of self-reported sensation seeking. Recently Breen and Zuckerman (1999) reported an association between the impulsivity component of the ImpSS and a laboratory analogue of pathological gambling.

Attention-Deficit/Hyperactivity Disorder

The *DRD4* long allele is associated with attention-deficit/hyperactivity disorder (ADHD) (Swanson et al. 1998). One might think that ADHD is a prototype of high sensation seeking, particularly the boredom susceptibility factor, in children. The greater restlessness of high sensation seekers during sensory deprivation or sensory restriction (Zuckerman et al. 1966) is also reminiscent of ADHD, but levels of sensation seeking in ADHD, using children's forms of the SSS (Russo et al. 1991), are mixed and inconsistent. Russo et al. (1991) found that children with conduct disorders scored higher on sensation seeking than did a group with anxiety disorders, and the group with ADHD scored lower than did the group with anxiety disorders, even on the Boredom Susceptibility scale. A second study with a revised child-SSS that included a Disinhibition scale produced similar results; children with conduct disorder scored high and those with ADHD and anxiety scored low (Russo et al. 1993).

Shaw and Brown (1990) developed another child-SSS, which more closely resembles the adult SSS, by directly adapting items from the adult scale to the child scale and found that children with ADHD scored higher than controls and also recalled fewer focally presented objects than controls, possibly because they were distracted by peripherally presented objects, which they had been instructed to ignore. Shaw and Giambra (1993) studied college students with histories of hyperactivity during childhood and found that they did score higher than controls on the adult SSS and had a higher incidence of task-unrelated thoughts during a vigilance task. Because the results on children with ADHD seem to depend on the specific SSS scales used, no definitive statement can be made about the relation between ADHD and sensation seeking, unless the latter is defined by behavioral rather than self-report responses.

Infant Behavior

In Chapter 7 (Dopamine D4 Receptor and Serotonin Transporter Promoter Polymorphisms and Temperament in Early Childhood) Ebstein and Auerbach discuss the association of DRD4 with infant behavior. Auerbach et al. (1998) took DNA from cord blood at birth and studied infants at 2 weeks, 2 months, and 1 year of age. At 2 weeks of age the infants with the long allele of *DRD4* were rated higher on orientation, motor organization, regulation of state, and range of state than infants with short alleles. At 2 months of age infants with the long *DRD4* allele showed less negative emotionality and less distress to limitations during daily care situations and to suddenly presented novel stimuli. At 1 year of age the infants with the long allele showed less negative emotionality, less distress to novel and sudden stimuli, and less social inhibition.

Of course, studies with the SSS have not been extended to infancy because of the impossibility of self-report at these ages. But some of the characteristics of the infants with the long *DRD4* allele resemble those of adult sensation seekers. For instance the interest in novel stimuli and strong orienting responses to such stimuli are characteristic of adult sensation seekers.

A study of newborn infants observed during the first 3 days of life showed that infants with low platelet monoamine oxidase B (MAO B) levels were more active, showed better motor integration, and were more aroused and cried more than infants with high MAO B levels (Sostek et al. 1981). Low levels of MAO B are found in high sensation seekers (Zuckerman 1994). It would be interesting to do a study of infant behavior assessing *DRD4* alleles, the genes for MAO B, *and* platelet MAO B levels.

Another Dopamine Receptor Gene Associated With Sensation Seeking

DRD4 accounts for only a small percentage of the trait of sensation seeking, so it is likely that other major genes are also involved. The dopamine D5 receptors are expressed in parts of the limbic system, particularly the hippocampus, and therefore may be involved in the response to novelty and the positive emotional arousal it produces in high sensation seekers. Vanyukov et al. (1998) found that one allele of DRD5 gene was more commonly found in substance abusers than in controls, and that this allele was also associated with the Experience Seeking subscale from the SSS. As an example of the candidate gene approach, a recent study has found an association between smoking and two alleles of the MAO B gene (Checkoway et al. 1998). Young sensation seekers are more likely to be smokers and have low levels of platelet MAO B (Zuckerman 1994). Young smokers also have low levels of MAO B. Given the trait and behavioral associations with the biochemical marker, the MAO B gene was a good candidate for association with smoking. No one has as yet studied the association between the MAO B gene and sensation seeking. DRD2 has also been associated with substance abuse, but so far it has not been related to novelty seeking.

Implications for Future Research in Molecular Genetics and Personality

The animal studies suggest that more than one monoamine is involved in sensation seeking. Evidence certainly exists for the involvement of serotonin receptors as well as dopamine receptors. Other genetic factors involving the noradrenergic and hypothalamus–pituitary–adrenal cortex (stress hormonal pathway) systems must also be considered. Noradrenaline and cortisol obtained from cerebrospinal fluid in humans showed that both the catecholamine and the hormone were negatively correlated with sensation seeking (Ballenger et al. 1983). Endorphin levels were also negatively related to sensation seeking in one study (Johansson et al. 1979), and other studies have shown relationships between sensation seeking and gonadal hormones (Daitzman and Zuckerman 1980). Plomin (1995) has criticized the *one gene, one disorder* idea. Considering the variety of biological correlates of a trait such as sensation seeking, it would be unlikely that only *one neurotransmitter* or *one hormone* would control *one trait.* Even within a single neurotransmitter system we must look at different genes for different receptors. *DRD2*, for instance, has been related to substance abuse in many studies. Neurotransmitters such as dopamine, noradrenaline, and serotonin interact at the neuronal level as well as the behavioral level. Effects of a gene interaction (between *D4DR* and the gene for the serotonin 2C receptor) on reward dependence have been reported by Benjamin et al. (1997). Once we get away from single-gene studies such interactions may become commonplace. At the behavioral level we could analogize that dopamine is the accelerator and serotonin is the brakes for reward-directed behavior. The interaction between the two determines approach versus inhibition.

The model I have proposed for the trait of impulsive sensation seeking incorporates all three monoamines as well as enzymes, such as MAO and dopamine β-hydroxylase, and other neurotransmitters, such as GABA, which regulate the monoamines (Zuckerman 1994, 1995). Between the levels of personality traits and biological systems lie the mechanisms mediated by the biological systems. Here we may find more one-to-one specificity, with *one neurotransmitter* for *one mechanism.* The tendency to approach rather than withdraw from novel or threatening stimuli may be involved in many personality traits, including extraversion, impulsivity, sensation seeking, and aggression. My model proposes that dopamine underlies the approach, serotonin the inhibition, and norepinephrine the arousal mechanisms. Impulsive sensation seekers are characterized by strong approach, weak inhibition, and weak arousal (related to fear). Therefore, we would expect impulsive sensation seekers to have highly reactive dopaminergic, and weakly reactive serotonergic and noradrenergic systems in response to stimuli associated with both reward and punishment.

Conclusions

Sensation seeking is a trait that has evolved in the mammalian line in the form of a readiness to approach novel stimuli or to explore new situations or places. It is probably an important component of adaptive foraging and hunting behaviors. It is highly heritable, being at the upper limits of heritability in personality traits. As with most other personality traits, the non-heritable component is almost entirely due to nonshared environment and/or errors of measurement. The subfactors of sensation seeking are influenced by a common genetic factor, or perhaps two major factors, plus some specific narrower factors. Although the Experience Seeking subscale is the best representative of the common genetic factor, the Disinhibition subscale shows a stronger or more consistent relationship to some of the biological correlates of sensation seeking such as testosterone levels, augmentation versus reduction of the cortical evoked potential, and MAO B activity. This latter relationship, as well as many direct brain studies in other species, suggests the involvement of the monoamine systems in sensation seeking. The discovery of a specific dopamine receptor gene *(DRD4)* associated with novelty seeking further reinforces the hypothesis of the involvement of the mesolimbic dopamine system in the trait. The other correlates of sensation seeking in humans and reactions to novelty in other species suggest additional candidate genes. A genomewide search may find the genes accounting for the other 90% of the genetic variance in novelty seeking.

Molecular genetics could provide the foundation for a science of personality. In a bottom-up approach we can move from the genes to their biological functions, to behavioral mechanisms mediated by these functions, and finally to the traits representing different combinations of these mechanisms. If we persist in this great gene hunt we may even find the gene that makes some believe that there is a gene for everything or that everything is due to genes. Or we may discover the gene that makes dogmatists on the social end believe that personality is entirely shaped by parents.

References

Auerbach J, Faroy M, Kahanna M, et al: Dopamine D4 receptor and serotonin transporter promoter in the determination of infant temperament. Poster presented at the 12th Occasional Temperament Conference, Philadelphia, PA, October 1998

Ballenger JC, Post RM, Jimerson DC, et al: Biochemical correlates of personality traits in normals: an exploratory study. Personality and Individual Differences 4:615–625, 1983

Bardo MT, Donohew RL, Harrington NG: Psychobiology of novelty seeking and drug seeking behavior. Behav Brain Res 77:23–43, 1996

Baron M: Mapping genes for personality: is the saga sagging? Mol Psychiatry 3:106–108, 1998

Benjamin J, Li L, Patterson C, et al: Population and familial association between the D4 dopamine receptor gene and measures of sensation seeking. Nat Genet 12:81–84, 1996

Berlyne DE: Conflict, Arousal, and Curiosity. New York, McGraw-Hill, 1960

Berlyne DE, Madsen KB: Pleasure, and Reward Preference: Their Nature, Determinants, and Role in Behavior. New York, Academic Press, 1973

Bouchard TJ Jr: Genes, environment, and personality. Science 264:1700–1701, 1994

Breen RB, Zuckerman M: "Chasing" in gambling behavior: personality and cognitive determinants. Personality and Individual Differences 27:1097–1111, 1999

Breuer J, Freud S: Studies in Hysteria (1895). Translated by Brill AA. New York, Nervous and Mental Disease Publishing, 1937

Castro IP, Ibanez A, Torres P, et al: Genetic association study between pathological gambling and a functional DNA polymorphism at the D4 receptor gene. Pharmacogenetics 7:345–348, 1997

Checkoway H, Frankin GM, Costa-Mallen P, et al. A genetic polymorphism of MAO-B modifies the association of cigarette smoking and Parkinson's disease. Neurology 50:1458–1461, 1998

Cloninger CR: A systematic method for clinical description and classification of personality variants. Arch Gen Psychiatry 44:573–588, 1987

Daitzman RJ, Zuckerman M. Personality, disinhibitory sensation seeking, and gonadal hormones. Personality and Individual Differences 1:103–110, 1980

Ebstein RP, Belmaker RH: Saga of an adventure gene: novelty seeking, substance abuse, and the dopamine D4 receptor (D4DR) exon III repeat polymorphism. Mol Psychiatry 2:381–384, 1997

Ebstein RP, Novick O, Umansky R, et al. Dopamine D4 receptor (D4DR) exon III polymorphism associated with the human personality trait of novelty seeking. Nat Genet 12:78–80, 1996

Eysenck HJ: The Biological Basis of Personality. Springfield, IL, Charles C Thomas, 1967

Eysenck HJ: A biometrical genetical analysis of impulsive and sensation seeking behavior, in Biological Bases of Sensation Seeking, Impulsivity, and Anxiety. Edited by Zuckerman M. Hillsdale, NJ, Erlbaum, 1983, pp 1–27

Fulker DW, Eysenck SBG, Zuckerman M: The genetics of sensation seeking. Journal of Personality Research 14:261–281, 1980

Hebb DO: The Organization of Behavior. New York, Wiley, 1949

Hebb DO: Drives and the C.N.S. (conceptual nervous system). Psychol Rev 62:243–254, 1955

Hur Y, Bouchard TJ Jr: The genetic correlation between impulsivity and sensation seeking traits. Behav Genet 27:455–463, 1997

Jinks JL, Fulker DW: Comparison of the biometrical genetical, MAVA, and the classical approaches to the analysis of human behavior. Psychol Bull 73:311–349, 1970

Johansson F, Almay BGL, von Knorring L, et al: Personality traits in chronic pain patients related to endorphin levels in cerebrospinal fluid. Psychiatry Res 1:231–239, 1979

Koopmans JR, Boomsa DI, Health AC, et al: A multivariate genetic analysis of sensation seeking. Behav Genet 25:349–356, 1995

Loehlin JC: Genes and Environment in Personality Development. Newbury Park, CA, Sage, 1992

McClearn GE: Genetics of mouse behavior in novel situations. Journal of Comparative and Physiological Psychology 52:62–67, 1959

Platt JJ, Labate C: Heroin Addiction: Theory, Research, and Treatment. New York, Wiley, 1976

Plomin R: Molecular genetics and psychology. Current Directions in Psychological Science 4: 114–117, 1995

Russo MF, Lakey BB, Christ MAG, et al: Preliminary development of a sensation seeking scale for children. Personality and Individual Differences 12:309–405, 1991

Russo MF, Stokes GS, Lakey BB, et al: A sensation seeking scale in children: further refinement and psychometric development. Journal of Psychopathology and Behavioral Assessment 15:69–86, 1993

Shaw GA, Brown G: Laterality and creativity concomitants of attention problems. Dev Neuropsychol 6:39–57, 1990

Shaw GA, Giambra L: Task-unrelated thoughts of college students diagnosed as hyperactive in childhood. Dev Neuropsychol 9:17–30, 1993

Siegel J, Sisson DF, Driscoll P: Augmenting and reducing of visual evoked potentials in Roman high- and low-avoidance rats. Physiol Behav 54:707–711, 1993

Simmel EC: Sensation seeking: Exploration of empty spaces or novel stimuli? Behav Brain Sci 3:449–450, 1984

Sostek AJ, Sostek AM, Murphy DL, et al: Cord blood amine oxidase activities relate to arousal and motor functioning in human newborns. Life Sci 28:2561–2568, 1981

Swanson JM, Sunohara GA, Kennedy JL, et al. Association of the dopamine receptor D4 (DRD4) gene with a refined phenotype of attention deficit hyperactivity disorder (ADHD): a family based approach. Mol Psychiatry 3:38–41, 1998

Vanyukov MM, Moss HB, Gioio AE, et al: An association between a microsatellite polymorphism at the DRD5 gene and the liability to substance abuse. Behav Genet 28:75–82, 1998

Wundt WM: Grundzuge der physiologischen Psychologie. Leipzig, Engleman, 1893

Yerkes RM, Dodson JD: The relation of strength of stimulus to rapidity of habit-formation. Journal of Comparative and Neurological Psychology 18:459–482, 1908

Zuckerman M: Theoretical formulations, in Sensory Deprivation: Fifteen Years of Research. Edited by Zubek JP. New York, Appleton-Century, 1969, pp 407–432

Zuckerman M: Dimensions of sensation seeking. J Consult Clin Psychol 36:45–52, 1971

Zuckerman M: Sensation Seeking: Beyond the Optimal Level of Arousal. Hillsdale, NJ, Erlbaum, 1979

Zuckerman M: Sensation seeking: A comparative approach to a human trait. Behav Brain Sci 7:413–471, 1984

Zuckerman M: The psychophysiology of sensation seeking. J Pers 58:313–345, 1990

Zuckerman M: Behavioral Expressions and Biosocial Bases of Sensation Seeking. New York, Cambridge University Press, 1994

Zuckerman M: Good and bad humors: biochemical bases of personality and its disorders. Psychol Sci 6:325–332, 1995

Zuckerman M, Cloninger CR: Relationships between Cloninger's, Zuckerman's, and Eysenck's dimensions of personality. Personality and Individual Differences 21:283–285, 1996

Zuckerman M, Kolin EA, Price L, et al: Development of a sensation seeking scale. Journal of Consulting Psychology 28:477–482, 1964

Zuckerman M, Persky H, Hopkins TR, et al: Comparison of stress effects of perceptual and social isolation. Arch Gen Psychiatry 14:356–365, 1966

Zuckerman M, Schultz DP, Hopkins TR: Sensation seeking and volunteering for sensory deprivation and hypnosis experiments. Journal of Consulting Psychology 31:358–363, 1967

Zuckerman M, Eysenck SBG, Eysenck HJ: Sensation seeking in England and America: cross-cultural, age, and sex comparisons. J Consult Clin Psychol 40:139–149, 1978

Zuckerman M, Kuhlman DM, Thornquist M, et al: Five (or three) robust questionnaire scale factors of personality without culture. Personality and Individual Differences 12:929–941, 1991

Zuckerman M, Kuhlman DM, Joireman J, et al: A comparison of three structural models for personality: the big three, the big five, and the alternative five. J Pers Soc Psychol 65:757–768, 1993

CHAPTER ELEVEN

Quantitative Trait Loci and General Cognitive Ability

Robert Plomin, Ph.D.

What Is *g*?

I refer to *g* rather than *intelligence* because intelligence means too many different things to different people (Jensen 1998). *g* is operationally defined as a general cognitive ability factor that represents what diverse tests of general cognitive ability have in common. That is, one of the most important facts about cognitive abilities, unlike noncognitive areas of personality, is that all reliable tests of cognitive ability intercorrelate. *g* is best assessed as an unrotated principal component among diverse cognitive tests—such as tests of spatial ability, verbal ability, processing speed, and memory—that weights the tests according to how highly they load on this general factor, which usually accounts for more than 40% of the variance of the tests. *g* is also indexed reasonably well by a total score on a diverse set of cognitive measures, as is done in IQ tests. It is less clear what *g* is, whether *g* is the result of a single general process such as executive function or a speedy brain, or whether it represents overlap among components of more specific cognitive processes (Mackintosh 1998). Whatever it is, *g* is one of the most stable, reliable, and predictive behavioral traits

(Gottfredson 1997). It is also one of the most heritable, as discussed in the section "Is *g* Heritable?"

Is *g* Personality?

Although psychology textbooks invariably have separate chapters on personality and intelligence, *g* fits under the rubric of trait theories of personality that focus on behavioral dimensions that are stable across time and situations. Cattell's 16 Personality Factor Inventory system (Cattell 1982) explicitly includes intelligence. In the Five Factor Model of personality (Costa and McCrae 1992), Openness to Experience is more than *g* in disguise in a self-report questionnaire, however; Openness correlates about 0.40 with *g* (McCrae 1996). For these reasons, it seems reasonable to include a chapter on *g* in a volume on personality.

Is *g* Heritable?

Although the genetic contribution to *g* has produced controversy in the media, especially following the publication of *The Bell Curve* (Herrnstein and Murray 1994), there is considerable consensus among scientists that *g* is substantially heritable—even among those who are not geneticists (e.g., Brody 1992; Mackintosh 1998). More data support the genetics of *g* than the genetics of any other human characteristic. Correlations for first-degree relatives living together average 0.43 for more than 8,000 parent-offspring pairs and 0.47 for more than 25,000 pairs of siblings. However, *g* might run in families for reasons of nurture or of nature. In studies involving more than 10,000 pairs of twins, the average *g* correlations are 0.85 for identical twins and 0.60 for same-sex fraternal twins. These twin data suggest a genetic effect size (heritability) that explains about half of the total variance in *g* scores. Adoption studies also yield estimates of substantial heritability. For example, in two studies, identical twins reared apart are almost as similar for *g* as are identical twins reared together, with an average correlation of 0.78 for 93 such pairs (Bouchard et al. 1990; Pedersen et al. 1992). Adoption studies of other first-degree relatives also indicate substantial heritability, as illustrated by results from the longitudinal 25-year Colorado Adoption Project (Plomin et al. 1997).

All the data converge on the conclusion that the heritability of *g* is about

50%, that is, genes account for about half of the variance in g scores (Bouchard and McGue 1981; Plomin et al. 2001). Even an attempt to explain as much of the variance of g as possible in terms of prenatal effects nonetheless yielded a heritability estimate of 48% (Devlin et al. 1997; McGue 1997). Although heritability could differ in different cultures, moderate heritability of g has been found, not only in twin studies in North American and western European countries, but also in Moscow, former East Germany, rural India, urban India, and Japan.

Additional Relevant Questions

Genetic research has moved beyond the rudimentary questions of whether and to what extent genetic differences are important in the origins of individual differences in g (Plomin and Petrill 1997). Rather than reviewing in detail the research already mentioned that converges on the conclusion that g is about 50% heritable, I believe it is of greater relevance to molecular genetic research to discuss three findings that go beyond merely estimating heritability.

Development

Research during the past decade has shown that the heritability of g increases steadily from infancy (20%) to childhood (40%) to adulthood (60%). For example, a recent study of twins aged 80 years and older reported a heritability of about 60% (McClearn et al. 1997). Studies of identical twins reared apart suggest that heritability may be as high as 80% in adulthood.

Why does heritability of g increase during the life span? It is possible that completely new genes come to affect g as more sophisticated cognitive processes come on line. However, a hypothesis that I prefer is that relatively small genetic effects early in life snowball during development, creating larger and larger phenotypic effects as individuals select or create environments that foster their genetic propensities. During the past decade, genetic research has pointed to such genotype-environment correlation for g in the sense that associations between environmental measures and cognitive development are mediated genetically to some extent (Plomin 1994). Another developmental finding of great importance concerns environmental influences on g: Shared family environments, which make siblings in a family similar, are important only until adolescence. In other words, in the long run, environmental influences on *g*, whatever they may be, make two children growing up in the same family different from one another. This type of environmental influence is called *non-shared environment* (Plomin and Petrill 1997).

This first finding suggests that adulthood might be a better target than childhood for attempts to identify genes. However, longitudinal genetic analyses indicate that although heritability of *g* is lower in childhood than in adulthood, the same genes largely operate in both childhood and adulthood (Plomin et al. 1997). In other words, although genes have a greater effect after childhood, the same genes can be expected to be associated with *g* in childhood and adulthood.

Additive Genetic Variance and Assortative Mating

A second finding about *g* that deserves to be better known, especially in relation to molecular genetics, concerns additive genetic variance and assortative mating. Most of the genetic variance for *g* is additive, that is, genetic effects add up rather than interact across loci. A hallmark of non-additive genetic variance is that identical twins (who are similar for all genetic effects no matter how complexly interactive the genes happen to be) are more than twice as similar as fraternal twins. Fraternal twins are said to be 50% genetically similar, but this is only in relation to additive genetic effects—they are not at all similar for epistatic effects (higher-order interactions among multiple genes). In contrast to *g*, noncognitive personality traits, especially the Big Five factor Extraversion, show some non-additive genetic influence (Loehlin 1992). The issue of additive versus nonadditive genetic variance is important in relation to attempts to identify specific genes responsible for genetic influence (see Chapter 18, Genes for Human Personality Traits).

The additivity of genetic effects on *g* may be due to the fact that there is far greater assortative mating for *g* than for any other behavioral trait. Correlations between spouses are only about 0.10 for other personality traits and about 0.20 for height and weight, but assortative mating for *g* is about 0.40. Assortative mating increases additive genetic variance cumulatively generation after generation (Plomin et al. 1997). If bright women mate with bright men, their offspring receive a double dose of genes for high *g*, and this spreads out the distribution of additive genetic effects in the population because parents share only additive genetic effects with their offspring.

Substantial Genetic Correlations Among Cognitive Abilities

The third quantitative genetic finding about *g* is of great importance for neurogenetic research on learning and memory. Specific cognitive abilities show substantial genetic influence, although less than for *g* (Plomin and DeFries 1998). To what extent do different sets of genes affect these different abilities? A technique called multivariate genetic analysis examines covariance among specific cognitive abilities and yields a statistic called the *genetic correlation*. The genetic correlation is an index of the extent to which genetic effects on one trait correlate with genetic effects on another trait independent of the heritability of the two traits. That is, although cognitive abilities are moderately heritable, the genetic correlations between them could be anywhere from zero, indicating complete independence of their genetic effects, to 1.0, indicating that the same genes are involved. Multivariate genetic analyses have consistently found that genetic correlations among specific cognitive abilities are very high—close to 1.0 (Petrill 1997). These quantitative genetic results make the strong molecular genetic prediction that genes found to be associated with one cognitive ability such as spatial ability will also be associated just as strongly with other cognitive abilities such as verbal ability or memory.

These multivariate genetic results also indicate a genetic reality to *g*. That is, genetic effects on cognitive abilities are general. A related interesting finding is that the *g* loadings of cognitive tests on a first unrotated principal component are highly correlated with their heritabilities. That is, the most highly loaded tests are the most heritable. In addition to indicating that *g* is a good target for molecular genetic research, this finding also has important implications for understanding the brain mechanisms that mediate genetic effects on cognitive ability. In contrast to the prevalent modular view of cognitive neuroscience that assumes that cognitive processes are specific and independent, these results suggest that genetic effects are general.

Can We Find Genes Associated With *g*?

Finding genes that affect personality broaches the same issues as molecular genetic research on any complex dimension or disorder influenced by multiple genes as well as by multiple environmental factors. The issues are more stark for personality than for disorders such as psychopathology because personality traits are clearly quantitative traits and the genes we are looking for are quantitative trait loci (QTLs) (Plomin et al. 1994b). Unlike single-gene effects, as in PKU, which are necessary and sufficient for the development of rare disorders, QTLs contribute interchangeably and additively, analogous to probabilistic risk factors. If multiple genes affect a trait, it is likely that the trait is distributed quantitatively as a dimension rather than qualitatively as a disorder; this was the essence of Fisher's classic 1918 paper on quantitative genetics (R. A. Fisher 1918). From a QTL perspective, there are no disorders, just the extremes of quantitative traits caused by the same genetic and environmental factors responsible for variation throughout the dimension. In other words, the QTL perspective predicts that genes found to be associated with complex disorders will also be associated with normal variation and vice versa.

Other chapters in this volume review the issues involved in finding QTLs for complex traits. My personal view is that far too many unknowns exist in this area at this time for anyone to be dogmatic about what will and will not work. I believe that the issues will be resolved empirically. For example, a few years ago, linkage was deemed to be the only acceptable approach, but now allelic association is widely accepted. Candidate gene approaches came and went as the flavor of the year. Today some argue that only within-family association designs are acceptable, but I think that worrying about ethnic stratification is like the tail wagging the dog. I would prefer to find replicable associations using more powerful case-control designs, matching cases and controls as epidemiologists have done for decades. After we have found replicable associations, we can explore whether ethnic stratification makes a difference.

My premise is that if additive genetic factors are important for complex traits, then we can identify the genes responsible if we have sufficient power to detect QTLs of small effect size. The critical question is the distribution of effect sizes of these QTLs: what is the average effect size of QTLs and how are QTL effect sizes distributed? My bet is that the distributions of QTL effect sizes for complex traits are positively skewed, with few QTLs accounting for more than 5% of the variance and having very long tails that fade out with QTL effect sizes so small that we will never detect them. If the average effect size is 1% we will eventually detect many QTLs given a heritability of at least 50%. However, if the average QTL effect size is 0.1%, we will detect very few QTLs, and they will be difficult to replicate. Time and much more empirical research will tell. The research described in this chapter begins to chart this territory by providing a systematic genome scan using more than 2,500 DNA markers throughout the genome.

It is interesting that the two best-replicated QTLs are both in the cognitive domain. Apolipoprotein E was first reported in 1993 to be related to late-onset dementia using allelic association (Corder et al. 1993), and this has since been replicated in scores of studies (Rubinstein et al. 1997). QTL sib-pair linkage designs were used to identify a linkage between chromosome 6p21 and reading disability (Cardon et al. 1994), a linkage that has been replicated in several subsequent studies (e.g., S. E. Fisher et al. 1999; Gayán et al. 1999; Grigorenko et al. 1997). The QTL perspective suggests that both dementia and reading disability are likely to be the quantitative extremes of continuous distributions.

In 1990, I decided that quantitative genetic research had gone about as far as it could in documenting genetic influence on *g*. Although quantitative genetics had much more to offer in terms of developmental, multivariate, and environmental analyses, as already mentioned, the most exciting prospect was to try to identify some of the QTLs responsible for the heritability of *g*. This led to a project called the IQ QTL Project.

The IQ QTL Project

The IQ QTL Project provides the first systematic genome scan for association using a new technique called DNA pooling. To my knowledge it is also the first molecular genetic study to focus on ability rather than disability. The goal is not to find genes for genius but to use very high functioning individuals to identify QTLs that operate throughout the entire distribution, including the low (mental retardation) end of the ability distribution. This is based on the simple hypothesis that, although any one of many genes can disrupt normal development, to be very high functioning requires most of the positive alleles and few of the negative alleles. This is just a hypothesis, but one that can be tested when QTLs are found because it predicts that QTLs found for high ability will have a similar effect throughout the rest of the distribution, including the low end of the distribution.

We chose to use an association design rather than linkage because we thought that association would be more powerful in detecting QTLs of small effect size (Plomin et al. 1994a; Risch and Merikangas 1996; Risch and Teng 1998). The major strength of linkage is that it is systematic in the sense that a few hundred DNA markers can be used to scan the genome. In contrast, because allelic association with a quantitative trait can be detected only if a DNA marker is itself the QTL or is very close to it, thousands of DNA markers would need to be genotyped in order to scan the genome. For this reason, allelic association has been used primarily to investigate associations with candidate genes. In earlier work on the IQ QTL Project, we genotyped high- and low-g individuals for 100 DNA markers in or near genes involved in brain functioning, primarily neurotransmitters, but no replicated associations were found (Plomin et al. 1995). We now make DNA from the IQ QTL Project available to other researchers who wish to test candidate genes so that we can focus on a systematic genome scan for association. The problem with the candidate gene approach is that any of the tens of thousands of genes expressed in the brain could be considered as candidate genes for g.

In summary, linkage is systematic but not powerful, and allelic association is powerful but not systematic. However, allelic association can be made more systematic by using a dense map of markers. In the IQ QTL Project, we used a dense map of markers on the long arm of chromosome 6 in an attempt to apply a more systematic association scan for QTL associations with g (Chorney et al. 1998). We found a replicated association for a marker that happened to be in the gene for the insulin-like growth factor 2 receptor (IGF2R), which has been shown to be especially active in brain regions most involved in learning and memory (Wickelgren 1998). We have subsequently genotyped another polymorphism in the IGF2R gene and found similar results (Hill et al. 1999b).

The problem with using a dense map of markers for a genome scan is the amount of genotyping required. In order to scan the entire genome at 1 million DNA base-pair intervals (1 Mb), about 3,500 DNA markers would need to be genotyped. This would require 700,000 genotypings in a study of 100 high-g individuals and 100 controls. With markers at 1 Mb intervals, no QTL would be farther than 500,000 (500 kb) from a marker. However, empirical data indicate that at least 10 times as many markers would be needed in order to detect all QTLs (e.g., Cambien et al. 1999). Despite the daunting amount of genotyping for such a systematic genome scan, there has recently been a sharp swing in favor of genome scans using association approaches that have the power to detect genes of small effect size operating throughout the distribution, as suggested by the QTL perspective. This change in attitude has been fueled by the promise of "SNPs on chips"—single-nucleotide polymorphisms (SNPs, often called *snips*) formatted as arrays of oligonucleotide primers on solid substrates

(DNA chips) that can quickly genotype thousands of DNA markers of the SNP variety.

DNA Pooling

As part of the IQ QTL Project, we developed a technique based on DNA pooling that provides a low-cost and flexible alternative to SNPs on chips for screening the genome for the simplest, largest, and oldest QTL associations, although it cannot detect all QTLs. DNA pooling greatly reduces the need for genotyping by pooling DNA from all individuals in each group and comparing the pooled groups so that only 7,000 genotypings are required to scan the genome in the previous example (Daniels et al. 1998). Unlike DNA chips and other high-throughput approaches, genotyping costs for DNA pooling are independent of sample size. The essence of our approach to DNA pooling is that comparison of two groups requires only an estimate of relative allelic frequencies in which individual errors are expected to cancel out. We focus on the difference in allele image patterns (ΔAIP) for the two groups seen when the AIPs for the two groups are overlaid (Daniels et al. 1998).

Proof of Principle for Chromosomes 4 and 22

The IQ QTL Project is applying DNA pooling to scan the genome for QTLs for *g*. Preliminary proof-of-principle papers have been published for a systematic search of chromosome 4 (P. J. Fisher et al. 1999) and chromosome 22 (Hill et al. 1999a). We use a three-stage strategy that seeks to balance false positive and false negative errors by permitting a more lenient significance criterion in the first stage (which reduces false negatives) and then removing false positives in later replications. In the first stage, ΔAIPs were assessed for 147 markers on chromosome 4 and 66 markers on chromosome 22 for DNA pooled from one group of children of high *g* (51 children with a mean IQ of 136) and from another group of controls of average *g* (51 children with a mean IQ of 105).

In the second stage, markers that yielded significant ΔAIPs in the first stage were replicated using DNA pooling in independent samples of children of extremely high *g* (50 children with IQs exceeding 160) and controls (50 children with a mean IQ of 101). In the third stage, markers that yielded significant ΔAIPs in both the original and replication samples were individually genotyped for all subjects in order to confirm the results of DNA pooling using traditional statistics.

Figure 11–1 illustrates DNA pooling results in the first stage for one of the markers (D4S2943) that showed a significant ΔAIP. Because the DNA is pooled, the AIPs generated by the DNA sequencer show all six alleles for D4S2943 rather than just the one or two alleles that would be seen when individuals rather than pools of individuals are genotyped. The relative height of each allele (each bump in Figure 11–1) is taken as a measure of its frequency. The overlaid AIPs for the original high g group and the original control group indicate that differences between the AIPs for the two groups are due primarily to the fourth allele.

Of the 213 markers on chromosomes 4 and 22, 17 yielded ΔAIPs with simulated P values less than 0.05 for the high-g and control groups in the original sample. With P set at less than 0.05, only 10 markers were expected to be significant by chance alone. Of the 17 markers with significant ΔAIPs in the original sample, 8 showed a significant difference for a specific allele. In addition, D4S2943 and D22S1170 showed trends ($P <$ 0.07) that warranted further exploration in the replication sample.

These 10 markers were tested for replication using DNA pooling in stage 2 DNA where none of the markers would be expected to be signifi-

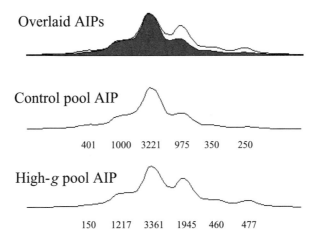

Figure 11–1　DNA sequencer–generated allele image patterns (AIPs) for D4S2943 for the original control group (middle), the original high-g group (bottom), and their overlaid images (top). The numbers represent peak heights representing the six alleles for this DNA marker expressed in fluorescence units. Although fluorescence units differ between the two groups because of polymerase chain reaction (PCR) differences in the amount of amplification and differences in loading the wells for the DNA sequencer, the overlaid AIPs calibrate for the AIPs for the two groups by equating their greatest peak heights.

cant by chance alone. Four of the 10 markers yielded a significant allele-specific difference in the replication sample that was in the same direction as the original sample.

These four markers were selected for the third stage of the design in which each high-g and control individual was genotyped separately. Three of the four markers showed significant differences between the groups in the original sample for the same alleles in the same direction as identified by DNA pooling. For these three markers (MSX1, D4S1607, D4S2943), the individual genotyping allele-specific directional test reached significance in the original sample. All three of these markers were also significant in the replication sample for the allele-specific directional test. These published results used original pools of 51 high-g and 51 control subjects and replication pools of 50 high-g and 50 control subjects, because we were still in the process of completing our new replication samples. However, our full genome scan has combined these subjects in a high-g pool of 101 subjects and a control pool of 101 subjects.

Ongoing Research

Rather than publishing results for other chromosomes, we have concentrated on finishing our three-stage genome scan. We have purchased 2,652 simple-sequence repeat (SSR) markers covering all 22 autosomes (the X chromosome requires sex-segregated pools), which represents the best 1 Mb SSR map that we can currently construct given gaps in the map. Coverage at 1 Mb is about 80% except for teleomeres, which show only about 30% coverage at 1 Mb. We plan to publish our genome scan results using the 2,652 SSR markers. However, SNPs are being identified at a fast rate, and we will be able to use SNPs to move closer to the planned 1 Mb density genome scan, now that it is possible to apply DNA pooling to SNPs (Hoogendoorn et al. 1999). Although it is generally accepted that 10 times more markers are needed to create a net sufficiently fine grained to scoop up most QTLs, our goal is more modest: to catch some, certainly not all, QTLs associated with g.

Because replication is critical for QTL associations, we are collecting several additional replication samples to test QTLs that survive our three-stage design. These include within-family comparisons using parents of our high-g children, which will remove the possibility that our QTL associations are due to ethnic stratification. These replication studies also extend the QTLs in several new directions. For example, we are obtaining large unselected samples of subjects assessed on g in order to test the hypothesis that QTLs identified at the high extreme of the distribution have similar effects throughout the distribution, including the low end of the distribution that represents mild mental retardation. One of these unselected samples involves older subjects, which will make it possible to test the hypothesis that the magnitude of genetic effects on g increases throughout the life span.

Once replicable QTLs are found and localized, the big question will concern functional genomics: what are the pathways between genes and g?

Behavioral Genomics: Top-Down Functional Genomics

Replicated QTL associations with g provide discrete windows through which to view pathways between genes and g. Functional genomics—understanding how genes affect traits—is generally viewed in terms of bottom-up molecular biological analyses of cellular function in which the gene product is identified and its effects studied at a molecular and cellular level. However, other levels of analysis are also likely to be useful in understanding how genes affect g, such as anatomical neuroimaging, functional neuroimaging, electrophysiology, psychophysiology, cognitive processing, and psychometrics (Deary 1999). As an antidote to the tendency to define functional genomics at the cellular level of analysis, the term *behavioral genomics* has been proposed (Plomin and Crabbe 2000).

The IQ QTL Project

Future plans for the IQ QTL Project include a top-down behavioral genomics approach to investigate how genes affect g at the psychological level of analysis. Although our QTL associations are identified in relation to g, the associations might be brought about by a gene's involvement in several component processes rather than by a single general process such as reasoning or speed of information processing (Mackintosh 1998). Are certain genes associated with g because they affect a core general process, or do they primarily affect specific cognitive processes that together contribute to individual differences in performance on tests of g? This issue will be explored in a cost-effective manner by collecting DNA from two samples from which collaborators have already obtained data for relevant information processing and electroencephalogram measures. We also plan to obtain new data that systematically address these issues.

Neurogenetics

The brain is where bottom-up molecular levels of analysis will eventually meet top-down behavioral levels of analysis. A highly productive area of cognitive neuroscience is neurogenetic research on learning and memory using animal models. This work largely uses artificially created mutations and targeted gene mutations (knockouts and conditional knockouts) in *Drosophila* (Dubnau and Tully 1998) and mice (Wahlsten 1999) to dissect the brain pathways that lie between genes and learning and memory. For example, one of the first knockout studies for mouse behavior was reported in 1992 (Silva et al. 1992). A gene *(Camk2)* was knocked out that normally codes for a protein (α-Ca^{2+}-calmodulin-dependent kinase II) that is expressed postnatally in the hippocampus and other forebrain areas critical for learning and memory. Mutant mice homozygous for the knockout gene learned a spatial task significantly more poorly than control mice, although otherwise their behavior seemed normal.

A recent summary lists 22 knockout mutations now known to affect learning and memory in mice (Wahlsten 1999), and scores of other knockout studies are in progress. For example, *N*-methyl D-aspartate (NMDA) gene products serve as a switch for memory formation by detecting coincident firing of different neurons. Overexpression of one particular NMDA gene (for NMDA receptor 2B) enhanced learning and memory in various tasks (Tang et al. 1999). A new type of targeted mutation called a conditional knockout was used to limit the mutation to a particular area of the brain, in this case the forebrain. Normally, expression of this gene is slowed down by adulthood, which may contribute to decreased memory in adults. In this research, the gene was altered so that it continued to be expressed in adulthood, which enhanced learning and memory in adulthood.

Naturally Occurring Genetic Variation

A future direction for neurogenetic research on learning and memory is to consider naturally occurring genetic variation rather than artificially created mutations. The two worlds of quantitative genetics and molecular genetics are coming together in the study of complex quantitative traits and QTLs. The new field of neurogenetics is largely an extension of molecular genetics, which has traditionally focused on artificially created single-gene mutations, in contrast to quantitative genetics, for which naturally occurring genetic variation is the center of attention. Although the advances made in neurogenetic mutational analyses of behavior during the 1990s have been extraordinary in the areas of circadian rhythms, learning and memory, and drug responses, this research is just beginning to consider naturally occurring genetic variation (Crusio 1999).

Work on naturally occurring genetic variation in learning and memory will be stimulated by recent research on mouse models of g (Locurto and Durkin, in press; Locurto and Scanlon 1998). We are beginning a study to test large numbers of mice from outbred stock derived from the cross of eight inbred strains on a diverse g battery of tests of learning and memory. Heterogeneous stock provide finer resolution for QTL mapping than the use of inbred strains or F2 crosses (Talbot et al. 1999) with other genetic variation randomized. DNA from these mice will be used as a resource for analyses of functional variants found to be associated with cognitive processes in human or mouse research. We also hope to test mice selected genotypically for candidate QTLs or selected phenotypically from the extremes of the g dimension on brain slice measures of long-term potentiation and long-term depression of hippocampal neurons, which are widely accepted as models of the synaptic events underlying the storage and erasure of associative memory information (Malenka and Nicoll 1999).

When neurogenetics turns to human cognition, the field will be confronted more starkly with naturally occurring genetic variation simply because it will not be possible to create mutations.

Human Neurogenetics

The 1990s were christened the "Decade of the Brain," and an enormous amount has been learned about the brain during the past 10 years. However, our knowledge about the brain has focused primarily on two distinct levels of analysis. On the one hand, the molecular basis of neural activity, including genetics, is understood today far better than one could have hoped 10 years ago. The mouse has become the favorite organism for such work (Battey et al. 1999). On the other hand, dramatic developments in neuroimaging technologies have illuminated the functions of specific areas of the human brain, primarily using positron emission tomography and functional magnetic resonance imaging as mentioned earlier. But an enormous gulf exists between these two domains of vigorous activity and rapid progress. Although there has been progress in understanding how simple genetic abnormalities underlie various types of diseases and cognitive disorders, remarkably little is known about the links between genetic mechanisms and the neural mechanisms that underlie normal human cognition. Bridging this gulf is the goal of human neurogenetics (Kosslyn and Plomin 2001).

Is the Sky Falling?

Finding QTLs for *g* has important implications for society as well as science (Plomin 1999). The grandest implication for science is that the functional (behavioral) genomics of *g* will serve as an integrating force across diverse disciplines with DNA as the common denominator, opening up new scientific horizons for understanding learning and memory. In terms of implications for society, it should be emphasized that no policies necessarily follow from finding genes associated with *g* because policy involves values. For example, finding genes for *g* does not mean that we ought to put all of our resources into educating the brightest children. Depending on our values, we might worry more about children falling off the low end of the bell curve in an increasingly technological society, and decide to devote more public resources to those who are in danger of being left behind.

Many ethical issues related to DNA are being broached at the level of single-gene disorders that are hardwired in the sense that a single gene is necessary and sufficient for the development of the disorder. This will benefit ethical deliberations about the genetics of *g*, which seems less pressing because genetic effects on *g* are probabilistic rather than deterministic for two reasons. First, heritability is closer to 50% than to 100%, which means that nongenetic factors make a major contribution. Second, because many genes contribute to the heritability of *g*, the system is inherently probabilistic. Potential problems related to finding genes associated with *g* have been discussed, such as prenatal and postnatal screening, discrimination in education and employment, and group differences (Newson and Williamson 1999; Plomin 1999).

The fear lurks in the shadows of such discussions that finding genes for *g* will limit our freedom and our free will. In large part such fears involve misunderstandings about how genes affect complex traits such as *g* (Rutter and Plomin 1997). Finding genes for *g* will not automatically open a door to a genetic version of Huxley's brave new world where babies are sorted out at birth (or before birth) into alphas, betas, gammas, and epsilons. Although the balance of risks and benefits to society of finding genes for *g* is not clear, basic science has much to gain from functional genomic studies of brain functions related to learning and memory. We need to be cautious and to consider carefully societal implications and ethical issues, but we need not take up the cry of Chicken Little that the sky is falling. There is much to celebrate here in terms of the increased potential for understanding our species' nonpareil ability to think and learn.

References

Battey J, Jordan E, Cox D, et al: An action plan for mouse genomics. Nat Genet 21:73–75, 1999

Bouchard TJ Jr, McGue M: Familial studies of intelligence: a review. Science 212:1055–1059, 1981

Bouchard TJ Jr, Lykken DT, McGue M, et al: Sources of human psychological differences: the Minnesota Study of Twins Reared Apart. Science 250:223–228, 1990

Brody N: Intelligence, 2nd Edition. New York, Academic Press, 1992

Cambien F, Poirier O, Nicaud V, et al: Sequence diversity in 36 candidate genes for cardiovascular disorders. Am J Hum Genet 65:183–191, 1999

Cardon LR, Smith SD, Fulker DW, et al: Quantitative trait locus for reading disability on chromosome 6. Science 266:276–279, 1994

Cattell RB: The Inheritance of Personality and Ability. New York, Academic Press, 1982

Chorney MJ, Chorney K, Seese N, et al: A quantitative trait locus (QTL) associated with cognitive ability in children. Psychol Sci 9:1–8, 1998

Corder EH, Saunders AM, Strittmatter WJ, et al: Gene dose of apolipoprotein E type 4 allele and the risk of Alzheimer's disease in late onset families. Science 261:921–923, 1993

Costa PT, McCrae RR: The Revised NEO Personality Inventory (NEO-PIR). Odessa, FL, Psychological Assessment Resources, 1992

Crusio WE: Using spontaneous and induced mutations to dissect brain and behavior genetically. Trends Neurosci 22:100–102, 1999

Daniels J, Holmans P, Plomin R, et al: A simple method for analyzing microsatellite allele image patterns generated from DNA pools and its application to allelic association studies. Am J Hum Genet 62:1189–1197, 1998

Deary IJ: Intelligence and visual and auditory information processing, in Learning and Individual Differences. Edited by Ackerman P, Kyllonen P, Roberts R. Washington, DC, American Psychological Association, 1999, pp 111–134

Devlin B, Daniels M, Roeder K: The heritability of IQ. Nature 388:468–471, 1997

Dubnau J, Tully T: Gene discovery in *Drosophila*: new insights for learning and memory. Annu Rev Neurosci 21:407–444, 1998

Fisher PJ, Turic D, McGuffin P, et al: DNA pooling identifies QTLs for general cognitive ability in children on chromosome 4. Hum Mol Genet 8:915–922, 1999

Fisher RA: The correlation between relatives on the supposition of Mendelian inheritance. Transactions of the Royal Society of Edinburgh 52:399–433, 1918

Fisher SE, Marlow AJ, Lamb J, et al: A quantitative-trait locus on chromosome 6p influences different aspects of developmental dyslexia. Am J Hum Genet 64:146–156, 1999

Gayán J, Smith SD, Cherny SS, et al: Quantitative-trait locus for specific language and reading deficits on chromosome 6p. Am J Hum Genet 64:157–164, 1999

Gottfredson LS: Why *g* matters: the complexity of everyday life. Intelligence 24:79–132, 1997

Grigorenko EL, Wood FB, Meyer MS, et al: Susceptibility loci for distinct components of developmental dyslexia on chromosomes 6 and 15. Am J Hum Genet 60:27–39, 1997

Herrnstein RJ, Murray C: The Bell Curve: Intelligence and Class Structure in American Life. New York, Free Press, 1994

Hill L, Craig IW, Ball DM, et al: DNA pooling and dense marker maps: a systematic search for genes for cognitive ability. Neuroreport 10:843–848, 1999a

Hill L, Craig IW, Chorney MJ, et al: IGF2R and cognitive ability in children. Paper presented at the World Congress on Psychiatric Genetics, October 14, Monterey, CA, 1999b

Hoogendoorn B, Owen MJ, Oefner PJ, et al: Genotyping single nucleotide polymorphisms by primer extension and high performance liquid chromatography. Hum Genet 104:89–93, 1999

Jensen AR: The *g* Factor: The Science of Mental Ability. Westport, CT, Praeger, 1998

Kosslyn S, Plomin R: Towards a neuro-cognitive genetics: goals and issues, in Psychiatric Neuroimaging Strategies: Research and Clinical Applications. Edited by Dougherty D, Rauch SL, Rosenbaum JF. Washington, DC, American Psychiatric Press, 2001, pp 491–515

Locurto C, Durkin E: Problem-solving and individual differences in mice *(Mus musculus)* using water reinforcement. J Comp Psychol (in press)

Locurto C, Scanlon C: Individual differences and a spatial learning factor in two strains of mice *(Mus musculus)*. J Comp Psychol 112:344–352, 1998

Loehlin JC: Genes and Environment in Personality Development. Newbury Park, CA, Sage, 1992

Mackintosh NJ: IQ and Human Intelligence. Oxford, UK, Oxford University Press, 1998

Malenka RC, Nicoll RA: Long-term potentiation: a decade of progress? Science 285:1870–1874, 1999

McClearn GE, Johansson B, Berg S, et al: Substantial genetic influence on cognitive abilities in twins 80+ years old. Science 276:1560–1563, 1997

McCrae RR: Social consequences of experiential openness. Psychol Bull 120:323–337, 1996

McGue M: The democracy of the genes. Nature 388:417–418, 1997

Newson A, Williamson R: Should we undertake genetic research on intelligence? Bioethics 13:327–342, 1999

Pedersen NL, Plomin R, Nesselroade JR, et al: A quantitative genetic analysis of cognitive abilities during the second half of the life span. Psychol Sci 3:346–353, 1992

Petrill SA: Molarity versus modularity of cognitive functioning? a behavioral genetic perspective. Current Directions in Psychological Science 6:96–99, 1997

Plomin R: Genetics and Experience: The Interplay Between Nature and Nurture. Thousand Oaks, CA, Sage, 1994

Plomin R: Genetics and general cognitive ability. Nature 402:C25–C29, 1999

Plomin R, Crabbe JC: DNA. Psychol Bull 126:806–828, 2000

Plomin R, DeFries JC: Genetics of cognitive abilities and disabilities. Sci Am May: 62–69, 1998

Plomin R, Petrill SA: Genctics and intelligence: what's new? Intelligence 24:53–77, 1997

Plomin R, McClearn GE, Smith DL, et al: DNA markers associated with high versus low IQ: the IQ Quantitative Trait Loci (QTL) Project. Behav Genet 24:107–118, 1994a

Plomin R, Owen MJ, McGuffin P: The genetic basis of complex human behaviors. Science 264:1733–1739, 1994b

Plomin R, McClearn GE, Smith DL, et al: Allelic associations between 100 DNA markers and high versus low IQ. Intelligence 21:31–48, 1995

Plomin R, Fulker DW, Corley R, et al: Nature, nurture and cognitive development from 1 to 16 years: a parent-offspring adoption study. Psychol Sci 8:442–447, 1997

Plomin R, DeFries JC, McClearn GE, et al: Behavioral Genetics, 4th Edition. New York, Worth, 2001

Risch N, Merikangas KR: The future of genetic studies of complex human diseases. Science 273:1516–1517, 1996

Risch N, Teng J: The relative power of family based and case-control designs for linkage disequilibrium studies of complex human diseases I. DNA pooling. Genome Res 8:1273–1288, 1998

Rubinstein M, Phillips TJ, Bunzow JR, et al: Mice lacking dopamine D4 receptors are supersensitive to ethanol, cocaine, and methamphetamine. Cell 90:991–1001, 1997

Rutter M, Plomin R: Opportunities for psychiatry from genetic findings. Br J Psychiatry 171:209–219, 1997

Silva AJ, Paylor R, Wehner JM, et al: Impaired spatial learning in α-calcium-calmodulin kinase mutant mice. Science 257:206–211, 1992

Talbot CJ, Nicod A, Cherny SS, et al: High-resolution mapping of quantitative trait loci in outbred mice. Nat Genet 21:305–308, 1999

Tang Y-P, Shimizu E, Dube GR, et al: Genetic enhancement of learning and memory in mice. Nature 401:63–69, 1999

Wahlsten D: Single-gene influences on brain and behavior. Annu Rev Psychol 50:599–624, 1999

Wickelgren I: Tracking insulin to the mind. Science 280:517–519, 1998

CHAPTER TWELVE

Genetic Polymorphisms and Aggression

Antonia New, M.D., Marianne Goodman, M.D.,
Vivian Mitropoulou, M.A., and Larry Siever, M.D.

Impulsive aggressive behavior presents a critical challenge in the treatment of patients with personality disorders. It accounts for a substantial portion of the morbidity and mortality associated with these disorders, as manifested by self-injurious behavior, domestic violence, assault, substance abuse, destruction of property, and suicide attempts. Furthermore, personality disorders (especially borderline and antisocial personality disorders) may be associated with an even greater risk for violent criminal behavior than Axis I diagnoses such as schizophrenia or substance abuse. It has become clear that genetic factors play a role in the development of impulsive aggressive symptoms, in that impulsive aggression has been shown to be partially heritable. The identification of genetic factors predisposing to impulsive aggression may prove a critical step in better understanding etiology and in developing new treatments for impulsive aggression.

Personality Disorders and Impulsive Aggression

Impulsive aggressive behavior in clinical populations of patients with personality disorders is a common clinical phenomenon and contributes to much of the dysfunction associated with these diagnoses. In particular, a high rate of repeated self-mutilation and episodic dyscontrol have been reported in patients with borderline, antisocial, and histrionic personality disorders, reflecting impulsive aggression (Pattison and Kahan 1983; Virkkunen 1976). This is not surprising because in DSM-IV-TR (American Psychiatric Association 2000), assaultiveness is one of the diagnostic criteria for antisocial personality disorder, and repetitive suicide attempts, self-mutilation, and impulsivity are among the diagnostic criteria for borderline personality disorder. Impulsive behaviors, which often lead to overt physical aggression, can also disrupt family relationships.

Certain forms of aggression, such as spousal abuse, are especially associated with personality disorders and are a frequent problem among individuals seeking psychiatric care (Hamberger and Hastings 1986; Mikolajczak and Hagen 1978). Suicidal behavior is common in patients with personality disorders, and in fact 9% of patients with borderline personality disorder die by suicide (Paris et al. 1987; Stone 1989). Data from our ongoing studies of individuals with personality disorders suggest that 51% of patients with personality disorder meet criteria for intermittent explosive disorder, revised research version; of these patients, 64% meet criteria for borderline or antisocial personality disorders (New et al. 1999). As pharmacological and other treatments for mood disorders and psychotic disorders have improved, an increasing proportion of patients requiring psychiatric hospitalization carry a primary personality disorder diagnosis (Breslow et al. 1993; Hansson 1989; Molinari et al. 1994). A common precipitant for psychiatric hospitalization in patients with personality disorders is an actual or threatened act of aggression directed toward self or others.

Further evidence of the significance of impulsive aggressive symptomatology in patients with personality disorders is demonstrated by the frequency of personality disorders in the forensic population. In one study of violent offenders and impulsive fire setters, 47% of the subjects were found to have a personality disorder diagnosis, especially borderline and antisocial personality disorders (Virkkunen et al. 1996). In a sample of wife batterers, higher scores on a measure of borderline personality organization (similar to scores seen in a sample of borderline patients diagnosed by DSM-III [American Psychiatric Association 1987] criteria) were found compared with controls (Dutton et al. 1996). Prison inmates in Quebec with antisocial personality disorder were found to have more convictions and an earlier onset of criminal activity than those without antisocial personality disorder (Hodgin and Cote 1993). Furthermore, the presence of antisocial personality disorder has been found to increase the likelihood of homicidal violence 10-fold in men and 50-fold in women (Eronen et al. 1996).

Evidence for Heritability of Impulsive Aggression and Suicidality

A partially heritable basis for impulsive aggression has been demonstrated by a number of observations from both twin (Coccaro et al. 1993) and adoption (Bohman et al. 1984) studies, suggesting heritability estimates from 20% to 62% (Coccaro et al. 1993). Preliminary data from monozygotic-dizygotic twin studies suggest that although the personality disorder diagnoses are not heritable, the traits of impulsive aggression or assertive aggressiveness are significantly heritable (Alnaes and Torgersen 1989; Coccaro et al. 1993; Torgersen 1994). Studies of adoptees with biological parents with antisocial personality disorder demonstrated a genetic contribution to the development of antisocial personality disorder characterized by antisocial aggressive behavior (Cadoret et al. 1985; Crowe 1974), and this heritable tendency appeared to be brought out by adverse home environment (Cadoret et al. 1995). Twin studies of suicide also demonstrate a greater concordance for suicidal behavior in monozygotic versus dizygotic twins, and adoption studies also suggest a heritable component to suicide that is independent from risk for affective illness itself (Egeland and Sussex 1985; Mitterauer 1990; Roy et al. 1997).

Impulsive Aggression and Serotonergic Studies

Abnormalities in central serotonergic activity have consistently been found to be associated with measures of impulsive aggression in patients with personality disorders (Coccaro et al. 1989; O'Keane et al. 1992; Siever and Trestman 1993). Studies of cerebrospinal fluid have shown a decrease in 5-hydroxyindolacetic acid (5-HIAA), a metabolite of serotonin, to be associated with impulsive aggression in patients with personality disorders, as well as in depressed patients, normal volunteers, and violent alcoholic offenders (Linnoila et al. 1989, 1994; Virkkunen et al. 1994). The prolactin response to fenfluramine, a serotonin releasing agent, can be viewed as a measure of net central serotonergic activity (Coccaro et al. 1989), and a blunted response has been associated with impulsive aggression in patients with personality disorders compared with normal controls (Coccaro et al. 1989, 1996). A blunted response to fenfluramine has also been demonstrated in patients with antisocial personality disorder, a diagnosis highly associated with impulsive aggression (O'Keane et al. 1992). Studies of serotonergic activity in relation to suicide demonstrate low cerebrospinal fluid 5-HIAA concentrations in patients with a history of violent suicide attempts (Asberg 1977; Asberg et al. 1976). Postmortem studies have demonstrated decreased imipramine binding in the brains of suicide victims and, more specifically, increases in 5-hydroxytryptamine A1 (5-HT1A) autoreceptors in the midbrain of suicide victims (Stockmeier et al. 1998), and alterations in binding to the serotonin transporter and to the 5-HT1A and 5-HT2A receptors in postmortem brains of suicide victims compared with controls (Arango et al. 1997). A blunted neuroendocrine response to serotonin stimulating agents has been found in patients with a history of suicide (Coccaro et al. 1989; Weiss and Coccaro 1997).

The relationship between reduced serotonergic function and impulsive aggression is, in fact, one of the most robust and replicable findings in biological psychiatry. The apparently heritable component of impulsive aggression, including suicidal behavior, compels the investigation of the role of genetic differences in determinants of serotonergic function (such as synthesis, metabolism, and receptor sensitivity or regulation) in the development of different susceptibilities to impulsive aggression. Indeed, studies demonstrate 1) an association between a polymorphism in the 5-HT1B gene *(HTR1B)* and antisocial alcoholics (Huang et al. 1999), 2) an association between a polymorphism in the tryptophan hydroxylase gene and suicide and particularly with violent suicide attempts (Nielsen et al. 1998), and 3) an association between allelic variation in the serotonin transporter gene *(SLC6A4)* (designated "5-HTTLPR" elsewhere in this volume) and variations in anxiety-related personality traits (Lesch et al. 1996). These studies demonstrate that genetic differences in the serotonin system may be associated with behavioral traits related to impulsive aggression. Further support for this hypothesis is found in the animal studies by Brunner et al. (1993) showing that a mutation in the MAO A gene can cause a syndrome including violence and impulsivity. In addition, enhanced aggressive behavior has been demonstrated in mice lacking the 5-HT1B receptor, which is comparable to the human 5-HT1B (Saudou et al. 1994).

Preliminary Studies From Our Research Group

We have elected to focus on the serotonin system in selecting candidate genes corresponding to the abnormalities most consistently associated with impulsive or aggressive behavior (Siever and Trestman 1993). The following candidate genes are discussed because they include polymorphisms in serotonin-related genes that are potentially functionally important:

Serotonin 1B receptor gene *(HTR1B):* G, C
Tryptophan hydroxylase gene *(TPH): 779A/218A* (U), *779C/218C* (L)
Serotonin transporter gene *(SLC6A4)* promoter l: s

HTR1B was chosen because it controls the synthesis and release of serotonin from the terminals. *TPH* was selected because it codes for the first enzyme involved in the synthesis of serotonin, and an association between the L *(218C/779C)* allele and suicidal behavior, at times a form of impulsive behavior, has been described (Nielsen et al. 1994). The serotonin transporter (SLC6A4) promoter polymorphism was chosen because allelic variation has been associated with variations in the personality traits of harm avoidance and impulsivity (Lesch et al. 1996).

Polymorphisms in Serotonin-Related Genes

Serotonin 1B Receptor

The serotonin 1B receptor (previously called 5-HT1Dβ) is a terminal autoreceptor involved in regulating serotonin synthesis and release. A common polymorphism in the coding region of the gene locus, *HTR1B*, has been described. The variant is caused by a G to C substitution (coding for the same amino acid) and has frequencies of 0.72 G and 0.28 C in a mixed population of controls and alcoholics (Lappalainen et al. 1995). The more common allele (G) lacks a site for *Hinc*II restriction endonuclease cleavage. Enhanced aggressive behavior has been demonstrated in mice lacking the 5-HT1B receptor, comparable to human 5-HT1B (Saudou et al. 1994). In a study of Finnish alcoholics and southwestern American Indians, antisocial alcoholism showed significant evidence of sib-pair linkage to *HTR1B*G816C* in both populations (Lappalainen et al. 1998). A functional significance for this polymorphism has not been established.

In preliminary data from our lab on 89 Caucasian patients with personality disorder, the G allele of *HTR1B* was associated with a history of suicide attempts (G alleles constituted 91% of the alleles in the 23 patients with suicide history, compared with 67% of the alleles in 66 patients without suicide history: $\chi^2 = 9.3$, $df = 1$, $P < 0.01$). In the sample to date, there is no significant association between the *HTR1B* genotype and self-reported measures of impulsive aggression as determined by Buss-Durkee Hostility Inventory irritability-assaultiveness subscale scores (Buss and Durkee 1957)(BDHI$_{irr-ass}$ GG = 11.7 ± 4.2, n = 52; GC = 9.9 ± 4.7, n = 31; CC = 11.3 ± 4.0, n = 6, P = not significant).

Tryptophan Hydroxylase

TPH is the first enzyme involved in the synthesis of serotonin. A biallelic intronic polymorphism in the gene on chromosome 11 coding for TPH has been identified, and the two alleles originally designated L and U (Nielsen et al. 1992) are found with frequencies of 0.40 and 0.60, respectively, in unrelated Caucasians. Subsequent sequencing of the TPH gene demonstrated two polymorphic sites: *A218C* and *A779C; A779A/A218A* corresponds to U and *A779C/A218C* corresponds to L (Nielsen et al. 1997). In two separate cohorts of Finnish violent alcohol offenders, the L *TPH* allele was associated with reduced cerebrospinal fluid 5-HIAA concentrations and a history of suicide attempts (Nielsen et al. 1994, 1995, 1998). Another study, however, reported that in patients with major depression, those with the U allele had a higher incidence of suicide attempts (particularly violent attempts) (Mann et al. 1997), whereas in a Japanese cohort no association between *TPH* genotype and suicide was found (Kunugi et al. 1999).

Preliminary evidence of an association between the L allele and aggressive behavior in a polymorphism in the TPH gene in primates has also been demonstrated (M. J. Raleigh, personal communication, May 1998). We have reported increased measures of impulsive aggression in 21 Caucasian men with personality disorders with the LL genotype as compared with the UL and UU genotypes (New et al. 1998). The LL genotype was associated with significantly higher total scores on the BDHI compared with Caucasian males with the UL or UU genotypes, as well as significantly higher scores on the BDHI Irritability/Assaultiveness Composite subscale. No significant association was found between the LL genotype and a history of suicide attempt or impulsive borderline personality disorder traits in this sample. Females with the LL genotype did not demonstrate higher BDHI scores nor a blunted prolactin response to fenfluramine (New et al. 1998).

This is in contrast to a recent study that reported an association between the U allele and measures of aggression and anger (Manuck et al. 1999). It should be noted, however, that the functional significance of this polymorphism has yet to be proven. Because it is an intronic polymorphism, the two alleles do not code for a different gene product. However, the association with clinical symptoms raises the possibility of linkage disequilibrium or a change in a regulatory region close to the TPH gene, and in fact another polymorphism closely linked to the *779A* polymorphism has been identified (Nielsen et al. 1997).

Serotonin Transporter

The serotonin transporter is important in serotonergic functioning in that it plays a central role in the termination of 5-HT neurotransmission by the presynaptic reuptake of 5-HT and represents a site of antidepressant activity (Amara and Kuhar 1993). Furthermore, twin studies suggest that platelet 5-HT uptake, mediated by the serotonin transporter, may be partially genetically controlled (Meltzer and Arora 1986). The serotonin transporter on the human platelet has been shown to be identical to the serotonin transporter in the human brain (Lesch et al. 1993).

A polymorphism in the promoter region of the serotonin transporter gene *(SLC6A4)* has been identified; this polymorphism has demonstrated *functional significance* in coding for high and low transporter production. Evidence suggests that the s allele may be associated with increased measures of harm avoidance and impulsivity, as measured by the NEO Personality Inventory (Costa and McCrae 1997), although other studies did not replicate this finding (Ebstein et al. 1997; Gelernter et al. 1998). Another study has reported that the s allele may confer susceptibility to severe alcohol abuse (Sander et al. 1997). Although one study demonstrated an association between the s allele and "dissocial alcoholics" (Sanders et al. 1998), another study did not demonstrate this association (Edenberg et al. 1998). Anxiety traits have been associated with the s allele (Nakamura et al. 1997), but no difference in allele frequency of the two common variants were found in patients with and without panic disorder (Deckert et al. 1997).

Conclusion

The well-established serotonergic abnormalities associated with aggression and the apparent heritable contribution to these behaviors compel genetic studies of serotonin-related genes and impulsive aggression. The approach of identifying the relationship between candidate genes and impulsive aggressive behavior is promising in that it may elucidate the mechanism underlying the susceptibility to impulsive aggression. Impulsive aggression in personality disorders is undoubtedly a complex behavior with a multifactorial etiology. This approach allows us to identify genes each with modest contributions to behavior. Including biological parents of probands in a subset of patients allows us to control for ethnic variability in allele frequencies. Because allelic variation in serotonin-related genes has been associated with impulsive aggressive behavior, the identification of behavioral differences by genotype in a specific receptor subtype may provide one tool to elucidate the specific pathophysiology underlying impulsive aggression. The clarification of the contribution of both inherited and environmental factors in the development of aggression could lead to a better understanding of treatment approaches. The identification of specific serotonin-related genes might lead to more-specific pharmacological strategies as an additional tool in the treatment of aggression. It is premature at this time to posit specific pharmacological interventions directed at receptor subtypes, but data on serotonergic abnormalities in impulsive aggression have already led to a successful trial of a selective serotonin reuptake inhibitor in the treatment of impulsive aggression (Coccaro and Kavoussi 1997). At this time, the observed relationships between specific serotonin-related genes and aggression by our group and others are preliminary. Our pilot data suggest an association between the *HTR1B-* G allele and suicide history, although another group has suggested an association between the C allele and impulsivity in antisocial alcoholic patients (Lappalainen et al. 1998). Our data also suggest an association between the L allele and impulsive aggression in Caucasian male patients with personality disorders, although this finding also differs from the findings of other groups (Manuck et al. 1999).

It is important to recognize that impulsive aggression is a complex behavior that is likely to be determined by multiple genetic factors as well as environmental factors. To date, association studies have demonstrated a relationship to specific serotonin-related genes, but these findings have been difficult to replicate between research groups. It is likely that the influence of genes of small effect is masked by factors such as ethnic variability in haplotype frequency. The employment of family-based association studies and the use of techniques such as the transmission dysequilibrium test coupled with the screening of larger samples will be helpful in resolving some of the ambiguity in results to date.

References

Alnaes R, Torgersen S: Clinical differentiation between major depression only, major depression with panic disorder, and panic disorder only:

childhood, personality and personality disorder. Acta Psychiatr Scand 79:370–377, 1989

Amara S, Kuhar M: Neurotransmitter transporters: recent progress. Annu Rev Neurosci 16:73–93, 1993

American Psychiatric Association: Diagnostic and Statistical Manual of Mental Disorders, 3rd Edition, Revised. Washington, DC, American Psychiatric Association, 1987

American Psychiatric Association: Diagnostic and Statistical Manual of Mental Disorders, 4th Edition, Text Revision. Washington, DC, American Psychiatric Association, 2000

Arango V, Underwood MD, Mann JJ: Postmortem findings in suicide victims. Implications for in vivo imaging studies. Ann N Y Acad Sci 836:269–287, 1997

Asberg M: Neurotransmitters and suicidal behavior: the evidence from cerebrospinal fluid studies. Ann N Y Acad Sci 836:158–181, 1997

Asberg M, Traskman L, Thoren P: 5-HIAA in the cerebrospinal fluid: a biochemical suicide predictor? Arch Gen Psychiatry 33:1193–1197, 1976

Bohman M, Cloninger CR, von Knorring A, et al: An adoption study of somatoform disorders, III: cross-fostering analysis and genetic relationship to alcoholism and criminality. Arch Gen Psychiatry 41:872–878, 1984

Breslow R, Klinger B, Erickson B: Crisis hospitalization on a psychiatric emergency service. General Hospital Psychiatry 15:307–315, 1993

Brunner HG, Nelen M, Breakefield XO, et al: Abnormal behavior associated with a point mutation in the structural gene for monoamine oxidase. Science 262:578–580, 1993

Buss AH, Durkee A: An inventory for assessing different kinds of hostility. Journal of Consulting Psychology 21:343–348, 1957

Cadoret RJ, O'Gorman TW, Troughton E, et al: Alcoholism and antisocial personality: interrelationships, genetic and environmental factors. Arch Gen Psychiatry 42:161–167, 1985

Cadoret RJ, Yates WR, Troughton E, et al: Genetic-environmental interaction in the genesis of aggressivity and conduct disorders. Arch Gen Psychiatry 52:916–924, 1995

Coccaro EF, Kavoussi RJ: Fluoxetine and impulsive aggressive behavior in personality-disordered subjects. Arch Gen Psychiatry 54:1081–1088, 1997

Coccaro EF, Siever LJ, Klar HM, et al: Serotonergic studies in patients with affective and personality disorders. Arch Gen Psychiatry 46:587–599, 1989

Coccaro EF, Bergman CS, McLean GE: Heritability of irritable impulsiveness: a study of twins reared together and apart. Psychiatry Res 48:229–242, 1993

Coccaro EF, Berman ME, Kavoussi RJ, et al: Relationship of prolactin response to d-Fenfluramine to behavioral and questionnaire assessments of aggression in personality disordered men. Biol Psychiatry 37:1–8, 1996

Costa PT Jr, McCrae RR: Stability and change in personality assessment: the revised NEO Personality Inventory in the year 2000. J Pers Assess 68:86–94, 1997

Crowe RR: An adoption study of antisocial personality. Arch Gen Psychiatry 31:785–791, 1974

Deckert J, Catalano M, Heils A, et al: Functional promoter polymorphism of the human serotonin transporter: lack of association with panic disorder. Psychiatr Genet 7:45–47, 1997

Dutton DG, Starzomski A, Ryan L: Antecedents of abusive personality and abusive behavior in wife assaulters. Journal of Family Violence 11:113–132, 1996

Ebstein RP, Gritsenko I, Nemanov L, et al: No association between the serotonin transporter gene regulatory region polymorphism and the tridimensional personality questionnaire (TPQ) temperament of harm avoidance. Mol Psychiatry 2:224–226, 1997

Edenberg HJ, Reynolds J, Koller DL, et al: A family based analysis of whether the functional promoter alleles of the serotonin transporter gene HTT affect the risk for alcohol dependence. Alcohol Clin Exp Res 22:1080–1085, 1998

Egeland JA, Sussex JN: Suicide and family loadings for affective disorders. JAMA 254:915–918, 1985

Eronen M, Hakola P, Tihonen J: Mental disorders and homicidal behavior in Finland. Arch Gen Psychiatry 53:497–501, 1996

Gelernter J, Kranzler H, Coccaro EF, et al: Serotonin transporter protein gene polymorphism and personality measures in African American and European American subjects. Am J Psychiatry 155:1332–1338, 1998

Hamberger LK, Hastings JE: Personality correlates of men who abuse their partners: a cross-validation study. Journal of Family Violence 1:323–341, 1986

Hansson L: Utilization of psychiatric inpatient care: a study of changes related to the introduction of a sectorized care organization. Acta Psychiatr Scand 79:571–578, 1989

Hodgin S, Cote G: Major mental disorder and antisocial personality disorder: a criminal combination. Bulletin of the Academy of Psychiatry and the Law 21:155–160, 1993

Huang Y, Grailhe R, Arango V, et al: Relationship of pathology to the human serotonin 1B genotype and receptor binding kinetics in postmortem brain tissue. Neuropsychopharmacology 21:238–246, 1999

Kunugi H, Ishida S, Kato T, et al: No evidence for an association of polymorphisms of the tryptophan hydroxylase gene with affective disorders of attempted suicide among Japanese patients. Am J Psychiatry 156:774–776, 1999

Lappalainen J, Dean M, Charbonneau L, et al: Mapping of the serotonin 5-HT1Db autoreceptor gene on chromosome 6 and direct analysis for sequence variants. Am J Med Genet 60:157–60, 1995

Lappalainen J, Long JC, Eggert M, et al: Linkage of antisocial alcoholism to the serotonin 5-HT1B receptor gene in two populations. Arch Gen Psychiatry 55:989–994, 1998

Lesch K, Wolozin B, Murphy D, et al: Primary structure of the human platelet serotonin uptake site: identity with the brain serotonin transporter. J Neurochem 60:2319–2322, 1993

Lesch K, Bengel D, Heils A, et al: Association of anxiety-related traits with a polymorphism in the serotonin transporter gene regulatory region. Science 274:1527–1531, 1996

Linnoila M, DeJong J, Virkkunen M: Family history of alcoholism in violent offenders and impulsive fire setters. Arch Gen Psychiatry 46:613–616, 1989

Linnoila M, Virkkunen M, George T, et al: Serotonin, behavior and alcohol, in Toward a Molecular Basis of Alcohol Use and Abuse. Edited by Jansson B, Jornvall H, Rydberg U, et al. Basel, Birkhauser Verlag, 1994, pp 155–164

Mann JJ, Malone KM, Nielson DA, et al: Possible association of a polymorphism of the tryptophan hydroxylase gene with suicidal behavior in depressed patients. Am J Psychiatry 154:1451–1453, 1997

Manuck SB, Flory JD, Ferrell RE, et al: Aggression and anger-related traits associated with a polymorphism of the tryptophan hydroxylase gene. Biol Psychiatry 45:603–614, 1999

Meltzer H, Arora R: Platelet markers of suicidality. Ann N Y Acad Sci 487:271–280, 1986

Mikolajczak J, Hagen D: Aggression in psychiatric patients in a VA hospital. Mil Med 143:402–404, 1978

Molinari V, Ames A, Essa M: Prevalence of personality disorders in two geropsychiatric inpatient units. J Geriatr Psychiatry Neurol 7:295–300, 1994

Nakamura T, Muramatsu T, Ono Y, et al: Serotonin transporter gene regulatory region polymorphism and anxiety-related traits in Japanese. Am J Med Genet 74:544–555, 1997

New AS, Gelernter J, Yovell Y, et al: Increases in irritable aggression associated with "LL" genotype at the tryptophan hydroxylase locus. Am J Med Genet 81:13–17, 1998

New AS, Gelernter J, Mitropoulou V, et al: Serotonin related genotype and impulsive aggression. Biol Psychiatry 45:120S, 1999

Nielsen DA, Dean M, Goldman D: Genetic mapping of the human tryptophan hydroxylase gene on chromosome 11, using an intronic conformational polymorphism. Am J Hum Genet 51:1366–1371, 1992

Nielsen DA, Goldman D, Virkkunen M, et al: Suicidality and 5-hydroxyindolacetic acid concentration associated with a tryptophan hydroxylase polymorphism. Arch Gen Psychiatry 51:34–38, 1994

Nielsen D, Stefanisko K, Virkkunen M, et al: Association of tryptophan hydroxylase genotype with suicidal behavior in Finns: a replication study. Paper presented at the 34th annual meeting of the American College of Neuropsychopharmacology, San Juan, PR, December 1995

Nielsen DA, Jenkins GL, Stefanisko KM, et al: Sequence, splice site, and population frequency distribution analyses of the polymorphic human tryptophan hydroxylase intron 7. Molecular Brain Research 45:145–148, 1997

Nielsen DA, Virkkunen M, Lappalainen J, et al: A tryptophan hydroxylase gene marker for suicidality and alcoholism. Arch Gen Psychiatry 55:593–602, 1998

O'Keane V, Moloney E, O'Neill H, et al: Blunted prolactin responses to d-fenfluramine in sociopathy: evidence for subsensitivity of central serotonergic function. Br J Psychiatry 160:643–646, 1992

Paris J, Brown R, Nowlis D: Long-term follow-up of borderline patients in a general hospital. Compr Psychiatry 28:530–535, 1987

Pattison E, Kahan J: The deliberate self-harm syndrome. Am J Psychiatry 140:867–872, 1983

Roy A, Rylabder G, Sarchiapone M: Genetic studies of suicidal behavior. Psychiatr Clin North Am 20:595–611, 1997

Sander T, Harms H, Lesch KP, et al: Association analysis of a regulatory variation of the serotonin transporter gene with severe alcohol dependence. Alcohol Clin Exp Res 21:1356–1359, 1997

Sander T, Harms H, Dufeu P, et al: Serotonin transporter gene variants in alcohol-dependent subjects with dissocial personality disorder. Biol Psychiatry 43:908–912, 1998

Saudou F, Amara DA, Dierich A, et al: Enhanced aggressive behavior in mice lacking 5-HT$_{1B}$ receptor. Science 265:1875–1878, 1994

Siever LJ, Trestman RL: The serotonin system and aggressive personality disorder. Int Clin Psychopharmacol 8:33–39, 1993

Stockmeier CA, Shapiro LA, Dilley GE, et al: Increase in serotonin-1A autoreceptors in the midbrain of suicide victims with major depression-postmortem evidence for decreased serotonin activity. J Neurosci 18:7394–7401, 1998

Stone MH: Long-term follow-up of narcissistic/borderline patients. Psychiatr Clin North Am 12:621–641, 1989

Torgersen S: Genetics in borderline conditions. Acta Psychiatr Scand Suppl 379:19–25, 1994

Virkkunen M: Reactive hypoglycemic tendency among habitually violent offenders. Nutritional Review 44 (suppl):94–103, 1976

Virkkunen M, Rawlings R, Tokola R, et al: CSF biochemistries, glucose metabolism, and diurnal activity rhythms in alcoholic violent offenders, fire setters, and healthy volunteers. Arch Gen Psychiatry 51:20–27, 1994

Virkkunen M, Eggert M, Rawlings R, et al: A prospective follow-up study of alcoholic violent offenders and fire setters. Arch Gen Psychiatry 53:523–529, 1996

Weiss D, Coccaro EF: Neuroendocrine challenge studies of suicidal behavior. Psychiatr Clin North Am 20:563–579, 1997

CHAPTER THIRTEEN

Molecular Genetics of Temperamental Differences in Children

Louis A. Schmidt, Ph.D.
Nathan A. Fox, Ph.D.

The study of individual differences in childhood temperament has received much attention over the last 30 years. Much of the focus surrounding research in this area was sparked by a change in the zeitgeist that occurred some three decades earlier in terms of how personality development was viewed. There was a movement away from the radical behavioral approaches of Watson and Skinner and a return to ideas of pragmatists such as James and Dewey. In the view of behaviorists, children were passive recipients of stimuli from the environment. Contextual factors were a major contributing source for personality formation. Pragmatists, such as James and Dewey, on the other hand, viewed individual differences in personality in children as emerging from innate predispositions, and these dispositions served to act on the environment. Temperamental differences, in this view, are rooted in biology, have a genetic basis, and serve important adaptive functions. Such notions are clearly

The longitudinal studies reported on in this chapter were supported in part by a grant from the National Institutes of Health (HD 17899) awarded to Nathan A. Fox.

evident in today's research on personality (see e.g., Cloninger et al. 1996; and the chapters contained in this volume).

In this chapter, we review evidence from longitudinal research concerned with the study of the origins of individual differences in temperament and social behavior. We have been following several cohorts of children from the opening months of postnatal life to the preschool years. To date, we have noted that children are of least two temperamental types: shy/socially withdrawn and bold/exuberant. We have found that these temperamental types are modestly preserved over the first 4 years of development; each is associated with distinct behavioral and physiological correlates during resting and emotionally challenging situations; and each is differentially affected by environmental experiences in the formation of personality. We review behavioral and physiological evidence of temperamental differences among children and recent molecular genetic data collected in our laboratory from these several cohorts of children.

Ongoing Longitudinal Studies of Childhood Temperament

Overview

One of the most striking features of individual differences in infant behavior is the manner with which infants react to novel sensory stimuli: some infants react immediately to the presentation of a novel stimulus whereas others do not. These individual differences, possibly in perceptual thresholds, are seen across species and appear to be clearly heritable (e.g., Blizard 1989). The two temperament types we have studied each differ in the pattern of their reactive response to sensory stimuli. Infants who exhibit a high degree of motor activity and distress in response to the presentation of novel auditory and visual stimuli during the first 4 months of postnatal life are likely to exhibit social withdrawal during the preschool and early school-age years. On the other hand, infants who exhibit a high degree of motor activity and positive affect in response to the presentation of novel auditory and visual stimuli during the first 4 months of postnatal life tend to display a high degree of exuberant and outgoing behavior during the preschool- and early school-age years. There is, in addition, at least some evidence to suggest that there may be a genetic etiology to shy behavior and social withdrawal. Kagan (DiLalla et al. 1994), for example, noted in an observational study of the behavior of 157 twenty-four-month-old twin pairs that monozygotic twins showed stronger intraclass correlations of shy/inhibited behavior to unfamiliar stimuli than did dizygotic and nontwin siblings.

We have been following four separate cohorts of children as part of a research program in which the focus is on the origins and development of temperament and social behavior in children. One cohort (1) was recruited 48 hours after birth and unselected for individual differences; two other cohorts (2, 3) were selected at 4 months of age for reactivity differences in motor activity and affect thought to predict shy or exuberant behavior in early childhood; and another cohort (4) was also unselected for individual differences in personality at age 4 (5). The children from cohorts 1, 3, and 4 were seen in our laboratory at ages 9, 14, 24, and 48 months, at which time their behavioral reactions to the presentation of novel social and nonsocial stimuli and regional brain electrical activity (electroencephalogram [EEG]) were collected during baseline and emotionally evocative conditions. The children were all healthy (i.e., without pre-, peri-, or postnatal complications), primarily Caucasian, and of middle-class background. All of the parents had completed high school, and a majority of the mothers and fathers were college graduates. The children were, for the most part, living with their families in or near College Park, Maryland.

Behavioral and Physiological Findings

To date, we have found a number of distinct patterns of behavioral, endocrine, and physiological activity during baseline and emotionally evocative situations in the two temperamental types (i.e., shy/socially withdrawn and bold/exuberant) of children, and these behavioral and physiological patterns tend to remain modestly preserved across the first 4 years of development (e.g., Fox et al. 2001). For example, we have found that infants who were easily distressed by the presentation of novel auditory and visual stimuli at age 4 months tended to exhibit greater relative right frontal EEG activity (a marker of a disposition toward avoidance) at 9 (Calkins et al. 1996) and 24 months (Fox et al. 1994) greater fear-potentiated startle at 9 months (Schmidt and Fox 1998) and were behaviorally inhibited at 14 months (Calkins et al. 1996) and shy at age 4 (Schmidt et al. 1997). On the other hand, infants who were easily aroused, but exhibited a greater degree of positive affect in response to the presentation of novel auditory and visual stimuli at age 4 months tended to exhibit greater relative left frontal EEG activity (a marker of a disposition toward approach) at 9 and 24 months and an attenuated startle response at 9 months and were outgoing and sociable at 14 and 48 months (Fox et al. 1995, 2001). In sum, the early appearance of temperamental differences among infants, in combination with the preservation of behavior and physiology in relation to these temperamental styles across development, raises the possibility that there may be a genetic basis to some temperamental traits in normal development.

Molecular Genetics Findings

In a recent collaboration with Dean Hamer at the National Institutes of Health, we have examined the molecular genetic basis of individual differences in temperament and social behavior in these four cohorts of children. In addition to the behavioral and physiological findings already noted, 244 (108 males, 136 females) children, comprising the four cohorts who we have been following as part of a larger longitudinal project, donated cheek cells that were subsequently genotyped. The genotyped data were examined in relation to behavioral and maternal report measures collected on the children during the preschool years. We were particularly interested in examining the associations of genes that regulate serotonin and dopamine with children's temperament and individual differences in social behaviors, given that these two key neurotransmitters have previously been implicated in individual differences in personality in adults (see chapters in this volume). Our study of the molecular genetics of child temperament and social behavior focuses on relevant candidate genes. The dopamine D4 receptor gene *(DRD4)*, which contains a functional repeated sequence polymorphism within its coding sequences, was originally studied for its role in personality traits related to novelty seeking. The initial two studies (Benjamin et al. 1996; Ebstein et al. 1996) found that adults with longer versions (6–8 repeats) self-reported higher novelty seeking scores compared with adults with shorter versions (2–5 repeats) of the coding sequence polymorphism. Dopamine has been implicated as a major neuromodulator of novelty seeking because of the role it plays in inducing euphoria in humans and approach behavior in animals (Cloninger 1987). The shorter alleles code for a receptor that is more efficient in binding dopamine compared with the larger alleles (see Plomin and Rutter 1998 for a review). Subsequently, the association between the DRD4 polymorphism and novelty seeking has been replicated in some populations (Ebstein et al. 1997; Noble et al. 1998; Ono et al. 1997; Strobel et al. 1999; Tomitaka et al. 1999). However, several other studies have found either no association (Gelernter et al. 1997; Goldman et al. 1996;

Jonsson et al. 1997; Pogue-Geile et al. 1998; Sander et al. 1997; Sullivan et al. 1998; Vandenbergh et al. 1997) or an association in the "wrong" direction relative to the initial reports (Malhotra et al. 1996).

The serotonin transporter gene was chosen as the second candidate locus for this study because of its role in anxiety-related personality traits in adults. Lesch et al. (1996) reported that adults carrying one or two copies of a short allele of a regulatory DNA sequence polymorphism in the serotonin transporter (5-HTTLPR) gene self-reported higher levels of neuroticism, anxiety, and depression compared with individuals homozygous for the long allele of this polymorphism. In vitro and in vivo expression studies have shown that the short allele leads to less gene transcription and protein production than does the long allele (Greenberg et al. 1999; Heils et al. 1996; Lesch et al. 1996; Little et al. 1998). Moreover, serotonin has been implicated as a major neurotransmitter of anxiety and withdrawal because of its effects on regulating mood and emotional states (see Westernberg et al. 1996 for a review). Subsequently the association between the serotonin transporter gene and anxiety-related states has been replicated in populations in the United States, Europe, Israel, and Japan, (e.g., Greenberg et al. 1999 and references therein), but still other studies have failed to find any association (Ball et al. 1997; Kumakiri et al. 1999).

There have been relatively few studies of the molecular genetics of complex human traits in children. Two recent studies (LaHoste et al. 1996; Swanson et al. 1998) noted an association of the DRD4 gene with attention-deficit/hyperactivity disorder (ADHD). Children with ADHD differed from controls in that the sevenfold repeat form of the DRD4 occurred more frequently in them than in the control group. Another recent study has noted a gene-gene interaction in determining neonatal temperament (Ebstein et al. 1998). Neonates with the short serotonin transporter promoter and who lack the long form of *DRD4* had a lower orientation score on the Brazelton Neonatal Assessment Scale compared with other neonates. In addition, a recent study (Auerbach et al. 2001) found that 1-month-old infants with seven-repeat *DRD4* allele showed less sustained attention and novelty preference than did infants without the seven-repeat *DRD4* allele.

To date, we have focused specifically on the associations of DRD4 and 5-hydroxytryptamine genes with behavior based largely upon the extant clinical and adult literatures implicating these genes in complex human traits (see chapters in this volume). We examined two questions: 1) is there an association of the DRD4 gene with bold/exuberant behavior and 2) is there an association of the serotonin transporter gene with shy/inhibited behavior?

We found modest support for the first hypothesis. We (Schmidt et al., in press) noted associations between the DRD4 receptor gene and a conceptually and statistically derived aggregate measure of exuberant behavior at age 4. The aggregate measure of exuberant behavior was derived using the sum of observed disruptive behavior (e.g., goofing-off) during peer play and problems with aggressive and delinquent behaviors as reported at age 4 by the subjects' mothers on the widely used Child Behavior Checklist (Achenbach and Edelbrock 1981). Children who scored high on the aggregate measure were likely to be impulsive—high in sensation seeking and novelty seeking behaviors. Children with long instead of short allelic repeats of the DRD4 receptor gene scored significantly higher on the aggregate measure of exuberant behavior at age 4. Overall, this finding is consistent with other studies in which relations between the DRD4 receptor gene and novelty seeking have been noted in adults (e.g., Benjamin et al. 1996; Ebstein et al. 1996) and suggests that children carrying the long version of the *DRD4* allele may be at risk for externalizing-related problems during the school-age years.

We did not find support for the second hypothesis. Contrary to our prediction, there was no significant association between the serotonin transporter gene and shy behavior in children at age 4. Here, we computed a conceptually and empirically derived aggregate measure of shyness at age 4. This aggregate measure comprised onlooking and unoccupied behaviors during free play with unfamiliar same age and gender peers plus a Child Behavior Checklist report of social problems. These behaviors are analogous to the anxious behaviors noted in studies of adults—studies that found an association between the serotonin transporter gene and anxiety.

A third question that we have recently begun to address concerns the role of the DRD4 gene in attention. Emerging evidence suggests a link between DRD4 and attention-related problems in children clinically diagnosed with ADHD (LaHoste et al. 1996; Swanson et al. 1998). Given the critical role that sustaining attention plays in the regulation of behavior and ultimately personality development, we were particularly interested in knowing whether there was an association of DRD4 with attention-related problems in normally developing children. We have found support for this hypothesis. We (Schmidt et al. 2001) have most recently noted an association of the DRD4 gene with attention problems in children. Children with long rather than short allelic repeats of the DRD4 gene scored significantly higher on attention problems at ages 4 and 7 (Table 13–1). This is consistent with recent work by LaHoste et al. (1996) and Swanson et al. (1998) with children diagnosed with ADHD and extends their data to attention problems in normally developing children, suggesting that DRD4 may play a role in a continuous range of attentional processes rather than a discrete category such as ADHD. This finding is also consistent with recent work that has implicated the long rather than short allelic repeats of the DRD4 gene in the ability of 1-month-old human infants to exhibit sustained attention to novel stimuli (Auerbach et al. 2000).

Conclusions

A major component of our research program has been devoted to understanding the origins of temperamental differences in normal childhood development. We have noted at least two temperamental types of children: shy/socially withdrawn and bold/exuberant. The origins of these two temperamental categories appear linked to infant reactivity. Given 1) the early appearance of these behavioral and physiological patterns, 2) their stability across development, 3) the substantive evidence for their importance from comparative, behavioral, and physiological studies, and 4) the emerging molecular genetics data reviewed in this chapter, the possibility is raised that there may be a genetic basis to some tempera-

Table 13–1   Differences between short and long DRD4 genotype on Child Behavior Checklist attention problems at ages 4 and 7 in normal children

Measure	DRD4 short group	DRD4 long group
	Age 4	
Z score Child Behavior Checklist attention problems	−0.14 (n = 97)	0.21 (n = 64)
	Age 7	
	−0.15 (n = 67)	0.25 (n = 40)

Source. Adapted from Schmidt et al. 2001.

mental features. Because genes stay the same while environment changes, the type of longitudinal studies described in this chapter may be useful to identify and analyze other genes and gene-gene combinations involved in normal variation in personality development, childhood behavioral problems, and ultimately psychiatric diseases.

References

Achenbach TM, Edelbrock CS: Behavioral problems and competencies reported by parents of normal and disturbed children aged four through sixteen. Monogr Soc Res Child Dev 46(1, serial no. 188):1–82, 1981

Auerbach JG, Benjamin J, Faroy M, et al: DRD4 related to infant attention and information processing: a developmental link to ADHD? Psychiatr Genet 11:31–35, 2001

Ball D, Hill L, Freeman B, et al: The serotonin transporter gene and peer-related neuroticism. Neuroreport 8:1301–1304, 1997

Benjamin J, Li L, Patterson C, et al: Population and familial association between D4 dopamine receptor gene and measures of novelty seeking. Nat Genet 12:81–84, 1996

Blizard DA: Analysis of stress susceptibility using the Maudsley reactive and non-reactive strains, in Coping With Uncertainty: Behavioral and Developmental Perspectives. Edited by Palermo DS. Hillsdale, NJ, Erlbaum, 1989, pp 75–99

Calkins SD, Fox NA, Marshall TR: Behavioral and physiological antecedents of inhibited and uninhibited behavior. Child Dev 67:523–540, 1996

Cloninger CR: A systematic method for clinical description and classification of personality variants. Arch Gen Psychiatry 44:573–588, 1987

Cloninger CR, Adolfsson R, Svrakic NM: Mapping genes for human personality. Nat Genet 12:3–4, 1996

DiLalla LF, Kagan J, Reznick JS: Genetic etiology of behavioral inhibition among 2-year-old children. Infant Behavior and Development 17:405–412, 1994

Ebstein RP, Novick O, Umansky R, et al: Dopamine D4 receptor (D4DR) exon III polymorphism associated with the human personality trait of novelty seeking. Nat Genet 12:78–80, 1996

Ebstein RP, Nemanov L, Klotz I, et al: Additional evidence for an association between the dopamine D4 receptor (D4DR) exon III repeat polymorphism and the human personality trait of novelty seeking. Mol Psychiatry 2:472–477, 1997

Ebstein RP, Levine J, Geller V, et al: Dopamine D4 receptor and serotonin transporter promoter in the determination of neonatal temperament. Mol Psychiatry 3:238–246, 1998

Fox NA, Calkins SD, Bell MA: Neural plasticity and development in the first two years of life: evidence from cognitive and socioemotional domains of research. Dev Psychopathol 6:677–696, 1994

Fox NA, Rubin KH, Calkins SD, et al: Frontal activation asymmetry and social competence at four years of age. Child Dev 66:1770–1784, 1995

Fox NA, Henderson HA, Rubin KH, et al: Stability and instability of behavioral inhibition and exuberance: psychophysiological and behavioral factors influencing change and continuity across the first four years of life. Child Dev 72:1–21, 2001

Gelernter J, Kranzler H, Coccaro E, et al: D4 dopamine-receptor (DRD4) alleles and novelty seeking in substance-dependent, personality-disorder, and control subjects. Am J Hum Genet 61:1144–1152, 1997

Goldman D, Malhotra A, Urbanek M, et al: The dopamine DRD2 and DRD4 receptors: lack of association to alcoholism, substance abuse and novelty seeking in Finnish Caucasians and southwestern American Indians (abstract). Psychiatric Genetics Abstracts 6:162, 1996

Greenberg BD, Tolliver TJ, Huang S-J, et al: Genetic variation in the serotonin transporter promoter region affects serotonin uptake in human blood platelets. Am J Med Genet 88:83–87, 1999

Heils A, Teufel A, Petri S, et al: Allelic variation of human serotonin transporter gene expression. J Neurochem 66:2621–2624, 1996

Jonsson EG, Nothen MM, Gustavsson JP, et al: Lack of evidence for allelic association between personality traits and the dopamine D4 receptor gene polymorphisms. Am J Psychiatry 154:697–699, 1997

Kumakiri C, Kodama K, Shimizu E, et al: Study of the association between the serotonin transporter gene regulatory region polymorphism and personality traits in a Japanese population. Neurosci Lett 263:205–207, 1999

LaHoste GJ, Swanson JM, Wigal SB, et al: Dopamine D4 receptor gene polymorphism is associated with attention deficit hyperactivity disorder. Mol Psychiatry 1:121–124, 1996

Lesch KP, Bengel D, Heils A, et al: Association of anxiety-related traits with a polymorphism in the serotonin transporter gene regulatory region. Science 274:1527–1531, 1996

Little KY, McLaughlin DP, Zhang L, et al: Cocaine, ethanol, and genotype effects on human midbrain serotonin transporter binding sites and mRNA levels. Am J Psychiatry 155:207–213, 1998

Malhotra AK, Virkkunen M, Rooney W, et al: The association between the dopamine D4 receptor (D4DR) 16 amino acid repeat polymorphism and novelty seeking. Mol Psychiatry 1:388–391, 1996

Noble EP, Ozkaragoz TZ, Ritchie TL, et al: D2 and D4 dopamine receptor polymorphisms and personality. Am J Med Genet 81:257–267, 1998

Ono Y, Manki H, Yoshimura K, et al: Association between dopamine D4 receptor (D4DR) exon III polymorphism and novelty seeking in Japanese subjects. Am J Med Genet 74:501–503, 1997

Plomin R, Rutter M: Child development, molecular genetics, and what to do with genes once they are found. Child Dev 69:1223–1242, 1998

Pogue-Geile M, Ferrell R, Deka R, et al: Human novelty-seeking personality traits and dopamine D4 receptor polymorphisms: a twin and genetic association study. Am J Med Genet 81:44–48, 1998

Sander T, Harms H, Dufeu P, et al: Dopamine D4 receptor exon III alleles and variation of novelty seeking in alcoholics. Am J Med Genet 74:483–487, 1997

Schmidt LA, Fox NA: Fear-potentiated startle responses in temperamentally different human infants. Dev Psychobiol 32:113–120, 1998

Schmidt LA, Fox NA, Rubin KH, et al: Behavioral and neuroendocrine responses in shy children. Dev Psychobiol 30:127–140, 1997

Schmidt LA, Fox NA, Hu S, et al: Association of dopamine D4 receptor (DRD4) gene with attention problems in normal childhood development. Psychiatr Genet 11:25–29, 2001

Schmidt LA, Fox NA, Rubin KH, et al: Molecular genetics of shyness and aggression in preschoolers. Personality and Individual Differences (in press)

Strobel A, Wehr A, Michel A, et al: Association between the dopamine D4 receptor (DRD4) exon III polymorphism and measures of novelty seeking in a German population. Mol Psychiatry 4:378–384, 1999

Sullivan PF, Fifield WJ, Kennedy MA, et al: No association between novelty seeking and the type 4 dopamine receptor gene (DRD4) in two New Zealand samples. Am J Psychiatry 155:98–101, 1998

Swanson JM, Sunohara GA, Kennedy JL, et al: Association of the dopamine receptor D4 (DRD4) gene with a refined phenotype of attention deficit hyperactivity disorder (ADHD): a family based approach. Mol Psychiatry 3:38–41, 1998

Tomitaka M, Tomitaka S, Otuka Y, et al: Association between novelty seeking and dopamine receptor D4 (DRD4) exon III polymorphism in Japanese subjects. Am J Med Genet 88:469–471, 1999

Vandenbergh DJ, Zonderman AB, Wang J, et al: No association between novelty seeking and dopamine D4 receptor (D4DR) exon III seven repeat alleles in Baltimore Longitudinal Study of Aging participants. Mol Psychiatry 2:417–419, 1997

Westernberg HG, Murphy DL, Den Boer JA (eds): Advances in the Neurobiology of Anxiety Disorders. New York, Wiley, 1996

CHAPTER FOURTEEN

Genetics of Sexual Behavior

Dean H. Hamer, Ph.D.

Human sexual behavior is wondrously variable. Probably no two people on the planet have exactly the same sexual desires, much less the same notion of how to consummate them. People differ greatly in terms of how frequently they have sex, how many different sexual partners they have had, and whether they prefer to have sex with members of the opposite sex, the same sex, or both.

Such individual differences in sexual behavior have many different causes. Some differences are purely cultural, others are due to particular circumstances, and yet others are developmental. However, some individual differences in sexual thoughts and behaviors appear to be more intrinsic to the individual.

Might a person's sexual preferences and peculiarities be influenced by heredity? In order to explore that possibility, researchers in our laboratory have been taking a molecular genetic approach to human sexual behavior. This chapter describes research on three candidate genes for human sexual behavior: a locus on the X chromosome that appears to be involved in male sexual orientation in some families; a dopamine receptor gene that may be related to sexual partner diversity; and the serotonin receptor gene, which appears to play a role in the frequency of sexual behavior. Portions of this material have appeared elsewhere (Hamer and Copeland 1994; LeVay and Hamer 1994).

Sexual Orientation

Most men are sexually attracted to women, whereas most women are sexually attracted to men. However, a significant minority of individuals prefer members of the same sex, and many others are drawn, to varying degrees, to both males and females (Bell et al. 1981; Kinsey et al. 1948, 1953). Attitudes to homo- and bisexuality have varied throughout history. It is only within the last few decades that scientists have begun to empirically explore the origins of sexual orientation using the tools of modern neurobiology and genetics.

My own laboratory's interest in sexual orientation began in 1992 as part of a study on risk factors for certain cancers that are more frequent in HIV-infected gay men. As we began to collect data, we soon realized that the men and their families would be a useful resource for examining the role of genes in sexual orientation. Because our cancer study focused on gay men, our initial studies were restricted to males (Hamer and Copeland 1994).

Previous twin and family tree studies consistently pointed in a genetic direction. Since 1985, six systematic studies on the twins and siblings of gay men have been reported (reviewed in LeVay and Hamer 1994). The pooled data show that approximately 57% of identical twins, 24% of fraternal twins, and 13% of brothers of gay men are also gay. By comparing this data to baseline rates of homosexuality, Bailey and colleagues calculated that the heritability of male sexual orientation—that proportion of the variance in the trait that comes from genetic variation—is roughly 50%. This considerable and yet incomplete genetic influence is typical of complex personality and behavioral traits (Bailey and Pillard 1991; Hamer and Copeland 1994).

We therefore initiated a family history study. Our survey included 114 extended families, 72 from random probands and 38 from gay sib-pair probands. Our data confirmed the sibling results of Pillard and Weinrich (1985). The brother of a randomly selected gay man had a 14% likelihood of being gay as compared with 2% for men without gay brothers. (The low baseline rate was due to the stringent definition of homosexuality used in this study.) Among more distant relatives, an unexpected pattern showed up. Maternal uncles had a 7% chance of being gay, sons of maternal aunts had an 8% chance, but all other male relatives including fathers, paternal uncles and other types of cousins had just the average rate. Moreover, in families selected on the basis of having two gay brothers, the rates of homosexuality increased to 10% in maternal uncles and 13% in cousins through a maternal aunt. This familial clustering, even in relatives outside the nuclear family, presents an additional argument for a genetic component to male sexual orientation (Hamer et al. 1993).

Why are most of the gay male relatives of gay men on the mother's side of the family? As a geneticist, the most obvious and interesting possibility is X chromosome linkage. Because males always inherit their X chromosome from their mother, any trait influenced by a gene on the X chromosome tends to be inherited through the mother's side and is preferentially observed in brothers, maternal uncles, and maternal cousins, which was exactly the observed pattern. An alternative possibility, that subjects somehow knew more about their maternal relatives, could be excluded because the lesbian relatives of gay male probands were equally distributed between both sides of the family. However, other possible explanations, such as female-specific cultural transmission, could not be ruled out by the family history method alone. It was therefore essential to look at DNA.

Because we had no strong candidate genes for sexual orientation, we elected to use the linkage approach. Linkage analysis is based on two principles. First, if a trait is genetically influenced, then relatives who share the trait share the gene more often than expected by chance, even if the gene plays only a small part. Second, genes that are close together on a chromosome are almost always inherited together. Therefore, if there is a gene that influences sexual orientation, it should be linked to a nearby DNA marker that tends to travel along with it in families.

We decided to conduct the linkage analysis on nuclear families with two gay sons. One advantage of this "trait expressing sib-pair method" is that individuals who say they are gay are unlikely to be mistaken. By contrast, individuals who identify as heterosexual might actually have a same-sex orientation but not realize it yet, or simply not want to acknowledge it because of the continuing social stigmatization of homosexuality. A second advantage of the method is that it is independent of penetrance. Therefore, it is especially useful for detecting a single linked gene even when other genes or nongenetic factors are involved.

Our first study involved 40 families with two gay brothers. Because we wanted to focus on the role of the X chromosome in males, families with obvious paternal or nonmale transmission or with multiple lesbians were excluded from the study. DNA samples were prepared from the gay brothers and, where possible, their mothers and sisters. The samples were typed for 22 markers that span the X chromosome from the tip of the short arm to the end of the long arm. At each marker, a pair of brothers was scored as concordant if they inherited identical marker alleles from their mother or as discordant if they inherited different ones. Fifty percent of the alleles were expected to be identical by chance. Statistical corrections were made for the possibility of the mother having two copies of the same marker.

The results of this study were striking (Hamer et al. 1993). Over most of the X chromosome the markers were randomly distributed between the gay brothers. But at the tip of the long arm, in region Xq28, there was a considerable excess of concordant brothers: 33 pairs shared the same markers whereas only 7 pairs did not. Although the sample size was small, the result was statistically significant ($P = 0.00001$).

When this study was published in *Science* in 1993 (Hamer et al. 1993), it caused quite a stir. Most of the controversy concerned the political and social implications of the study, but there were two legitimate questions about the science: could the results be replicated, and what was the status of the locus in heterosexual men? To answer these questions, we collected a new group of families with two gay brothers, and this time obtained DNA from all available heterosexual brothers as well. The new study replicated the finding of excess DNA marker sharing in the Xq28 region. This time 22 out of 32 pairs, or 67%, shared alleles. Two independent statisticians examined the data in detail and concluded that there was significant linkage to Xq28 ($P = 0.04$) and that the results of the first and second studies were indistinguishable (Hu et al. 1995).

Examination of the families with heterosexual brothers also gave the expected result. Most of them had different DNA markers than their gay siblings. Our statistical experts estimated that the degree of DNA sharing of the straight brothers with the gay brothers was 22%, significantly less than the 50% expected by chance ($P < 0.05$). This was an independent confirmation that Xq28 was involved in sexual orientation, and strengthened the overall linkage findings ($P = 0.004$).

Since 1995, two other groups of researchers have conducted linkage studies of male sexual orientation. Sanders and colleagues performed an X chromosome linkage analysis of 54 pairs of gay brothers. They found 66% Xq28 allele sharing, which had a significance level of $P = 0.04$ (Sanders et al. 1998). Sander's results were indistinguishable from our replication study (Hu et al. 1995) both in terms of the degree of allele sharing (66% vs. 67%) and the precise chromosomal location of maximum sharing (locus DXS1108). By contrast, Rice and colleagues, working in Canada, studied 52 pairs of gay brothers and found no evidence for linkage to Xq28; they reported approximately 46% allele sharing, a nonsignificant result (Rice et al. 1999).

Given the modest sample sizes of the above studies, the most accurate estimate of Xq28 linkage can be obtained by combining the data from each of the four data sets. This meta-analysis gives an estimated level of allele sharing of 64%, which is significant at the $P = 0.0001$ level (Figure 14–1). Basically the same result is obtained if one discards the highest and lowest reported allele sharing values and uses only the Hu et al. (1995) and Sanders et al. (1998) data, which gives estimated allele sharing of 66% at a significance level of $P = 0.001$. A 64% allele sharing level corresponds to an S value of 1.4, where S is the ratio for homosexual orientation in the brothers of a gay index subject, as compared with the population fre-

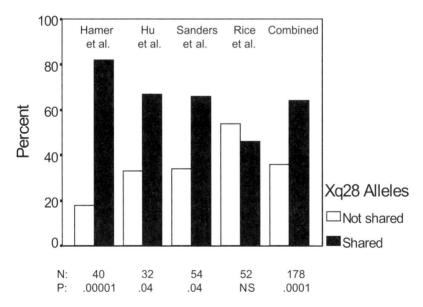

Figure 14–1   Summary of linkage studies of male sexual orientation and X chromosome DNA markers. The percentage of Xq28 allele sharing in four studies of gay male sib pairs is shown. Meta-analysis (last set of columns) shows overall estimated allele sharing of 64% at a significance level of 0.0001. N = sample size. P = statistical significance.

quency that is attributable to a gene in this region. This modest level of influence is typical for the effect of a single locus on a complex behavioral trait such as sexual orientation.

What might be the pertinent differences between the work of Rice et al. (1999) and the previous three studies, which did find linkage (Hamer et al. 1993; Hu et al. 1995; Sanders et al. 1998)? One possibility is derived from the fact that only 48 (26%) of the 182 families originally interviewed for the Rice et al. (1999) study were actually studied at the DNA level. Apparently the subset of genotyped families was not a representative subset of the starting population because they displayed an excess of paternal rather than maternal gay relatives, which was exactly the opposite pattern found in the total data set. One would not logically expect such a non-representative subset of the families to display any X-chromosome linkage.

A second possible explanation for the failure of Rice et al. (1999) to observe linkage is the modest statistical power of their sample. A population of 52 sib pairs has 65% power to detect 64% allele sharing at the 0.05 level of significance; thus there was a 35% chance that Rice et al. would have failed to detect linkage simply by chance.

A third consideration is the lack of defined criteria for homosexuality in the article by Rice et al. (1999). Instead of using objective criteria, such as Kinsey scale scores, Rice et al. depended on the investigator's judgement, in some cases based on a single question to the research subject.

A final difference between the linkage studies is that Rice et al. (1999) did not methodically exclude families inconsistent with the hypothesis of X chromosome linkage. The use of defined inclusion and exclusion criteria to select appropriate families for the study of a putative X-linked locus was a key feature of our two studies. Indeed, Hu et al. (1995) showed that families that did not meet the defined inclusion criteria failed to show linkage to Xq28. It is therefore not surprising that Rice et al. were able to find a subgroup of families that did not display linkage. The idea that *every* instance of homosexual orientation is due to Xq28 is nothing but a straw man hypothesis.

In summary, a meta-analysis of all available DNA linkage data supports a modest but significant role of the Xq28 region in male sexual orientation. We do not think that Xq28 is the only source of genetic variability in male sexual orientation; indeed, we are currently conducting a genomewide search for additional loci that may contribute to this complex phenotype. We also understand very little about female sexual orientation; we did not find any linkage to Xq28 in lesbian sisters, and there is currently some question about the degree to which female orientation is genetically influenced (Hamer and Copeland 1994; Pattatucci and Hamer 1995). Finally, and most importantly, we have no idea what type of proteins are coded for by the Xq28 region; our understanding of sexual orientation ultimately depends on the identification of functionally relevant polymorphisms in molecularly defined genes rather than on the purely statistical evidence afforded by linkage analysis. Only when the actual genes are identified will it begin to be possible to trace the undoubtedly complex pathways from a person's genes and proteins to the direction of their sexual desire.

Partner Number and Diversity

There is tremendous variability in the number of sexual partners that men have or would like to have. The typical American man has six sexual partners over a lifetime. However, some men have none or one, and others claim as many as 20,000. Is there any genetic basis to this variability, and if so what are the genes?

An important clue for our research came from studying personality, specifically the trait of novelty seeking. Having a varied sex life is one way for high novelty seekers, also known as thrill seekers, (see Chapter 10, Genetics of Sensation Seeking) to satisfy their need for change and variety. Zuckerman and colleagues studied college students during the so-called sexual revolution during the early 1970s. High novelty seekers said it was fine to have intercourse with someone they just met, even if they weren't sure they liked each other. Low thrill seekers were more likely to endorse sex only when deeply in love and preferably married. Novelty seeking even affected the type of sex people have. For example, in Zuckerman's college survey, high and low novelty seekers were about equally likely to engage in kissing, but the high thrill seekers were much more likely to engage in oral sex and positions other than missionary style (Hamer and Copeland 1994; reviewed in Zuckerman 1994).

This information led us to hypothesize that genes involved in novelty seeking would influence sexual partner diversity. We had an opportunity to test this idea in 1995 when Ebstein and colleagues discovered an association between a coding sequence polymorphism in the dopamine D4 receptor gene and the Novelty Seeking scale of the Tridimensional Personality Questionnaire (Ebstein et al. 1996). Specifically, they found that individuals carrying the seven-repeat allele of a 48-bp variable number of tandem repeats sequence in exon III of the DRD4 gene had average Novelty Seeking scores that were approximately 0.5 standard deviations higher than individuals carrying only the more common four-repeat version of the gene. Although this was exciting news, the evidence was less than completely convincing. For one thing, this study looked at only one group of rather modest size ($N = 124$). A more serious concern was the possibility of population stratification, that is, that the subject population included ethnic or racial subgroups that just happened to have different variations of the gene and different levels of novelty seeking.

In the hope of overcoming these limitations, we attempted to replicate their findings by studying the association of the DRD4 gene with personality traits in a population of 315 U.S. subjects, most of whom were members of sibling pairs (Benjamin et al. 1996). We used this design so that we could measure association both in the population at large and in siblings with different forms of the gene. This discordant sib-paired t-test is a test of linkage and association that is immune to population stratification. This was the first description of using sib pairs to test for linkage and association in a manner analogous to the use of parent-child trios in the transmission disequilibrium test. Subsequently, several different statistical techniques for using sib pairs in this way have been described, but all of them use the same basic strategy of analyzing genotype-discordant pairs.

Because we did not have Tridimensional Personality Questionnaire (Cloninger 1991) data on these subjects, we estimated novelty seeking scores by regression analysis of their data for a different personality instrument, the NEO Personality Inventory, Revised (Costa and McCrae 1992). When the calculations were complete, the results were supportive of Ebstein et al.'s (1996) findings. Individuals with long alleles of the DRD4 gene (more than five repeats) scored on average 0.4 standard deviations higher for estimated novelty seeking scores than did individuals with short versions of the gene, which is a statistically significant difference. Importantly, the effect of the gene was just as large when the comparison was made between siblings with different forms of the gene as when it was made between unrelated individuals, which indicated that the observed association was not due to population stratification (Benjamin et al. 1996). Subsequent attempts to replicate the association between DRD4 and novelty seeking have given variable results (reviewed in Chapter 5, *DRD4* and Novelty Seeking); however, there appears to be a more consistent association to the presumably related trait of attention deficit disorder (Chapter 13, Molecular Genetics of Temperamental Differences in Children).

Given that an association between the DRD4 gene and novelty seeking was observed in the particular population we were studying, we could ask an interesting question: does the dopamine receptor gene influence sexual partner diversity? Fortunately, we had obtained detailed sexual histories on many of the participants of the study, including both sexual orientation and their lifetime number of male and female partners. We found that men with different forms of the gene had different numbers of sexual partners, but in an unexpected way (Figure 14–2).

Looking first at the heterosexual men in the study, those with a long allele of the DRD4 gene (the form associated with high novelty seeking) had slightly more female partners than those with the short form, but the difference was small and not significant. Although these subjects classified themselves as heterosexual, some of them had had sex with another man, usually just once when they were young. In these cases the DRD4 gene had a strong and statistically significant effect ($P = 0.008$). Heterosexual men with a long allele (the form associated with high novelty seeking) were sixfold more likely to have had sex with another man than those

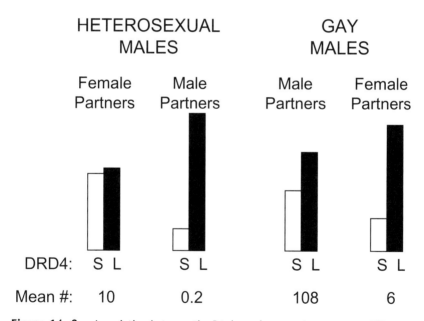

Figure 14–2 Association between the D4 dopamine receptor gene exon III polymorphism and number of sexual partners. Shown are the relative numbers of male and female sexual partners of heterosexual and homosexual males with either short or long DRD4 genes ($N = 251$). For genotyping details see Benjamin et al. (1996). DRD4: S indicates short/short exon III genotypes; L indicates long/short and long/long exon III genotypes. Mean # = average number of indicated gender of sexual partners for subjects of both genotypes.

who were homozygous for the short form. About half of the subjects with the long gene had ever had a male sexual partner compared with only 8% of those with the short gene.

Just the converse was true for gay men. As expected, the gay men had far more male partners than the heterosexual men did female partners; most of the subjects in this study were middle aged, and thus had begun their sexual careers prior to the AIDS epidemic. For these subjects, the main effect of the DRD4 gene was the number of female partners. Gay men with a long allele (the form associated with high novelty seeking) had sex with more than five times as many woman as men carrying only short alleles, a significant difference ($P = 0.02$). Although many of these men may have had sex with women in part because of social pressures, it appears that a desire for novel experiences also played a role. The long allele was also associated with having more male partners, but the difference was less pronounced.

These results suggest that the DRD4 gene does influence male sexual behavior, but indirectly, through personality, rather than directly. For a heterosexual man, sex with another man is considered very novel. For a gay man, sex with a woman is equally unique. The gene is not important as to whether people prefer males or females, but rather whether they like novelty.

Frequency

Different people have different ideas about how much sex is enough. Some people never have sex during their whole lives, whereas for others once a day is barely enough. Most of us fall somewhere in between these two extremes.

How often a person has sex depends on many variables, and the frequency also changes. Most people have more sex when they are younger than when they are older, and when they have a partner than when they are single. Despite the popular notion of "swinging singles," married people have the most sex; about 40% of married people have sex twice a week compared with 25% of singles. For married couples, frequency tends to decrease over time, but on the other hand, bursts of sexual activity can occur at any stage of a relationship, such as during vacations. But despite changes that occur as a person ages, marries, divorces, or has periods of stress, the level of sex drive is a relatively stable part of a person's makeup. Might it have a genetic component?

In this case, serotonin was the logical neurotransmitter to examine. Experiments in rats showed that alteration of serotonin transmission can cause hypersexuality. In humans, the best evidence came from side effects of the drug Prozac, which is a specific serotonin reuptake inhibitor. Although Prozac is a popular and effective antidepressant, it does have a negative side effect in some individuals: it can inhibit sexuality. A significant fraction of people taking the drug report a loss of sexual desire. In men, Prozac's effect is not just psychological; it may also cause trouble getting erections or ejaculating.

Once again, we had a logical gene to look at: the serotonin transporter gene. The serotonin transporter regulates the brain's supply of serotonin by sopping up excess neurotransmitter from the space between nerve cells. We had previously found that a common DNA sequence polymorphism in the control region for the serotonin transporter gene (5-HTTLPR) influences how well the gene works in people. The evidence came from both biochemical experiments and from analyzing the effect of the gene on personality; people with a poorly expressed version of the gene had increased levels of anxiety, depression, and other traits typically associated with serotonin (Lesch et al. 1996). This effect of the serotonin transporter gene polymorphism on personality has now been replicated in many different populations using a variety of personality measures (Greenberg et al. 2000; see also Chapter 6, Serotonin Transporter, Personality, and Behavior).

The obvious question was whether the serotonin transporter gene influences sexual desire. It was fairly easy to use our male research subjects to compare frequency of sex with the version of the gene. There was a significant correlation: men with the poorly expressed short genotype had sex more often than those with the better-expressed long genotype (Figure 14–3). When the population was divided into two types of men— those who have sex once or more a week and those who have sex less than once a week—there was a clear-cut relationship to genotype. Approximately two-thirds of the short genotype group were in the frequent sex category compared with one-third of the long genotype group, a highly significant difference ($P = 0.0004$). The effect of the gene on sexual frequency was even stronger when age, education level, ethnic group, and sexual orientation were statistically corrected for ($P = 0.0002$). To make sure that the observed association was not an artifact of population stratification, the analysis was also performed on sib pairs, and again there was a significant difference between subjects with the short and long genotypes ($P = 0.008$). Of course there were many exceptions to the rule

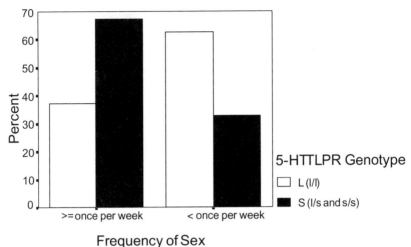

Figure 14–3 Association between the serotonin transporter gene promoter polymorphism and frequency of sex. Shown are the relative proportions of men with short and long 5-HTTLPR genotypes having sex at least once a week or less than once a week (*N* = 241). For genotyping details see Lesch et al. (1996). 5-HTTLPR genotype: L indicates long (l/l) genotypes; S indicates short (s/l and s/s) genotypes.

because the gene accounts for only a small portion of the variability in sexual frequency, just as it does for anxiety and depression.

Do people with the short gene have more sex because they are anxious, perhaps to relieve stress? This appears not to be the case; there was no significant correlation between anxiety and sexual frequency in this population. Furthermore the association between the serotonin transporter gene polymorphism and sexual frequency remained just as strong after statistically correcting for personality scores. The serotonin transporter must be influencing personality and sexuality by independent routes, which is not surprising given the many different functions and localizations of serotonin in the brain.

The role of the serotonin transporter gene in sexual frequency solves an interesting riddle. Namely, why should nature burden approximately half of the human population with a genetic polymorphism that causes people to feel sad, worried, and even miserable? The answer is that evolution couldn't care less about how you feel. As long as you are having sex and passing on the gene, it survives.

Sexual Science

Our work on the genetics of male sexual orientation was one of the first attempts to identify specific DNA sequences involved in a normal variation in human behavior. When the linkage results were announced in 1993, many people seemed shocked that such a complex trait might be swayed by genes. To biologists, however, the results came as no surprise. Because sex is the way that genes are passed from one generation to the next, sexual behavior must certainly be under very intense natural selection and therefore have a substantial genetic component. And because the human genome is highly variable, individual differences in sexual behavior are also likely to be based, at least in part, on genetic variability.

Indeed, there is no logical reason to think that sexual behavior in humans should be any less biologically or genetically influenced than in any other species. Although some critics contend that humans can think and make choices, therefore their sexual behavior is less hardwired than in other species, they overlook the obvious fact that our thinking devices are also constructed of and by gene products. One might even make the counterargument that precisely because we can think, we can control our own environment, and therefore our behavior should be even more genetically channeled. Suppose that a lab rat had the "gay gene"; he might prefer males to females, but if he were never placed in a cage with other males, he'd never have a chance to show it. By contrast, consider a human male with the "gay gene"; even if he were born into a strict family in a remote area, he would have the opportunity to overcome his environment when he grew up.

This is not the say that genes are the *only* determinants of human sexual behavior. The environment also plays an important role, as is most clearly demonstrated by the large changes in sexual attitudes and practices that have occurred over just the course of this century, a period far too short to accommodate any major changes in our genetic makeup. And certainly no individual gene can either predict or dictate a person's unique suite of sexual preferences and peculiarities. Each of the three loci discussed in this chapter account for only a fraction of the genetic variance, which in turn is only a portion of total variability.

What I find shocking is the continuing dearth of scientific research on the genetics of sexual behavior, or indeed on any aspect of human sexuality that is not directly related to reproduction or sexually transmitted disease. In the 7 years since our article on the genetics of male sexual orientation was published (Hamer et al. 1993), only three experimental studies of this topic have been undertaken, and only two of those were published. By contrast, in the 4 years since the publication of the article on the serotonin transporter gene and anxiety (Lesch et al. 1996), more than 100 studies examining role of this gene on various aspects of personality, behavior, and psychopathology have been published. Anxiety is not any more important or any easier to study than sexuality; but perhaps sexuality is still considered too private, too controversial, and too embarrassing to be studied scientifically.

Within the next few years, we will know the complete sequence of the human genome and the 100,000 or so genes it contains. It can confidently be predicted that many of these genes—perhaps more than half—will be involved in the development and functioning of the brain and therefore in behavior. It also seems likely, judging from the information that our preliminary studies have revealed, that many of these genes either directly or indirectly influence sexuality, which from an evolutionary standpoint is one of the most important domains of behavior. It would be sad not to learn what these genes are doing for reasons as silly as embarrassment or prudery.

Acknowledgments

I am grateful to my friends Simon LeVay and Peter Copeland for their contributions to previously published portions of this article. I also thank the many talented colleagues who collaborated on the research described here, especially Stella Hu, Angela Pattatucci, and Chavis Patterson. This work would not have been possible without the interest and generosity of the many volunteers who participated in our research.

References

Bailey JM, Pillard RC: A genetic study of male sexual orientation. Arch Gen Psychiatry 48:1089–1096, 1991

Bell AP, Weinberg MS, Hammersmith SK: Sexual Preference: Its Development in Men and Women. Bloomington, Indiana University Press, 1981

Benjamin J, Li L, Patterson C, et al: Population and familial association between the D4 dopamine receptor gene and measures of novelty seeking. Nat Genet 12:81–84, 1996

Cloninger CR: The Tridimensional Personality Questionnaire: U.S. normative data. Psychol Rep 69:1047–1057, 1991

Costa P, McCrae R: Revised NEO Personality Inventory (NEO PI-R) and NEO Five Inventory (NEO-FFI) Professional Manual. Odessa, FL, Psychological Assessment Resources, 1992

Ebstein RP, Novick O, Umansky R, et al: Dopamine D4 receptor (D4DR) exon III polymorphism associated with the human personality trait of novelty seeking. Nat Genet 12:78–80, 1996

Greenberg BD, Li Q, Lucas F, et al: Association between the serotonin transporter promoter polymorphism and personality traits in a primarily female population sample. Am J Med Genet 96:202–216, 2000

Hamer DH, Copeland P: The Science of Desire. New York, Simon and Schuster, 1994

Hamer DH, Hu S, Magnuson VL, et al: A linkage between DNA markers on the X chromosome and male sexual orientation. Science 261:321–327, 1993

Hu S, Pattatucci AML, Patterson C, et al: Linkage between sexual orientation and chromosome Xq28 in males but not in females. Nat Genet 11:248–256, 1995

Kinsey AC, Pomeroy WB, Martin CE: Sexual Behavior in the Human Male. Philadelphia, PA, WB Saunders, 1948

Kinsey AC, Pomeroy WB, Martin CE, et al: Sexual Behavior in the Human Female. Philadelphia, PA, WB Saunders, 1953

Lesch KP, Bengel D, Heils A, et al: Association of anxiety-related traits with a polymorphism in the serotonin transporter gene regulatory region. Science 274:1527–1531, 1996

LeVay S, Hamer DH: Evidence for a biological influence in male homosexuality. Sci Am 270:44–49, 1994

Pattatucci AML, Hamer D: Development and familiality of sexual orientation in females. Behav Genet 25:407–420, 1995

Pillard RC, Weinrich JD: Evidence of familial nature of male homosexuality. Arch Gen Psychiatry 43:808–812, 1985

Rice G, Anderson C, Risch N, et al: Male homosexuality: absence of linkage to microsatellite markers at Xq28. Science 284:665–667, 1999

Sanders AR, Cao Q, Zhang J, et al: Genetic linkage study of male homosexual orientation. Poster presentation 149 at the annual meeting of the American Psychiatric Association, Toronto, ON, June 1998

Zuckerman M: Behavioral Expressions and Biosocial Bases of Sensation Seeking. Cambridge, UK, Cambridge University Press, 1994

CHAPTER FIFTEEN

From Phenotype to Gene and Back

A Critical Appraisal of Progress So Far

David Goldman, M.D.
Chiara Mazzanti, Ph.D.

It has been widely acknowledged that genetic research strategies are critical to an understanding of the etiology of genetically influenced psychiatric disorders and behavior. However, only recently have advances in DNA technology, statistical linkage methods, genome information, phenotype, and data set collection begun to make it possible to realize this widely recognized potential. For example, because of the multiyear timeframe of large genetic studies it is now worthwhile considering study designs suitable for a whole-genome linkage disequilibrium analysis, requiring many thousands of genetic markers, at the conclusion of data collection.

The purpose of this review is to critically summarize progress in identification of genes and gene variants that play crucial roles in human behaviors and common, severe behavioral diseases such as alcoholism, schizophrenia, and bipolar disorder. We see that in several cases the difficult step of proving the relationship of a DNA sequence variant to a complex behavioral trait has actually been completed (proven). On the other hand, the statistical and functional evidence is incomplete for numerous other linkages of genes to behavior, and at the opening of the new century these linkages may be regarded as probable, putative or possible (Table 15–1).

Table 15–1   Genes for human neuropsychiatric diseases and phenotypes by the candidate gene approach

Gene[a]	Protein	Disease or condition	
Proven			
ALDH2	ALDH2	Alcoholism	Harada et al. 1981
ADH2	ADH2	Alcoholism	Harada et al. 1981
APP	Amyloid precursor protein	Alzheimer's disease	Tanzi et al. 1992
PSEN1	Presenilin	Alzheimer's disease	Cruts and Van Broeckhoven 1998
MAOA	MAO A	Brunner syndrome	Brunner et al. 1993
HPRT1	HPRT	Lesch-Nyhan syndrome	Rossiter et al. 1991
Probable			
SLC6A4	5-HTT	Anxiety-related traits	Lesch et al. 1996
HTR2A	5-HT2A	Anorexia nervosa	Collier et al. 1997
		Anorexia nervosa	Enoch et al. 1998
		Obsessive-compulsive disorder	Enoch et al. 2001
COMT	COMT	Cognitive executive function	Egan et al. 2001
Putative			
TPH	TPH	Suicidality	Nielsen et al. 1994
HTR1B	5-HT1B	Antisocial alcoholism	Lappalainen et al. 1998
HTR2A	5-HT2A	Clozapine response	Arranz et al. 1998
HTR5A	5-HT5A	Schizophrenia	Iwata et al. 2001
SLC6A4	5-HTT	Psychosis/schizophrenia	Malhotra et al. 1998b; Hranilovic et al. 1999
DRD4	D4 receptor	Novelty seeking	Benjamin et al. 1996
		Attention-deficit/hyperactivity disorder	Faraone et al. 1999
SLC6A3	DAT	Attention-deficit/hyperactivity disorder	Cook et al. 1995
		Alcohol withdrawal	Sander et al. 1997
COMT	COMT	Obsessive-compulsive disorder	Karayiorgou et al. 1997
		Bipolar disorder	Kirov et al. 1998
		Aggressive behavior	Lachman et al. 1996, 1998
		Schizophrenia	Egan et al. 2001

MAOA	MAO A	Panic	Deckert et al. 1999
APOE	ApoE	Schizophrenia	Malhotra et al. 1998a
NPY	Neuropeptide Y	Obesity	Bray et al. 1999
		Obesity	Karvonen et al. 1998

Possible (partial listing)

SLC6A3	DAT	Tourette syndrome	Rowe et al. 1998
		Generalized anxiety	Rowe et al. 1998
DRD2	D2 receptor	Substance abuse	Goldman et al. 1997
		Obesity	Comings et al. 1996
		Alcoholism	Goldman et al. 1997
		Impulsive, addictive, and compulsive behavior	Blum et al. 1995
		Schizophrenia	Jonsson et al. 1999
DRD3	D3 receptor	Schizophrenia	Dubertret et al. 1998
DRD4	D4 receptor	Tourette syndrome	Comings et al. 1999
TH	Tyrosine hydroxylase	Schizophrenia	Meloni et al. 1995
		Bipolar disorder	Bellivier et al. 1998
HTR1B	5-HT1Dβ	Obsessive-compulsive disorder	Mundo et al. 1999
HTR2C	5-HT2C	Clozapine response	Sodhi et al. 1999
OPRM1	Opioid receptor μ	Opioid addiction	Kranzler et al. 1998
GABRA6	GABAA6	Benzodiazepine sensitivity	Iwata et al. 1999
CCKAR	Cholecystokinin receptor	Alcoholism	Harada et al. 1998
		Panic	Kennedy et al. 1999
ARSA	Arylsulfatase-A	Alcoholism	Ricketts et al. 1996
CALLA	Neutral endopeptidase	Attachment behavior	Huss et al. 1999
CCR5	Chemokine receptor	Schizophrenia	Malhotra et al. 1999
KCNN3	Calcium-activated potassium channel	Schizophrenia	Cardno et al. 1999
CHRNA7	α7 nicotinic receptor	Autism	Betancur et al. 1999
INPP1	Inositol polyphosphate 1-phosphatase	Lithium response	Lovlie et al. 1999
IMPA1	Myo-inositol monophosphatase 1	Bipolar disorder/schizophrenia	Birkett et al. 1999
ADRA2C	α2C adrenergic receptor	Cocaine abuse	Feng et al. 1999
PAX6	Paired box gene 6	Bipolar disorder	Okladnova et al. 1998a

The focus of this review is on candidate genes and candidate (functional) alleles, rather than on linkage findings to anonymous markers. This sequence and sequence-variation-oriented approach has become more salient because of the impending availability of the sequences of all human genes and the prospect of knowledge of their expression and function. As a result of methodological advances it is also now feasible to scan a set of genes for genetic variation across a large number of affected subjects, and in this way identify uncommon functional variants that contribute to a phenotype. The information on gene sequences, sequence variants, and function enables more specific targeting of studies on genetically influenced phenotypes toward the candidate genes and alleles that are most likely to be etiological. It also enables a more direct and rapid exploration of whole-genome linkage findings, which generally implicate broad regions of chromosomes.

Finally, it has become recognized that identification of specific gene variants in behavior has multiple potential implications, and that the divergent examples that are available teach us that we cannot extrapolate from any one example to the empirical outcome of genetic studies on each new phenotype. However, the overall impact of identification of genes in behavior is a scientific revolution in the study of brain and behavior in health and disease. Once a disease-causing allele is identified, 1) therapeutic drugs can be designed to target the gene, gene product, or biochemical pathway; 2) the disease may be redefined, with genetic markers serving as one new tool to identify subgroups that may differ in etiology, pathology, treatment response, and other aspects of prognosis; 3) genetic tests for vulnerability to the disease may be found; 4) new mechanisms in brain function and development may be identified through correlation of variation with function; and 5) the study of gene-environment interaction in behavior can essentially begin.

Gene Action Versus Phenotype

Almost all phenotypes reflect the concerted action of many genes, but complex genetic phenotypes reflect the action and environmental interaction of different alleles either alone (creating a pattern of genetic heterogeneity) or in concert (creating a pattern consistent with polygenicity). Unlike classical disease gene variants, which appear to act deterministically, many genes for complex behavioral disease are observed to act probabilistically. When important interactions of gene variant with gene variant and gene variant with environment have yet to be identified, or when the genetic phenotype has been imprecisely defined, causal genetic factors may be better understood as variance components. Later it may be recognized that a gene variant (say *ALDH2* Lys487) that was probabilistically related to a broadly defined phenotype (i.e., alcoholism) is deterministically related to a more precisely defined phenotype, or an *endophenotype* (i.e., alcohol-induced flushing) (reviewed by Gotteman and Erlenmeyer-Kimling 2001; see also Chapter 18, Genes for Human Personality Traits) that can also be thought of as an intermdiate phenotype.

Owing to genetic complexity, whether due to heterogeneity or polygenicity, methods are required that can identify genes responsible for a small component of the variance. There are essentially three options: 1) increase the variance component attributable to a particular gene by redefining (narrowing) the phenotype or by studying a genetic isolate or family in which phenotype-associated genetic variation is restricted; 2) collect a larger sample; and 3) use candidate gene and candidate (functional) allele approaches, which offer more power to detect small effects.

Positional Cloning (Reverse Genetics) in Psychiatry

A scientific revolution was initiated by the observation by White et al. (Botstein et al. 1980), that in principle the gene for any Mendelian trait might be chromosomally localized and positionally cloned through the use of a genetic map comprising a discrete number of genetic markers arrayed across the human genome. In 1980, these genetic markers were serological markers, enzyme polymorphisms, and restriction fragment length polymorphisms, a human beta-globin restriction fragment length polymorphism having been discovered by Kan et al. in 1978 (Kan et al. 1978). Positional cloning was immediately recognized as a potentially universal solution to the problem of gene identification: the analysis can be conducted with no prior biological clue to disease origin or chromosomal localization. An additional breakthrough was the rediscovery of sib-pair and affected-relative-pair comparisons as robust, nonparametric linkage approaches for instances in which the mode of genetic transmission was unknown. One result of these insights in mapping was that for the first time large genetic disease data sets suitable for whole-genome identity by descent linkage were collected for most of the major psychiatric diseases, for example, schizophrenia, bipolar disorder, alcoholism, and panic disorder.

The paradigmatic success stories for positional cloning were Huntington's disease (Gusella et al. 1993, 1996) and cystic fibrosis (Riordan et al. 1989). An increasing number of promising whole-genome linkage findings are under investigation in diverse psychiatric diseases, especially schizophrenia (Antonarakis et al. 1995; Kendler et al. 1996), bipolar disorder (Berrettini 1998), and alcoholism (Long et al. 1998; Williams et al. 1999). However, for psychiatric diseases and behavioral phenotypes, positional cloning is characterized by the very large genomic regions that have been identified and by failures to replicate statistically substantial linkages including bipolar disorder and schizophrenia (Owen and Craddock 1998; Shaw et al. 1998). Because of these failures, it was realized that the problems in this area included the need for rigorous methodology and criteria (Kruglyak 1999; McCarthy et al. 1998) and the low power of linkage analysis to detect genes of small effect (Risch and Teng 1998). However, because of the excitement created by the positional cloning approach, a series of large data sets were collected, which are foundational for candidate gene studies and linkage studies using new technology and information resources.

Association Studies: Forward Genetics

The vast majority of disease genes have been identified through a careful consideration of physiology, pharmacology, and biochemical clues and comparison of cases and controls at the genes implicated. For the brain, new targets are arising at an increasing rate because of whole-genome sequencing (Normile and Pennisi 1999), large-scale detection of sequence variation (Cargill et al. 1999; Cravchik and Goldman 2000; Haluska et al. 1999), comprehensive mapping and expression studies of genes in brain, and new methods for multiplex analysis of gene expression (Eisen and Brown 1999), including expression studies at the single-cell level (O'Dell et al. 1999). This discussion on the application of these findings in the candidate gene/allele approach joins other perspectives on progress and pitfalls in the association approach (Malhotra et al. 1999). Case-control comparisons are also a final common pathway for positional cloning studies when a gene is successfully identified. From a genetic perspective, the essential difference between positional cloning and association studies using candidate genes and candidate (functional) alleles is that association studies are identity-by-state analyses. A test of association of a candidate allele to a phenotype is typical hypothesis testing in that the independent variable is genotype and the dependent variable is phenotype.

If the allele is nonfunctional, association may be due to linkage disequilibrium of the marker allele with a functional allele elsewhere. Indeed large-scale disequilibrium mapping prospectively offers a finer-scale version of the whole-genome positional cloning approach (Risch and Merikangas 1993, 1996). The linkage disequilibrium approach has the potential to identify ancestral chromosomes on which specific alleles were introduced to populations via mutation or migration. A method for objective phylogenetically informed analysis of combinations of linked genetic markers has been introduced by Templeton and colleagues (Templeton et al. 1987), and such cladistic association approaches will be increasingly applied across combinations of linked loci (Kittles et al. 1999). In addition, it has become recognized that linkage varies greatly in strength across populations and is highest and found across larger chromosomal regions in recently admixed populations (Dean et al. 1994). Differences between populations in linkage disequilibrium relationships (Goldman et al. 1993) imply that associations to nonfunctional genetic markers may be particularly vulnerable to nonreplication in other populations.

As in all hypotheses testing, Type I errors (false positive) and Type II errors (false negative) occur in case-control comparisons. It has come to be recognized that the likelihood of these errors can be predicted through a consideration of sample size, expected effect size of genotype on phenotype, genotype frequency, and the number of hypotheses tested. Multiple testing is increasingly the norm because of the availability of multiple candidate genes, multiple polymorphisms at genes, and the various combinations of these, which can be tested against multiple phenotypes. Failure to correct for multiple testing has led to an underestimation of the likelihood of Type I errors. Also, although the number of hypotheses that imaginably could be tested is infinite, we believe that correction should be made for the number of tests actually made rather than the imaginary number. Frequently the phenotypes that are evaluated are intercorrelated or even nested, so that correction is overly conservative. Sometimes a prior analysis could have objectively narrowed and improved the range of dependent variables. In similar fashion, certain new genotyping methodologies (e.g., DNA chip) will provide large numbers of marker typings, and it will be possible to identify certain genotypes as targets and others as exploratory.

For genetic hypothesis testing, the hidden variable of greatest concern as a source for systematic positive and negative errors has been population stratification, creating or masking differences between patient and control samples (Goldman et al. 1993). Many approaches to this problem, including the use of population isolates and transmission disequilibrium test (parent-child trios and sib–unaffected sib) structures (Spielman et al. 1993, 1996, 1998), have been proposed. The recent availability of large numbers of genetic markers, including markers that are relatively population specific, may now enable a sufficient test of ethnic matching between cases and controls (Pritchard and Rosenberg 1999), or the construction of an ethnically matched control subsample. Finally, evaluation tests of genetic association can be strongly guided by the Bayesian principle that the post hoc likelihood of a biological association between gene and phenotype is strongly influenced by the original plausibility of the hypothesis (Gordis et al. 1990). In Table 15–1, genetic associations are grouped (approximately) by likelihood of eventual validation. Likelihoods were assigned in part on the basis of plausibility of the original gene hypothesis: was the gene involved in a component of the physiological or pharmacological pathway to the behavior? Likelihoods were also assigned based on the gene variant: does the gene variant alter gene expression or gene product function in vitro or in vivo?

A signal achievement of the last decade has been the discovery of a panel of genetic variants that are themselves functional in vitro or in vivo. These have been termed *candidate alleles*. A partial listing of common candidate alleles for neurobehavior is presented in Table 15–2, which lists gene, polymorphism, allele frequency, and the effect of the polymorphism on function. This table is a precursor of an emerging detailed picture of neurochemical individuality for the human. For example, polymorphisms affecting primary amino acid sequence have already been found in 10 of 18 G-protein-coupled dopamine and serotonin receptors, and approximately 94% of people express at least one structural variant even across this relatively small subset of brain-expressed genes. The level of genetic variation is also such that the average level of heterozygosity (genotype in which two alleles are present at the locus) across these genes is about 15% (Cravchik et al. 1999). Large-scale scanning for sequence variation using automated sequencing and denaturing high-performance liquid chromatography is revealing comparable levels of variation at other loci. Wang and colleagues (Wang and Fan 1998) have systematically searched for sequence variants in approximately 2.3 Mb of anonymous and 3' untranslated region (UTR) DNA and report more than 3,200 candidate single-nucleotide polymorphisms (SNPs). In two other large-scale studies (Cargill et al. 1999; Haluska et al. 1999) similar results were obtained on different sets of genes. Halushka et al. reported (Haluska et al. 1999) 874 SNPs in 74 samples over 190 kb of DNA (87 kb of coding, 25 kb of intron, and 77

Table 15–2 A partial listing of common, candidate alleles for neurobehavior

Gene	Variant	Allele frequency	Functional significance	
SLC6A3	VNTR (ins/del)	0.40 (del)	Transcription	Lesch et al. 1996
HTR2A	His452Tyr	0.09	Signal transduction	Ozaki et al. 1997
HTR2C	Cys23Ser	0.13	Ligand affinity	Lappalainen et al. 1995
DRD2	Ser311Cys	0.03–0.16	Ligand affinity/signal transduction	Cravchik et al. 1999
DRD4	16–amino acid repeat	0.64 (4 repeat) 0.20 (7 repeat) 0.08 (2 repeat)	Ligand affinity	Asghari et al. 1995
	Val194Gly	0.12	Ligand affinity/signal transduction	Liu et al. 1996
	13-bp del	0.02	Translation	Nothen et al. 1994
COMT	Val158Met	0.04	Enzyme activity	Lachman et al. 1996
PAX6	VNTR	0.5 (26 repeat) 0.11 (28 repeat) 0.10 (25 repeat)	Transcription	Okladnova et al. 1998b

Note. VNTR = variable number tandem repeat.

kb of 5' and 3' UTR sequences) with a frequency of 1 SNP per 217 bp. Of these 874 candidate SNPs, 44% were in coding sequences (cSNPs), 17% in introns, and 39% in 5' and 3' UTRs. Of the cSNPs, 54% lead to replacement of an amino acid residue and probably affect protein function.

Thus far the functional alleles for genes expressed in brain have been largely identified by in vitro measures, principally transfection of mammalian cell lines or *Xenopus* oocytes followed by studies of the gene product. Examples include studies of receptor ligand affinity (Jovanovic et al. 1999), signal transduction (Ozaki et al. 1997) and downregulation (Rotondo et al. 1997), and differential ability of alleles to drive transcription of reporter genes (*SLC6A4* [serotonin transporter; 5-HTT], *PAX6*, Table 15–2) or the authentic gene. An advantage of these studies is that allele function can be compared within a constant genetic and environmental milieu. However, the role of in vivo measures of gene expression and gene product function is increasing and is especially important at the point where the gene has been identified and it is necessary to retrace the pathway in physiology from gene to behavior.

Phenotype: Tip of a Genetic Iceberg

Genetic redefinition of the behavioral phenotypes has been a major stimulus for genetic research in behavior. Gottesman recognized the utility of endophenotype, intervening physiological variables, which may more closely reflect gene action. A paucity of phenotypes is one of the most notable features of Table 15–1, which provides a summary status of candidate gene/allele associations to behavior. Furthermore, an important element in each validated (proven) relationship of gene to behavior was phenotypic definition providing clues to physiology (i.e., alcoholism → flushing response → alcohol metabolism → *ALDH2*; Brunner syndrome → chromosomal localization and disturbed monoamine function → *MAOA*; self-mutilation → Lesch-Nyhan syndrome → hyperuricemia → *HPRT1*). Thus, although human behavioral phenotypes visible in Table 15–1 include clinical diagnosis, measures of temperament (for example novelty seeking [Benjamin et al. 1996] and cognitive function), psychophysiological differences, and pharmacogenetic differences (clozapine → *HTR2A* [Arranz et al. 1998]), the largest obstacle to behavioral genetic research continues to be a lack of phenotypes.

As described in the introduction, an important alternative to the more precise resolution of the phenotype is the use of phenotypes that facilitate the collection of extremely large data sets, discarding the collection of expensive data that will not be utilized. It is important to point out that the first efforts in this direction, involving for example measures of IQ (Plomin 1999) across populations and sampling at the extremes (e.g., comparison of highly discordant sib pairs [Horvath and Laird 1998; Risch and Zhang 1996]), are recent in their inception, and therefore the results of such studies are not represented in Tables 15–1 and 15–2.

References

Antonarakis S, Blouin J, Pulver A, et al: Schizophrenia susceptibility and chromosome 6p24–22. Nat Genet 11:235–236, 1995

Arranz M, Munro J, Sham P, et al: Meta-analysis of studies on genetic variation in 5HT2a receptors and clozapine response. Schizophr Res 32:93–99, 1998

Asghari V: Modulation of intracellular cyclic AMP levels by different human dopamine D4 receptor variants. J Neurochem 65:1157–1165, 1995

Bellivier F: Methodological problems in meta-analysis of association studies between bipolar affective disorder and the tyrosine hydroxylase gene. Am J Med Genet 81:349–350, 1998

Benjamin J, Li L, Patterson C, et al: Population and familial association between the D4 dopamine receptor gene and measures of novelty seeking. Nat Genet 12:81–84, 1996

Berrettini W: Progress and pitfalls: bipolar molecular linkage studies. J Affect Disord 50:287–297, 1998

Betancur C, Moulard B, Philippe A, et al: TDT and affected sib-pair analyses of the nicotinic receptor alpha 7 subunit gene in autism (abstract). Mol Psychiatry 4 (suppl 1):s63, 1999

Birkett J, Kirov G, Arranz M, et al: Association between a 2030-G/A substitution in the human myo-inositol monophosphatase gene (IMPA) and bipolar disorder and schizophrenia (abstract). Mol Psychiatry 4 (suppl 1):s103, 1999

Blum K, Sheridan P, Wood R, et al: Dopamine D2 receptor gene variants: association and linkage studies in impulsive-addictive-compulsive behavior. Pharmacogenetics 5:121–141, 1995

Botstein D, White R, Skolnik M, et al: Construction of a genetic linkage map in man using restriction fragment length polymorphisms. Am J Hum Genet 32:314–331, 1980

Bray M, Boerwinkle E, Hanis C, et al: Linkage analysis of candidate obesity genes among the Mexican-American population of Starr County, Texas. Genet Epidemiol 16:397–411, 1999

Brunner H, Nelen M, Breakefield XO, et al: Abnormal behavior associated with a point mutation in the structural gene for monoamine oxidase A. Science 262:578–580, 1993

Cardno A, Bowen T, Guy C, et al: CAG repeat length in the hKCa3 gene and symptom dimensions in schizophrenia. Biol Psychiatry 45:1592–1596, 1999

Cargill M, Altshuler D, Ireland J, et al: Characterization of single-nucleotide polymorphism in coding regions of human genes. Nat Genet 22:231–238, 1999

Collier D, Arranz M, Li T, et al: Association between 5-HT2a gene promoter polymorphism and anorexia nervosa (abstract). Lancet 350:412, 1997

Comings D, Gade R, MacMurray J, et al: Genetic variants of the human obesity (OB) gene: association with body mass index in young women, psychiatric symptoms, and interaction with the dopamine D2 receptor (DRD2) gene. Mol Psychiatry 1:325–335, 1996

Comings D, Gonzales N, Wu S, et al: Studies of the 48 repeat polymorphism of the DRD4 gene in impulsive, compulsive, addictive behaviors: Tourette syndrome, ADHD, pathological gambling, and substance abuse. Am J Med Genet 88:358–368, 1999

Cook E, Stein MA, Krasowski M, et al: Association of attention deficit disorder and the dopamine transporter gene. Am J Hum Genet 56:993–998, 1995

Cravchik A, Goldman D: Neurochemical individuality: genetic diversity of human dopamine and serotonin receptors and transporters. Arch Gen Psychiatry 57: 1105–1114, 2000

Cravchik A, Sibley D, Gejman P, et al: Analysis of neuroleptic binding affinities and potencies for different human D2 dopamine receptor missense variants. Pharmacogenetics 9:17–23, 1999

Cruts M, Van Broeckhoven, C: Presenilin mutations in Alzheimer's disease. Hum Mutat 11:183–190, 1998

Dean M, Stevens J, Winkler C, et al: Polymorphic admixture typing in human ethnic populations. Am J Hum Genet 55:788–808, 1994

Deckert J, Catalano M, Syagailo Y, et al: Excess of high activity monoamine oxidase A gene promoter alleles in female patients with panic disorder. Hum Mol Genet 8:621–624, 1999

Dubertret C, Gorwood P, Ades J, et al: Meta-analysis of DRD3 gene and schizophrenia: ethnic heterogeneity and significant association in Caucasians. Am J Med Genet 81:318–322, 1998

Egan MF, Goldberg TE, Kolachana BS, et al: Effect of COMT Val 108/158 Met genotype on frontal lobe function and risk for schizophrenia. Proc Natl Acad Sci U S A 98:6917–6922, 2001

Eisen M, Brown, P: DNA arrays for analysis of gene expression. Methods Enzymol 303:179–205, 1999

Enoch M, Kaye W, Rotondo A, et al: 5-HT2A promoter polymorphism 1438G/A, anorexia nervosa, and obsessive-compulsive disorder. Lancet 351:1785–1786, 1998

Enoch MA, Greenberg BD, Murphy DL, et al: Sexually dimorphic relationship of a 5-HT2A promoter polymorphism with obsessive-compulsive disorder. Biol Psychiatry 49:385–388, 2001

Faraone S, Biederman J, Weiffenbach B, et al: Dopamine D4 gene 7-repeat allele and attention deficit hyperactivity disorder. Am J Psychiatry 156:768–770, 1999

Feng J, Zheng J, Gelernter J, et al: A common in-frame deletion in the a2c adrenergic receptor (a2cAR): possible association with cocaine abuse (abstract). Mol Psychiatry 4 (suppl 1):s106, 1999

Goldman D, Brown G, Albaugh B, et al: DRD2 dopamine receptor genotype, linkage disequilibrium and alcoholism in American Indians and other populations. Alcohol Clin Exp Res 17:199–204, 1993

Goldman D, Urbanek M, Guenther D, et al: Linkage and association of a functional variant (Ser311Cys) and DRD2 markers to alcoholism, substance abuse, and schizophrenia in southwestern American Indians. Am J Med Genet 74:386–394, 1997

Gordis E, Tabakoff B, Goldman D, et al: Finding the gene(s) for alcoholism. JAMA 263:2094–2095, 1990

Gottesman II, Erlenmeyer-Kimling L: Family and twin strategies as a headstart in defining prodromes and endophenotypes for hypothetical early interventions in schizophrenia. Schizophr Res 51:93–102, 2001

Gusella J, MacDonald M, Ambrose C, et al: Molecular genetics of Huntington's disease. Arch Neurol 50:1157–1163, 1993

Gusella J, McNeil S, Persichetti F, et al: Huntington's disease. Cold Spring Harb Symp Quant Biol 61:615–626, 1996

Haluska M, Fan J, Bentley K, et al: Patterns of single-nucleotide polymorphisms in candidate genes for blood-pressure homeostasis. Nat Genet 22:239–247, 1999

Harada S, Agarwal D, Goedde H, et al: Aldehyde dehydrogenase deficiency as cause of flushing reaction to alcohol in Japanese. Lancet 2:982, 1981

Harada S, Okubo T, Tsutsumi M, et al: A new genetic variant in the Sp1 binding cis-element of cholecystokinin gene promoter region and relationship to alcoholism. Alcohol Clin Exp Res 22:93s–96s, 1998

Horvath S, Laird N: A discordant-sibship test for disequilibrium and linkage: no need for parental data. Am J Human Genet 63:1886–1897, 1998

Hranilovic D, Schawb S, Jernej B, et al: Serotonin transporter gene and schizophrenia: evidence for association/linkage disequilibrium in families with affected siblings as obtained by transmission disequilibrium test (abstract). Mol Psychiatry 4 (suppl 1):s23, 1999

Huss M, MacMurray J, Dietz G, et al: Opioids and attachment behavior: studies of the neutral endopeptidase gene (abstract). Mol Psychiatry, 4 (suppl 1):s45, 1999

Iwata N, Cowley D, Radel M, et al: Relationship between a GABAa a6 Pro385Ser substitution and benzodiazepine sensitivity. Am J Psychiatry 156:1447–1449, 1999

Iwata N, Ozaki N, Inada T, et al: Association of a 5-HT(5A) receptor polymorphism, Pro15Ser, to schizophrenia. Mol Psychiatry 6:217–219, 2001

Jonsson E, Nothen M, Neidt H, et al: Association between a promoter polymorphism in the dopamine D2 receptor gene and schizophrenia. Schizophr Res 40:31–36, 1999

Jovanovic V, Guan H, Van Tol H: Comparative pharmacological and functional analysis of the human dopamine D4.2 and D4.10 receptor variants. Pharmacogenetics 9:561–568, 1999

Kan Y, Dozy A: Polymorphisms of DNA sequence adjacent to human betaglobin structural gene: relationship to sickle mutation. Proc Natl Acad Sci U S A 75:5631–5635, 1978

Karayiorgou M, Altemus M, Galke BL, et al: Genotype determining low catechol-O-methyltransferase activity as a risk factor for obsessive-compulsive disorder. Proc Natl Acad Sci U S A 94:4572–4575, 1997

Karvonen M, Pesonen U, Koulu M, et al: Association of a leucine(7)-to-proline(7) polymorphism in the signal peptide of neuropeptide Y with high serum cholesterol and LDL cholesterol levels. Nat Med 4:1434–1437, 1998

Kendler K, MacLean C, O'Neill F, et al: Evidence for a schizophrenia vulnerability locus on chromosome 8p in the Irish Study of High-Density Schizophrenia Families. Am J Psychiatry 153:1534–1540, 1996

Kennedy J, Bradwejn J, Koszycki D, et al: Investigation of cholecystokinin system genes in panic disorder. Mol Psychiatry 4:284–285, 1999

Kirov G, Murphy K, Arranza M, et al: Low activity allele of catechol-O-methyltransferase gene associated with rapid cycling bipolar disorder. Mol Psychiatry 3:342–345, 1998

Kittles R, Long J, Bergen A, et al: Cladistic association analysis of Y chromosome effects on alcohol dependence and related personality traits. Proc Natl Acad Sci U S A 96:4204–4209, 1999

Kranzler H, Gelernter J, O'Malley S, et al: Association of alcohol or other drug dependence with alleles of the mu opioid receptor gene (OPRM1). Alcohol Clin Exp Res 22:1359–1362, 1998

Kruglyak L: Prospects for whole-genome linkage disequilibrium mapping of common diseases genes. Nat Genet 22:139–144, 1999

Lachman H, Papolos D, Saito T, et al: Human catechol-O-methyltransferase pharmacogenetics: description of a functional polymorphism and its potential application to neuropsychiatric disorders. Pharmacogenetics 6:243–250, 1996

Lachman H, Nolank A, Mohr P, et al: Association between catechol-O-methyltransferase genotype and violence in schizophrenia and schizoaffective disorder. Am J Psychiatry 55:835–837, 1998

Lappalainen J, Zhang L, Dean M, et al: Identification, expression, and pharmacology of a Cys23–Ser23 substitution in the human 5HT2c receptor gene (HTR2C). Genomics 27:274–279, 1995

Lappalainen Y, Long J, Eggert M, et al: Linkage of antisocial alcoholism to the serotonin 5HT1B receptor gene in 2 populations. Arch Gen Psychiatry 55:989–994, 1998

Lesch K, Bengel D, Heils A, et al: Association of anxiety-related traits with a polymorphism in the serotonin transporter gene regulatory region. Science 274:1527–1531, 1996

Liu I: Dopamine D4 receptor variant in Africans D4Val194Glycine is insensitive to dopamine and clozapine: report of a homozygous individual. Am J Med Genet 61:277–282, 1996

Long J, Knowler W, Hanson R, et al: Evidence for genetic linkage to alcohol dependence on chromosome 4 and 11 from autosome-wide scan in an American Indian population. Am J Med Genet 81:216–221, 1998

Lovlie R, Berle J, Steen V: A role of the human inositol polyphosphate 1-phosphatase gene (INPP1) in lithium-treated bipolar disorder (abstract). Mol Psychiatry 4 (suppl 1):s68, 1999

Malhotra A, Goldman, D: Benefits and pitfalls encountered in psychiatric genetic association studies. Biol Psychiatry 45:544–550, 1999

Malhotra A, Breier A, Goldman D, et al: The apolipoprotein E epsilon 4 allele is associated with blunting of ketamine-induced psychosis in schizophrenia: a preliminary report. Neuropsychopharmacology 19, 445–448, 1998a

Malhotra A, Goldman D, Mazzanti C, et al: A functional serotonin transporter (5-HTT) polymorphism is associated with psychosis in neuroleptic-free schizophrenics. Mol Psychiatry 3:328–332, 1998b

Malhotra A, Dean M, Buchanan R, et al: Chemokine receptor variation in schizophrenia: support for the retroviral hypothesis (abstract). Mol Psychiatry 4 (suppl 1):s38, 1999

McCarthy M, Kruglyak L, Lander E, et al: Sip-pair collection strategies for complex diseases. Genet Epidemiol 15:317–340, 1998

Meloni R, Laurent C, Campion D, et al: A rare allele of a microsatellite located in the tyrosine hydroxylase gene found in schizophrenic patients. C R Acad Sci III 318:803–809, 1995

Mundo E, Richter M, Hood K, et al: Evidence for linkage disequilibrium between 5ht1db receptor gene and obsessive compulsive disorder (abstract). Mol Psychiatry 4 (suppl 1):s8, 1999

Nielsen D, Goldman D, Virkunnen M, et al: Suicidality and 5-hydroxyindoleacetic acid concentration associated with a tryptophan hydroxylase polymorphism. Arch Gen Psychiatry 51:34–38, 1994

Normile D, Pennisi E: Team wrapping up sequence of first human chromosome. Science 285:2038–2039, 1999

Nothen M: Human dopamine D4 receptor gene: frequent occurrence of a null allele and observation of homozygosity. Hum Mol Genet 3:2207–2212, 1994

O'Dell D, McIntosh T, Eberwine J, et al: Single-cell molecular biology: implications for the diagnosis and treatment of neurological disease. Arch Neurol 56:1453–1456, 1999

Okladnova O, Syagaylo Y, Meyer J, et al: Association analysis of the dinucleotide repeat polymorphism in the regulatory region of the human PAX-6 gene with psychiatric disorders (abstract). Am J Med Genet 81:518, 1998a

Okladnova O, Syagailo Y, Tranitz M, et al: A promoter-associated polymorphic repeat modulates PAX-6 expression in human brain. Biochem Biophys Res Commun 248:402–405, 1998b

Owen M, Craddock N: Chromosome 11 workshop. Psychiatr Genet 8:89–92, 1998

Ozaki N, Manji H, Lubierman V, et al: A naturally occurring amino acid substitution of the human serotonin 5-HT2A receptor influences amplitude and timing of intracellular calcium mobilization. J Neurochem 68:2186–2193, 1997

Plomin R: Genetics and general cognitive ability. Nature 402 (6761 suppl):c25–c29, 1999

Pritchard J, Rosenberg N: Use of unlinked genetic markers to detect population stratification in association studies. Am J Hum Genet 65:220–228, 1999

Ricketts M, Goldman D, Long J, et al: Arylsulfatase a pseudodeficiency-associated mutations: population studies and identification of a novel haplotype. Am J Med Genet 67:387–392, 1996

Riordan J, Rommens J, Kerem B, et al: Identification of the cystic fibrosis gene: cloning and characterization of complementary DNA. Science 245:1066–1073, 1989

Risch N, Merikangas K: Linkage studies of psychiatric disorders. Eur Arch Psychiatry Clin Neurosci 243:143–149, 1993

Risch N, Merikangas K: The future of genetic studies of complex human diseases. Science 273:1516–1517, 1996

Risch N, Teng J: The relative power of family based and case control designs for linkage disequilibrium studies of complex human diseases, I: DNA pooling. Genome Res 8:1273–1288, 1998

Risch N, Zhang H: Mapping quantitative trait loci with extreme discordant sib pairs: sampling considerations. Am J Hum Genet 58:836–843, 1996

Rossiter B, Edwards A, Caskey C: HPRT Mutation and the Lesch-Nyhan syndrome. New York, Academic Press, 1991

Rotondo A, Nielsen D, Nakhai B, et al: Agonist-promoted down-regulation and functional desensitization in two naturally occurring variants of the human serotonin 1A receptor. Neuropsychopharmacology 17:18–26, 1997

Rowe D, Stever C, Gard J, et al: The relation of the dopamine transporter gene (DAT1) to symptoms of internalizing disorders in children. Behav Genet 28:215–225, 1998

Sander T, Harms H, Podschus J, et al: Allelic association of a dopamine transporter gene polymorphism in alcohol dependence with withdrawal seizures or delirium. Biol Psychiatry 41:299–304, 1997

Shaw S, Kelly M, Smith A, et al: A genome-wide search for schizophrenia susceptibility genes. Am J Med Genet 81:364–376, 1998

Sodhi M, Kerwin R, Campbell I, et al: A pharmacological study of variant 5HT2c receptor proteins (abstract). Mol Psychiatry 4 (suppl 1):s94, 1999

Spielman R, Ewens W: The TDT and other family based tests for linkage disequilibrium and association. Am J Hum Genet 59:983–989, 1996

Spielman R, Ewens W: A sibship test for linkage in the presence of association: the sib transmission/disequilibrium test. Am J Hum Genet 62:450–458, 1998

Spielman R, McGinnis R, Ewens W: Transmission test for linkage disequilibrium: the insulin gene region and insulin dependent diabetes mellitus (IDDM). Am J Hum Genet 52:506–516, 1993

Tanzi R, Vaula G, Romano D, et al: Assessment of amyloid beta-protein precursor gene mutations in a large set of familial and sporadic Alzheimer disease cases. Am J Human Genet 51:273–282, 1992

Templeton A, Boerwinkle E, Sing C: A cladistic analysis of phenotypic associations with haplotypes inferred from restriction endonuclease mapping, I: basic theory and an analysis of alcohol dehydrogenase activity in *Drosophila*. Genetics 117:343–351, 1987

Wang D, Fan J, Siao C, et al: Large scale identification, mapping, and genotyping of single-nucleotide polymorphisms in the human genome. Science 280:1077–1082, 1998

Williams J, Begleiter H, Porjesz B, et al: Joint multipoint linkage analysis of multivariate qualitative and quantitative traits, II: alcoholism and event related potentials. Am J Human Genet 65:1148–1160, 1999

CHAPTER SIXTEEN

Human Correlative Behavioral Genetics

An Alternative Viewpoint

Evan Balaban, Ph.D.

What Is the Problem?

As someone who has publicly criticized the design, interpretation, presentation, and rationale of the genre of studies represented in this volume (Balaban 1996, 1998, 2000; Balaban et al. 1996; Fausto-Sterling and Balaban 1993), I respect the editors' decision to include at least one dissenting viewpoint. I do research on behavior and genetics and perceive the correlative-genetics-of-human-behavior community as being too isolated from the discourse that has occurred in related fields with similar interests. I would like to convince my fellow authors and interested readers that such isolation is scientifically disadvantageous. There is much about human biology that correlative molecular techniques combined with a rigorous study of behavioral variation may teach us. But there must be willingness to accept the possibility that the lessons gained could have little to do with the clinical and theoretical reasons why a particular topic

The preparation of this chapter was supported by the Neurosciences Research Foundation.

was pursued in the first place. There must also be a willingness to adhere to the same standards of scientific rigor that prevail in other areas of behavioral biology.

I write as a research biologist with training in genetics (classical, molecular, population, and developmental), neurobiology, and behavior, who studies the evolutionary and developmental neurobiology underlying inborn species differences in behavior (Balaban 1990, 1997; Balaban et al. 1988; Gahr and Balaban 1996; Long et al. 2001; Park and Balaban 1991). In the past I have also studied the relationship between population genetic variation and culturally transmitted behavioral variation in natural populations (Balaban 1988a, 1988b, 1988c).

My laboratory studies animals (currently chickens and quail) because one can control the developmental environment subjects experience, both prenatally and postnatally. By rearing members of two different species together in particular environments, we find that certain behavioral differences are reliably obtained between all individuals of different species, in spite of the fact that the behaviors involved can show considerable interindividual variation within a species. We can study the developmental causation of such reliable differences by performing embryonic brain transplants between individuals of the two bird species to locate cellular populations that transfer a behavioral difference from donor to host individuals. Because these transplants are done before embryonic cells have decided upon their eventual fate(s), this boils down to studying the mechanisms by which genetic differences confer chicken-ness or quail-ness, in particular, behaviorally relevant, neural circuits. Once the cells are located, we can study the developmental pathways through which such gene differences manifest their effects and identify the gene differences implicated in the developmental differences.

We study directly measurable differences in physical behavioral acts such as vocalizations and body movements, as well as differences in less tangible behavioral attributes such as auditory perception (Long et al. 2001). The perceptual differences can be quite subtle. In a world where physical stimuli do not have labels that say "ignore me" or "pay attention to me," how can an individual brain be prepared to pay more attention to (and to learn) certain sounds and virtually ignore others? We are also developing methods for studying neurobiological correlates of auditory perception in humans using noninvasive brain imaging (Patel and Balaban 2000, 2001).

One can directly learn a great deal about the mechanistic details underlying biases in developmental organization that make chickens pay more attention to chicken sounds than to quail sounds. This is because we can do manipulative developmental, physiological, and molecular experiments using chickens and quail. We will never get such a direct wealth of knowledge about similar biases in the development of human brains that may make human fetuses and infants especially responsive to speech sounds. The knowledge we acquire will come primarily from correlative data. The question is what should be concluded from such data and how this knowledge should be represented to others. This question is especially important when decisions affecting people's lives and well-being are involved, as in many of the more medically oriented questions discussed by the other authors in this volume.

It should by now be clear that 1) I think it is possible to learn something useful about how genetic differences contribute to the development and variation of behavior, and 2) that I do not have a knee-jerk reaction against the value of correlative research in humans. Why, then, do I criticize much of the work on correlative genetics and human behavioral variation?

Simplistic Assumptions

One reason I am critical of human correlative behavior genetics is that many investigators make simplifying assumptions about heredity, genetics, development, and behavior that I find biologically questionable.

Heredity

A lot of quantitative-trait-locus (QTL) and linkage-oriented researchers seem to think that heredity means genetics. It has been a truism in biology for a long time that biological traits can be passed on from parents to offspring and not be inherited as independently assorting, chromosomal factors with intrinsic effects on an organism's phenotype. That is, familiality does not necessarily equal genetics of the sort envisioned by people looking for QTLs. There are a few known alternative biological pathways through which familial effects can be mediated, as shown by recent research in animals.

The first, and least well documented pathway, is via epigenetic modifications of the chemical structure of DNA that can alter the expression of particular alleles without altering the DNA sequence of the expressed gene product. A concise introduction to research in this area can be found in a series of recent reviews (Grunstein 1998; Henikoff and Comai 1998; Lewin 1998; Panning and Jaenisch 1998; Pirrotta 1998; Surani 1998; Wakimoto 1998; Wiens and Sorger 1998). A rigorous demonstration of such an effect has been provided by Morgan et al. (1999), who documented the inheritance of an epigenetic modification at the agouti locus of mice, which affects coat color, obesity, diabetes, and tumor susceptibility. By ingenious manipulation of embryos, Morgan et al. were able to show that an effect formerly attributed to metabolic differences in the intrauterine environment or to factors in the cytoplasm of maternal oocytes is instead due to a DNA methylation modification that can be transmitted intergenerationally. The modification is subsequently erased in male germ lines but incompletely erased in female germ lines. This phenomenon differs from parental genetic imprinting in that phenotypic modifications are not strictly based on parental sex and genotype. Parental genetic imprinting is being studied by Keverne, Surani, and colleagues, who have examined differences in neural phenotypes using chimeric mice made up of androgenetic and parthenogenetic/gynogenetic cells (Allen et al. 1995; Keverne et al. 1996). This same group is also examining the effects of mutations in different parentally imprinted genes on maternal behavior and offspring growth (Lefebvre et al. 1998; Li et al. 1999).

A second pathway for nongenetic familial effects is the uterine environment. It has been classically considered that human twin studies rule out such effects with analysis-of-variance models. Devlin et al. (1997) reanalyzed 212 previous twin studies of IQ using an alternative analysis-of-variance model with different maternal-womb environment terms for twins and siblings and found evidence for a significant contribution of maternal-womb effects to phenotypic variance, significantly reducing the component assigned to genetic variance. However, Devlin et al.'s model may itself be too simplistic, because it assumes that all twins have the same maternal-womb environment. As noted previously (Balaban 1998), twins that share the same chorionic compartment (as do many monozygotic twins) and twins that are in different chorionic compartments (many dizygotic twins) may have different intrauterine environments. Fetuses sharing the same chorionic compartment can act as diffusion sources of developmentally active substances for each other, which would tend to synchronize their development to a greater extent than in twin pairs that are diffusionally isolated from each other in separate chorionic compartments.

Recent animal research has shown important maternal effects on behavior in mammalian species. Denenberg et al. (1998) placed genetically identical eight-cell-stage mouse embryos into either same-strain recipient mothers or into foster mothers of a hybrid strain. They found consistent and significant differences in performance of these groups on six standard laboratory cognitive tests (open-field activity, water escape learning, discrimination learning in a T maze, Lashley type III maze learning, Morris water maze learning, and shock avoidance learning). The groups did not differ significantly in noncognitive tests such as paw preference or swimming performance in a cylinder. The exact causal attribution of these behavioral differences is problematic, because same-strain and hybrid-strain foster animals also differed in their mode of birth (caesarian section in same-strain animals, vaginal birth in hybrid-strain animals). The mice delivered through caesarian section appeared to have slightly higher activity scores, even though the authors presented corollary evidence this had no effect on the animals' performance in cognitive tests.

Caldji et al. (1998) and Francis et al. (1999) have examined the biological effects of subtle postnatal differences in maternal behavior on behavioral and endocrine responses to stress throughout the life of rat offspring. Offspring of mothers who showed differential amounts of licking/grooming (LG) and arch-backed nursing (ABN) (where the mother's body is hovering over, rather than lying on top of her pups) were assayed later in life for their behavioral and endocrine responses to a novel, stressful situation. Offspring were classified into two groups, those of high-LG-ABN mothers, and those of low-LG-ABN mothers. In two different behavioral tests, the performance of the two groups differed significantly, and there were significant correlations across animals between offspring and maternal behavioral measures (Caldji et al. 1998). Adult offspring of the high-LG-ABN mothers also showed increased central benzodiazepine receptor density in the amygdala and locus coeruleus, increased hippocampal glucocorticoid receptor mRNA expression, and decreased corticotropin releasing hormone mRNA expression in the locus coeruleus (relative to adult offspring from the low-LG-ABN group) when placed in a stressful situation. Francis et al. (1999) performed a postnatal cross-fostering study between pups of high- and low-LG-ABN mothers, carefully monitoring foster mothers to assure that there was no effect of pup's origin on maternal behavior. Biological offspring of low-LG-ABN mothers reared by high-LG-ABN females showed the same behavioral profile as biological offspring of high-LG-ABN mothers reared by high-LG-ABN mothers, and vice versa.

When the maternal behavior of the female offspring used in the cross-fostering study was examined, it was found that the biological offspring of low-LG-ABN mothers raised by high-LG-ABN females showed the maternal behavior of their foster mother's type (and vice versa). Francis et al. (1999) also examined the expression of central benzodiazepine receptor mRNA, hippocampal glucocorticoid receptor mRNA, and corticotropin releasing factor mRNA in these animals in response to stress and found that the patterns corresponded to the behavior shown by the animal (and its foster mother) rather than to its biological origin. They concluded that "individual differences in fearfulness to novelty could be transmitted from parent to offspring through a nongenomic mechanism of inheritance . . . [that] involves differences in maternal care during the first week of life. In humans, social, emotional, and economic contexts influence the quality of the relationship between parent and child and can show continuity across generations" (Francis et al. 1999, p. 1158).

It is notable that the behavioral paradigms used in the Denenberg et al. (1998), Caldji et al. (1998), and Francis et al. (1999) studies are all used by research groups looking for QTLs affecting rodent behavior, none of whom employ the controls that would be necessary to separate an assorting genetic "factor" from one transmitted biologically in the womb or as a result of postnatal maternal behavior. A genetic effect that manifests itself indirectly through its effects on a mother's uterine environment, behavior, or physiology can be either incorrectly ascribed to a direct effect operating within individual offspring, or missed altogether, depending on the design of the experiment.

Do alternative trait transmission pathways that are not biologically autonomous to individual subjects necessarily create complications for human correlative behavior genetics? They do if you want to use QTL and linkage data as facts, for instance, to say that you have located a genetic contributor to some behavior that can serve as a predictor or risk factor. The establishment of gene-behavior links in this factual sense depends on goodness-of-fit arguments that in turn depend on the fair specification and evaluation of alternative models. Much of the work in human correlative behavior genetics seems to assume that phenotypes that do not show clear patterns of Mendelian segregation in a study population will yield evidence for single genes of discernable effect with the application of more derived statistical averaging techniques. Given the sample size and quality of most human data sets, evaluating alternative transmission models fairly may be a challenge that proves difficult or impossible to meet.

If, on the other hand, QTL and linkage results are treated, both in the laboratory and in print, as highly preliminary preludes to locating a candidate gene and studying its role in development (Balaban 1998; Balaban et al. 1996; Flint 1999), then such considerations may be less important. If you are willing to gamble on a transmission genetics interpretation by investing time and money in an attempt to actually locate genes and specify their functions, then the eventual results will speak for themselves. If the putative behavioral linkage does not pan out, you have another potential explanation for why this was the case. This implies that the human correlative behavior genetics community should be very wary of investigators who regard themselves as "specialized" correlationists whose only job is to find and publish associations in which they have no further professional stake. The real work is not finding correlations, but placing the functional consequences of DNA sequence variation into some sort of meaningful biological context.

Genetics

Let us say you have your hands on a putative candidate gene. Let us also say that you accept the point of view that to make any statement about a gene's role in behavioral variation you need to understand something about its role in the development and function of the nervous system (Balaban 1998, 2000; Balaban et al. 1996; Flint 1999). There are many complications to be dealt with when analyzing the contribution of a single genetic factor to an organism's phenotype, which have either been ignored or poorly dealt with by the human correlative behavior genetic community. These include the contributions of genetic background, variation imposed by developmental regulation, and the importance of documenting the full, pleiotropic range of phenotypic effects associated with allelic differences rather than effects on one or a few behavioral phenotypes (Balaban 1998, 2000; Balaban et al. 1996). A recent animal study examining locomotor activity in D2 dopamine receptor–deficient mice illustrates the potential importance of these complicating factors quite nicely (Kelly et al. 1998). The first point is additionally underscored by a recent study on the effects of naturally occurring genetic variation in cellular signal-transduction pathways on photoreceptor determination in *Drosophila* (Polaczyk et al. 1998). Pleiotropy is still one of the areas most poorly handled by both the animal and human molecular behavior genetics communities, where investigators continue to tout "specific" effects of gene variants without advancing sufficient data to support them.

The confounding effects of genetic background should be of special concern to people conducting studies in humans. Such effects are frequently used as a throwaway explanation for why particular alleles may have behavioral effects in some lineages and not in others. But they raise a number of problems for data collection and interpretation that have not been widely addressed. How robust must the effect of an allele be across different human lineages in order for it to be considered significant? Particular alleles could affect behavior in a particular way in a very small number of lineages—how can we tell a real but rare effect from a false positive correlation? What kind of population sampling methods should one use to test the consistency of an allele's behavioral effects? Alleles that have effects on behavior in only some lineages can either be missed entirely or overinterpreted depending on the design of any particular study.

As already indicated, many practitioners of human correlative behavior genetics have claimed that linkage or QTL information is translatable into risk factors or predictors that may someday be useful for clinical intervention. Problems with such interpretations in the realm of normal phenotypic variation are discussed by Balaban (1998), and problems in the realm of pathological variation are discussed by Templeton (1998). While agreeing that some coarse predictive power may be obtained in the realm of pathologies, both authors were rather pessimistic about the possibility of fine-scale predictability for reasons each goes into in detail. It is interesting to note in this regard that recent human studies focusing on psychopathology such as those by Ginns et al. (1998) are casting their phenotypic nets ever more widely, looking for single-factor linkages associated with the presence or absence of any psychiatric disorder. At the same time, increasingly detailed studies correlating molecular variants and phenotypes for particular, classical monogenic disorders such as PKU are concluding that there is no close correlation between the mutant genotype and the type or severity of the phenotype. Monogenic disorders are, at a finer level of phenotypic and genetic resolution, multifactorial and complex (Scriver and Walters 1999).

The difficulties encountered in chasing down the phenotypic effects of even single "simple" genetic factors need not deter research on human genetic and behavioral variation. But the kinds of objectives that it is realistic to achieve depend on the direction in which correlative human behavioral geneticists want to take their studies. If you are looking to "predict" individual variation in personality attributes, novelty seeking, substance abuse, sexual orientation, or performance on IQ tests, then I think that effects of genetic background, regulation, and phenotypic specificity loom quite large and must now be dealt with more effectively. If you are simply using variation in behavioral phenotypes as a new way of gaining entry into more subtle cellular developmental or functional pathways rather than trying to make immediate statements about behavioral causation, then these problems are not of immediate concern.

Development

As far as correlative human behavior genetics is concerned, development seems to be the love that dare not speak its name (Balaban 1998, 2000). When people want to explain how gene differences among individuals are translated into behavioral differences, they are implicitly asking about developmental and functional processes that go on in those individuals, and not about average gene effects on an average population phenotype. Variations in transcribed and nontranscribed regions of the genome (which can alter gene expression) affect behavior in the context of these processes. Because we are talking about behavior, the primary locus for our attention is the nervous system. In essence, behavior-genetic questions are questions about the roles that particular gene sequences play in neural development or ongoing neural function, and how changes in the sequences themselves can either compromise those roles or change them altogether. It is strange that developmental-biological concepts, processes, and thinking are so conspicuously absent from the discourse of human correlative behavior geneticists.

One of the consequences of this absence has been a tendency to regard historic contributions to development that come from sources external to the organism itself as somehow not a part of biology. They are treated as a source of uninteresting "noise," and there is also a tendency to downplay stochastic components of developmental processes intrinsic to organisms as sources of interindividual variation. Documenting stochastic and historical contributions to development will be very difficult in humans. In animal studies this can be partially accomplished by empirically assessing norms of reaction for behavioral traits (Balaban 1998, in press). An exemplary illustration of a behavioral norm-of-reaction was recently provided in a heroic study by Crabbe et al. (1999). Using mice from seven inbred strains and one null mutant strain for the 5-HT1B receptor obtained from the same source colonies, they conducted simultaneous tests of six mouse behaviors at three separate laboratories (Portland, Oregon, USA; Edmonton, Alberta, Canada; Albany, New York, USA): locomotor activity in an open field, exploration of a plus maze, walking and balancing on a rotating rod, a water maze, locomotor activation following cocaine administration, and ethanol preference. They went to a great deal of trouble to equate test apparatus, protocols, and animal care.

Despite all of these efforts, significant and large "site" effects were found for six of the eight behavioral measures, and the pattern of strain differences varied substantially among the test sites. The null-mutant

5-HT1B strain, previously shown to prefer ethanol more than control mice in four separate test replications at the Portland site (Crabbe et al. 1996), did not have a different ethanol preference from controls in all three laboratories (Enserink 1999). Conclusions of this study were that very large, well-established strain differences in behavior were generally robust, but that "for behaviors with small genetic effects, there can be important influences of environmental conditions specific to individual laboratories. . . . We further recommend that, if possible, genotypes should be tested in multiple labs and evaluated with multiple tests of a single behavioral domain before concluding that a specific gene influences a specific behavioral domain" (Crabbe et al. 1999, p. 1672).

It will probably never be possible to rigorously document effects of this sort in human studies. However, the practitioners of human correlative behavior genetics should take the results of the Crabbe et al. (1999) study to heart in their thinking (and writing). The genes that correlative studies evaluate usually have "small genetic effects" on particular behaviors, and the particular subject pools used in an individual study are rarely, if ever, "tested in multiple labs and evaluated with multiple tests of a single behavioral domain before concluding that a specific gene influences a specific behavioral domain."

There appears to be some variance of opinion in the human correlative behavior genetics community about the latter issue. When the same lab looks at a different sample using the same techniques but relying on one-tailed instead of the two-tailed statistical tests used in their earlier study (Hu et al. 1995), does this constitute an independent replication? In this case a recently published study by another group with a larger sample and grossly similar methods excluded the chromosomal region in question from any linkage to the same phenotypic trait, male sexual orientation (Rice et al. 1999a). This set off an exchange of letters about purported methodological differences (Hamer 1999; Rice et al. 1999b) but no apparent change in views from the head of the original study (Wickelgren 1999). Similarly, Benjamin (1998) recounts a "replication" of a result by his own laboratory in the face of at least six external failed attempts at replication, which he seems very sanguine about. Failed attempts at replication by other labs should be taken more seriously than they appear to be at present.

Retrospective information about individual developmental environments will probably never be detailed enough to fully accept or reject the assumption that environmental contributions to behavioral differences have been either randomized or are unimportant. But more detailed information on the way that individuals with the same allele(s) differ from each other may provide some kind of rough proxy that can be worked with. I have yet to find a human correlative behavior genetic study examining phenotypic differences within an allelic group in detail.

Paying attention to development also means using as much information as possible about gene effects, be they small or large, behavioral or nonbehavioral, to try to put a DNA sequence's function into the context of a whole set of cellular developmental and functional pathways. This is not well served by the single-behavior-specific or single-clinical-syndrome-specific mindset of much of the human correlative behavior genetics community reflected in this volume.

Behavior

Perhaps the biggest conceptual gulf that separates human correlative behavior genetic researchers from other behavioral biology researchers exists in the realm of quantifying behavior to make it appropriate for biological analyses. Many different training backgrounds divide behavioral researchers and heavily influence the ways they choose to measure behavior (Balaban 1998, 2000). In the world of animal research, there has always been a large difference between researchers from a more psychological background, who devise controlled situations in which simple measurements can be taken, and more ethologically oriented researchers, who focus on measurement of natural behaviors or behavioral attributes (Balaban 2000). These differences are emphasized in the context of recent work on transgenic mice by Gerlai and Clayton (1999), who spiritedly argue for more ethologically relevant tasks to be used in genetic work on hippocampal function.

However, these arguments pale when we examine the type of behavioral measures employed in much of the work discussed in this book. With reference to *virtual reality,* the term *virtual behaviors* is an appropriate shorthand for human measures such as questionnaires, IQ and personality tests, and tests that inappropriately apply population behavioral measures back to individuals (Balaban 1998, 2000). I accept that such tests can serve a useful purpose in the realms they were originally designed for—indicating when a particular individual is grossly different in some way from socially or empirically determined norms of population variation and in need of some sort of help. What I cannot fathom is their use in the context of biological research.

If we were trying to relate pig genetics and pig morphology, an approach that took snout length, added it to the number of kinks in the tail, divided this by anus width, multiplied the result by the square root of the number of peristaltic contractions of the rostral two-thirds of the esophagus during the force-feeding of 1/2 liter of water, and then added the arcsine transform of the number of papillae in the front third of the tongue divided by the number of hairs within 1 cm^2 of the navel would seem to require special justification beyond the fact that such a series of operations gives a reliable result and that the number might roughly agree with some arbitrary concept such as the subjectively perceived tastiness or cleanliness of the pig. Yet as far as I can tell such measures can fly in human correlative behavior genetics. A lot of the discussion in the literature seems to regard the finding of any correlation between a biological variable and these behavioral tests as some sort of philosophical or scientific triumph.

Spurred by recent work on the molecular genetics of human personality, I delved into one of its main instruments, the NEO Personality Inventory (Benjamin 1998; Benjamin et al. 1996; Cloninger et al. 1996; Ebstein et al. 1996). After struggling through literature on the rationale, development, and validation of this instrument (Block 1995; Costa 1991; Costa and McCrae 1986, 1988, 1992a, 1992b, 1995, 1997; Costa et al. 1986, 1991; McCrae and Costa 1987, 1989, 1992; McCrae et al. 1996), I had the opportunity of looking over the question set itself (the 1992 NEO Personality Inventory, Revise, Form S, 1992), as well as a copy of the Tridimensional Personality Questionnaire (Cloninger 1987, version 4, 10/26/87 revision, scoring key revised February 1, 1988). I presume these tests are useful in defining individuals who could benefit from therapeutic intervention. Yet there is nothing in their design or construction to indicate that we should regard a 7% mean change in an "extraversion" score (from 53.4 to 57.3), or a 6% mean change in "conscientiousness" score (from 45.9 to 43.2) between two groups of individuals sorted by their genotype as differences on which to found a realistic research program looking for biological effects at the level of individuals. From the construction of the test, it appears that these differences can result from answers to very few questions, which have the form of "I often crave excitement" and "I am easily frightened."

There is an apocryphal story about a well-known evolutionary biologist, noted for his intolerance of the foibles of others. At the conclusion of one of his lectures, he asked, "Are there any questions?" and a young gentleman in the front row proceeded to pose a long, pompous, and convoluted query, to which the speaker replied, without skipping a beat, "Are there any *pertinent* questions?" Because even the most derived behavioral variables contain measures that depend on the activity of the nervous system and bodily organs whose function depends on developmental and ongoing action of gene products, and because there are an awful lot of A's, C's, G's, and T's in everyone's genome and a lot of ways in which their variation can affect brain and bodily function, correlations do not mean a lot. Putting DNA variation and behavioral variation into particular causal pathways does. The trick is not to ask *any* question, but to ask the pertinent ones—the ones from which you can hope to learn something meaningful about the biology of an organism.

Maybe investigators should initially pick more limited, definable aspects of human behavior than IQ tests, personality inventory scores, or even broad clinical disorders or personal attributes—aspects that have a clearer relationship to biological variables that are already known. An alternative suggestion would be to consider a variant of the approach advocated by Dryja (1997), who presented an argument for a gene-based, rather than a phenotype-based approach to human gene-phenotype correlations. Investigators in this volume who have already settled on candidate genes may find this a more scientifically productive course than limiting their view to allelic correlations in groups of subjects. Investigators who are wedded to a particular type of behavior or pathology and who initially want to identify all of the genes that have any impact on their object of study should consider how unstable a foundation this may provide for future research. It may be better to concentrate efforts on genes whose products are involved in a particular biological pathway strongly implicated in behavioral or pathological causation. It is probably better to have a few sure bases from which to proceed than a lot of unsure ones.

There is one realm in which I concede that even virtual behaviors can serve a useful purpose, and that is the case mentioned at the end of each of the previous sections—using gene effects found by any kind of phenotypic screen to provide entry points into some aspect of cellular or developmental physiology. This requires investigators to be more interested in understanding an aspect of development than in one particular phenotypic outcome of that aspect of development.

Simplistic Interpretations

Many authors have spilled a lot of ink disapproving of simple gene-behavior linkages. Although most practicing biologists agree with Plasterk (1999) and Scriver and Waters (1999) that genes speak biochemistry and not phenotypes, labeling genes by particular behaviors or calling them genes *for* particular behaviors shows no signs of vanishing from the literature. For example, Benjamin (1998) retained these usages even after admitting that they are essentially meaningless and can be misleading. But I know from the experience of talking with the people who use these shorthands that they are much more sophisticated: they do not mechanistically believe that special genes regulate homosexuality or novelty seeking, and they do not believe in simple pathways from genes to behavior. These are not the "simplistic interpretations" that bother me.

What bothers me is more subtle and will require more discussion with human correlative behavior geneticists than space in this volume permits. It can briefly be raised by considering the following quote:

> The point I wish to make is that if DRD4 really does affect all these conditions . . . , then it behooves us to try to understand the possible common psychological consequence of what may be a common biochemical effect. This psychological consequence may be a common link in the chains of psychological cause and effect that lead to these various conditions. A second possibility is that the same potential biochemical consequence of having a long allele for the gene for this receptor has *in reality very different* biochemical consequences when the DRD4 polymorphism is inherited *in conjunction* with one or another different biochemical conditions [sic] unique to each of the following: "normality". . . , hyperactivity, Tourette's disorder, and panic disorder; and each of these different biochemical results leads to different psychological results. But as a research strategy we will presumably first pursue the first possibility. So we must rethink what we know of the psychology, and seek commonalities among the conditions described. (Benjamin 1998, pp. 363–364, emphases in original)

There are two things here that I have trouble with, which can have an appreciable impact on the design and interpretation of research. The first is a sentiment that is expressed with incredible frequency by human correlative behavior geneticists: that both "normal" and "abnormal" behavior can be somehow better understood, systematized or united by information on allelic variation. This seems to be the catechism of many biological psychiatrists. I understand that the basic notion comes from pathology. In metabolic "diseases" such as PKU, abnormal function of a single gene product brings together a bewildering variety of systemic failures in diverse bodily systems under one comprehensive explanatory umbrella. I grant that when we are talking about genes contributing to brain pathologies that are causally associated with behavioral ones, this statement may not be simplistic (but see Templeton 1998). But when talking about pathological conditions with multiple causal components and "normal" variation, such a view seems as inadvisable as the second thing which bothers me: the direct link between psychology and genes.

Neural development intervenes between genes and psychology. Here it is not enough to "speak biochemistry," because brains are not just bags of biochemicals. They have anatomy, intracellular and intercellular physiology, and lots of cell-cell signaling. Their development in some cases can make up for (regulate) changes in biochemical components and sometimes cannot (for both stochastic and genetic background reasons). To get from genes to psychology, we need to get from genes to biochemical pathways, from biochemical pathways to cell physiology, from cell physiology to development and ongoing cell function, from functioning cells to their anatomical organization and physiological cooperation in brain structures, and from systems brain function to whole-brain and whole-organism attributes such as psychology. How about placing DRD4 receptors into particular biochemical pathways that play key roles in particular cell lineages where the structural differences encoded by different alleles will influence the development of brain anatomy and physiology in particular ways, which may bear quite a variable relationship to whole-organism behavioral attributes, before we start talking about psychology and how DRD4 changes interact with other gene products?

Misleading Representations and the Dark Side of Human Correlative Behavior Genetics

Before concluding this chapter, there is one more issue that needs to be addressed that is potentially very divisive: the conflicts of interest that all biologically oriented scientists face when communicating our work to other scientists and the public at large (Balaban 1996, 1998; Balaban et al. 1996). When you work on biological aspects of things that scare, matter to, or titillate people, there is always a temptation to play to the crowd for individual gain, which can all too easily be rationalized as playing to the crowd for collective gain. Whether our work is publicly or privately funded, publicity usually translates into more funding. Although making controversial statements and claiming the existence of new revolutions in understanding and controlling behavior may attract attention and funding to the field in the short term, it is not a good long-term strategy. Many of us tend to ignore the fact that what may be good for conventional career advancement of particular individuals (not only within science but also in the realm of personal wealth via popular book contracts and paid public appearances), may not be good for establishing public and scientific confidence in the veracity and solidity of behavioral biology.

If you believe in what is being promulgated in the press or in popular writings, then there is no problem: the public and one's scientific peers can consider what sort of confidence they want to have in your research programs. The problem comes about when people want to promulgate certain ideas for the sake of publicity, yet maintain a respectable distance from the same ideas for the sake of their scientific credibility.

I believe that most people doing human correlative behavior genetics do not have a simplistic view about linking genes to behavior. What, then, accounts for the almost universally simplistic treatment of human correlative behavior genetic work when its proponents write popular books, and in press accounts of their work? The unanimous answer of the scientists is that this is due to the ignorance or willful misrepresentation of their work on the part of the press, and/or decisions of editors or journalist cowriters who want to make material more "accessible" to a general audience.

In discussing this problem with science writers at major national newspapers, I have the idea that they face the same conflicts of interest we scientists do. Science writers get paid for covering "important" news stories, and they try to be independent and critical. Yet anything that they decide to cover for whatever reason needs to have its "importance" justified. This sets up a common interest with the scientist whose work is being covered, where journalists become eager conduits for any tidbit that makes work more revolutionary and more topical. However, they are adamant that they do not put words in people's mouths, and in hearing what many scientists actually say to them I believe this is generally true. Some scientists may have the idea that they can play both sides of the fence: say or imply things to journalists that they would not say to other scientists to get more attention, and then deny to other scientists that they said these things in order to maintain their credibility with their peers.

The only way to combat this is to take some personal responsibility for how your work is portrayed in the press. If you do not like how it is portrayed, be very vocal about it. Journalist's bosses generally listen to problems scientists have about the portrayal of their work. Any publicity is not necessarily good publicity. You do a service to all behavioral biologists when you promote a realistic vision on the part of other scientists and the public of what behavioral biology is about.

The Future Is Interdisciplinary

Relating genetics and behavior is an intensely interdisciplinary endeavor, encompassing different fields and research in both humans and animals. The more frequently that human correlative behavioral geneticists speak the language, think the concepts, and appreciate the complexities facing their brethren in other areas of biology who will help them make linkages between genetic and behavioral variation, the better it will be for everyone. I am willing to accept that increased contact with people doing human correlative behavior genetics may change my opinions and reservations about a lot of the work. I am also convinced that increased scientific contact with cellular, developmental, and systems neurobiologists will have a positive impact on the way that problems are chosen, followed, and presented by the human correlative behavior genetics community. I hope that the foregoing remarks will be heard in this spirit.

Acknowledgments

I thank Drs. Benjamin, Ebstein, and Belmaker for their invitation to contribute to this volume, and Seymour Benzer for access to materials.

References

Allen N, Logan K, Lally G, et al: Distribution of parthenogenetic cells in the mouse brain and their influence on brain development. Proc Natl Acad Sci U S A 92:10782–10786, 1995

Balaban E: Bird song syntax: learned intraspecific variation is meaningful. Proc Natl Acad Sci U S A 85:3657–3660, 1988a

Balaban E: Cultural and genetic variation in swamp sparrows (Melospiza georgiana), I: song variation, genetic variation, and their relationship. Behaviour 105:250–291, 1988b

Balaban E: Cultural and genetic variation in swamp sparrows (Melospiza georgiana), II: behavioral salience of geographic song variants. Behaviour 105:292–322, 1988c

Balaban, E. Avian brain chimeras as a tool for studying species behavioral differences, in The Avian Model in Developmental Biology: From Organism to Genes. Edited by Le Douarin N, Dieterlen-Lièvre F, Smith J. Paris, CNRS Press, 1990, pp 105–118

Balaban E: Reflections on Wye Woods: crime, biology, and self-interest. Politics and the Life Sciences 15:86–88, 1996

Balaban E: Changes in multiple brain regions underlie species differences in a complex, congenital behavior. Proc Natl Acad Sci U S A 94:2001–2006, 1997

Balaban E: Eugenics and phenotypic variation: to what extent is biology a predictive science? Science in Context 11:331–356, 1998

Balaban E: Behavior genetics: Galen's prophecy or Malpighi's legacy? in Thinking about Evolution: Historical, Philosophical, and Political Perspectives. Edited by Singh R, Krimbas C, Paul D, et al. Cambridge, UK, Cambridge University Press, 2000, pp 429–466

Balaban E: A biological perspective on innateness, in Growth, Development and Learning. Edited by Bonatti L, Carey S, Mehler J. Cambridge, MA, MIT Press (in press)

Balaban E, Teillet M-A, Le Douarin N: Application of the quail-chick chimeric system to the study of brain development and behavior. Science 241:1339–1342, 1988

Balaban E, Alper JS, Kasmon YL: Mean genes and the biology of aggression: a critical review of recent animal and human research. J Neurogenet 11:1–43, 1996

Benjamin J: Genes for human personality traits. Science in Context 11:357–372, 1998

Benjamin J, Li L, Patterson C, et al: Population and familial association between the D4 dopamine receptor gene and measures of novelty seeking. Nat Genet 12:81–84, 1996

Block J: A contrarian view of the five-factor approach to personality description. Psychol Bull 117:187–215, 1995

Caldji C, Tannenbaum B, Sharma S, et al: Maternal care during infancy regulates the development of neural systems mediating the expression of fearfulness in the rat. Proc Natl Acad Sci U S A 95:5335–5340, 1998

Cloninger CR: A systematic method for clinical description and classification of personality variants. Arch Gen Psychiatry 44:573–588. 1987

Cloninger C, Adolfsson R, Svrakic N: Mapping genes for human personality. Nat Genet 12:3–4, 1996

Costa P (ed): Special series: clinical use of the five-factor model of personality. J Pers Assess 57:393–464, 1991

Costa P, McCrae R: Cross-sectional studies of personality in a national sample, I: development and validation of survey measures. Psychol Aging 1:140–143, 1986

Costa P, McCrae R: Personality in adulthood: A six-year longitudinal study of self-reports and spouse ratings on the NEO Personality Inventory. J Pers Soc Psychol 54:853–863, 1988

Costa P, McCrae R: Four ways five factors are basic. Personality and Individual Differences 13:653–665, 1992a

Costa P, McCrae R: Trait psychology comes of age, in Psychology and Aging: Current Theory and Research in Motivation. (Nebraska Symposium on Motivation, Vol 39) Edited by Sonderegger T. Lincoln, University of Nebraska Press, 1992b, pp 169–204

Costa P, McCrae R: Domains and facets: hierarchical personality assessment using the Revised NEO Personality Inventory. J Pers Assess 64:21–50, 1995

Costa P, McCrae R: Stability and change in personality assessment: the Revised NEO Personality Inventory in the year 2000. J Pers Assess 68:86–94, 1997

Costa P, McCrae R, Zonderman A, et al: Cross-sectional studies of personality in a national sample, II: stability in neuroticism, extraversion, and openness. Psychol Aging 1:144–149, 1986

Costa P, McCrae R, Dye D: Facet scales for agreeableness and conscientiousness: a revision of the NEO Personality Inventory. Personality and Individual Differences 12:887–898, 1991

Crabbe J, Phillips T, Feller D, et al: Elevated alcohol consumption in null mutant mice lacking 5-HT-1B serotonin receptors. Nat Genet 14:98–101, 1996

Crabbe, J, Wahlsten D, Dudek B: Genetics of mouse behavior: interactions with laboratory environment. Science 284:1670–1672, 1999

Denenberg V, Hoplight B, Mobraaten L: The uterine environment enhances cognitive competence. Neuroreport 9:1667–1671, 1998

Devlin B, Daniels M, Roeder K: The heritability of IQ. Nature 388:468–471, 1997

Dryja T: Gene-based approach to human gene-phenotype correlations. Proc Natl Acad Sci U S A 94:12117–12121, 1997

Ebstein R, Novick O, Umansky R, et al: Dopamine D4 receptor (D4DR) exon III polymorphism associated with the human personality trait of novelty seeking. Nat Genet 12:78–80, 1996

Enserink M: Fickle mice highlight test problems. Science 284:1599–1600, 1999

Fausto-Sterling A, Balaban E: Genetics and male sexual orientation (letter). Science 261:1257, 1993

Flint J: The genetic basis of cognition. Brain 122:2015–2031, 1999

Francis D, Diorio J, Liu D, et al: Nongenomic transmission across generations of maternal behavior and stress response in the rat. Science 286:1155–1158, 1999

Gahr M, Balaban E: The development of a species difference in the local distribution of brain estrogen receptive cells. Developmental Brain Research 92:182–189, 1996

Gerlai R, Clayton N: Analysing hippocampal function in transgenic mice: an ethological perspective. Trends Neurosci 22:47–51, 1999

Ginns EI, St Jean P, Philibert RA, et al: A genome-wide search for chromosomal loci linked to mental health wellness in relatives at high risk for bipolar affective disorder among the Old Order Amish. Proc Natl Acad Sci U S A 95:15531–15536, 1998

Grunstein M: Yeast heterochromatin: regulation of its assembly and inheritance by histones. Cell 93:325–328, 1998

Hamer D: Genetics and male sexual orientation (letter). Science 285:797, 1999

Henikoff S, Comai L: Trans-sensing effects: the ups and downs of being together. Cell 93:329–332, 1998

Hu S, Pattatucci A, Patterson C, et al: Linkage between sexual orientation and chromosome Xq28 in males but not in females. Nat Genet 11:248–256, 1995

Kelly M, Rubinstein M, Phillips T, et al: Locomotor activity in D2 dopamine receptor-deficient mice is determined by gene dosage, genetic background, and developmental adaptations. J Neurosci 18:3470–3479, 1998

Keverne E, Fundele R, Narasimha M, et al: Genomic imprinting and the differential roles of parental genomes in brain development. Developmental Brain Research 92:91–100, 1996

Lefebvre L, Viville S, Barton S, et al: Abnormal maternal behavior and growth retardation associated with loss of the imprinted gene Mest. Nat Genet 20:163–169, 1998

Lewin B: The mystique of epigenetics. Cell 93:301–304, 1998

Li L, Keverne E, Aparicio S, et al: Regulation of maternal behavior and offspring growth by paternally expressed Peg3. Science 284:330–333, 1999

Long K, Kennedy G, Balaban E: Transferring an inborn auditory perceptual preference with interspecies brain transplants. Proc Natl Acad Sci U S A 98:5862–5867, 2001

McCrae R, Costa P: Validation of the five-factor model of personality across instruments and observers. J Pers Soc Psychol 52:81–90, 1987

McCrae R, Costa P: Rotation to maximize the construct validity of factors in the NEO Personality Inventory. Multivariate Behavioral Research 24:107–124, 1989

McCrae R, Costa P: Discriminant validity of NEO-PIR facet scales. Educational and Psychological Measurement 52:229–237, 1992

McCrae R, Zonderman A, Costa P, et al: Evaluating replicability of factors in the Revised NEO Personality Inventory: confirmatory factor analysis versus Procrustes rotation. J Pers Soc Psychol 70:552–566, 1996

Morgan H, Sutherland H, Martin D, et al: Epigenetic inheritance at the agouti locus in the mouse. Nat Genet 23:314–318, 1999

Panning B, Jaenisch R: RNA and the epigenetic regulation of X chromosome inactivation. Cell 93:305–308, 1998

Park T, Balaban E: Relative salience of species maternal calls in neonatal Gallinaceous birds: a direct comparison of Japanese quail *(Coturnix coturnix japonica)* and domestic chickens *(Gallus gallus domesticus)*. J Comp Psychol 105:45–54, 1991

Patel A, Balaban E: Temporal patterns of human cortical activity reflect tone sequence structure. Nature 404:80–84, 2000

Patel A, Balaban E: Human pitch perception is reflected in the timing of stimulus-related cortical activity. Nat Neurosci 4:839–844, 2001

Pirrotta V: Polycombing the genome: PcG, trxG, and chromatin silencing. Cell 93:333–336, 1998

Plasterk R: Hershey heaven and *Caenorhabditis elegans.* Nat Genet 21:63–64, 1999

Polaczyk P, Gasperini R, Gibson G: Naturally occurring genetic variation affects *Drosophila* photoreceptor determination. Development, Genes and Evolution 207:462–470, 1998

Rice G, Anderson C, Risch N, et al: Male homosexuality: absence of linkage to microsatellite markers at Xq28. Science 284:665–667, 1999a

Rice G, Risch N, Ebers G: Genetics and male sexual orientation: response (letter). Science 285:797, 1999b

Scriver C, Waters P: Monogenic traits are not simple: lessons from phenylketonuria. Trends Genet 15:267–272, 1999

Surani M: Imprinting and the initiation of gene silencing in the germ line. Cell 93:309–312, 1998

Templeton AR: The complexity of the genotype-phenotype relationship and the limitations of using genetic "markers" at the individual level. Science in Context 11:373–389, 1998

Wakimoto B: Beyond the nucleosome: epigenetic aspects of position-effect variegation in *Drosophila.* Cell 93:321–324, 1998

Wickelgren I: Discovery of "gay gene" questioned (news item). Science 284:571, 1999

Wiens G, Sorger P: Centromeric chromatin and epigenetic effects in kinetochore assembly. Cell 93:313–316, 1998

CHAPTER SEVENTEEN

Genetics of Human Personality

Social and Ethical Implications

Jon Beckwith, Ph.D.
Joseph S. Alper, Ph.D.

Grumpy, fearful neurotics appear to be short on a gene.
(Angier 1996)

Research points toward a "gay" gene. (Bishop 1993)

Man's genes made him kill, his lawyers claim. (Felsenthal 1994)

These headlines reflect the renewed interest in the genetics of human personality traits that has resulted from the revolution in genetic research of the last 25 years. This interest parallels events of almost one hundred years ago that followed the rediscovery of Mendel's laws of inheritance. Geneticists moved beyond the simple traits of fruit flies and pea plants to speculate about the genetic basis of personality traits characteristic of various racial and ethnic groups. For example, in "The Biological Effects of Race Movements" published in the magazine *Popular Science Monthly*, David Starr Jordan, evolutionist and Stanford University president, spoke of "lower races" that were immigrating into the United States from Europe and Asia and lowering "our own average" (D. S. Jordan 1915). This same magazine, in 1913 alone, featured articles by J. G. Wilson (1913) and H. E. Jordan (1913) discussing the genetic inferiority of Jews and "the Mulatto."

German geneticists Fritz Lenz and Erwin Baur and anthropologist Eugen Fischer also used genetics to explain personality characteristics of racial and ethnic groups in their widely used 1921 *Human Genetics* text: "Fraud and the use of insulting language are commoner among Jews" (Bauer et al. 1931, p. 681). "In general, a Negro is not inclined to work hard" (p. 628). "The Mongolian character . . . inclines to petrifaction in the traditional" (p. 636). "The Russians excel in suffering and in endurance" (p. 639).

These pronouncements from scientists provided some of the rationale for oppressive social policies, ranging from eugenic sterilization laws in the United States and many western European countries to the extermination programs of the Nazis (Butler 1997; Kevles 1985; Muller-Hill 1988).

As we enter the twenty-first century, the genetics community has largely moved beyond the stereotyping of groups (except see Herrnstein and Murray 1994). Scientists and the media no longer attribute particular personality traits to racial or ethnic minorities. Today, behavioral geneticists are interested primarily in individual and familial characteristics. Nevertheless, just as with the earlier claims put forth by scientists, the ways in which contemporary findings are communicated to the public can exert a harmful influence on social policy and public attitudes.

In this chapter, we point out these problems in the context of the scientific approaches that are being used to study the genetics of personality traits. We describe some of the limitations of the science, contrasting it with its presentation to the public. We outline some of the social consequences of the public misrepresentation of the significance of new genetic findings. Finally, we suggest how geneticists in this field might best communicate their results to avoid these consequences.

Limitations and Problems in the Genetics of Personality Traits

In recent years the power of the tools available to geneticists has dramatically increased. Medical researchers using these new approaches have identified genes associated with both "simple" genetic diseases such as cystic fibrosis and with complex multifactorial diseases such as breast cancer and colon cancer. Yet despite this remarkable progress in human medical genetics, all the reports to date of genes for mental illnesses have encountered scientific difficulties. For example, many genetic loci have been reported to be associated with schizophrenia or manic depression. None of these associations has, to date, been definitively confirmed, some have been retracted and others have been dropped from consideration when attempts at replication of the original studies failed (Kelsoe et al. 1989; Robertson 1989; Watt and Edwards 1991). Similarly, flaws have been found in all the reports of genes for normal personality traits (Baron 1998; Gelernter et al. 1991; Pato et al. 1993; Rice et al. 1999).

Why is the genetics of mental illness and personality traits so difficult?

The problems in studying the genetics of mental illness and personality traits can be conveniently divided into three categories: the characterization of the traits, the complexity of the genetics, and the methods of genetic analysis.

Characterizing Traits

An important assumption underlying genetic studies is that the trait as defined by its observable or clinical manifestations corresponds to an actual biological entity that is influenced by genes. In the language of the social sciences, we must assume that the illness is not simply a reification. In studying somatic diseases, this assumption is usually, though not always, correct. However, when studying a mental illness, for example, schizophrenia, we cannot be certain that the grouping of a set of symptoms under the heading *schizophrenia* corresponds to the same discrete causal mechanism (possibly involving both genetic and environmental factors) in all cases. Two people with seemingly identical symptoms may be suffering from illnesses caused by two entirely different sets of genes. Or, conversely, the same set of genes operating in different environments may result in very different sets of symptoms.

Even assuming that there is biological validity to a particular definition of an illness, it is often difficult to decide whether a specific individual's set of symptoms matches the established criteria for the illness. This difficulty is exaggerated in the study of personality traits because these traits are measured on a quantitative scale rather than a dichotomous scale (either/or). Psychological testing is by no means an exact science, and so we cannot be confident that quantitative tests of personality actually measure the trait as it has been defined. If we simply define the trait as that which is measured by the test (e.g., defining intelligence by IQ scores), then we are in grave danger of reifying the trait.

Genetic Complexity

Even if a trait is well defined and even if the trait runs in families, the causal mechanism may be so complicated that the task of finding genes associated with the trait will prove to be exceedingly difficult. A list of the difficulties resulting from genetic complexity includes: 1) Several or many genes may be involved. 2) Environmental factors may be as important as genes. 3) The contributions of the individual genes and the environment may not be additive. The nonadditive contributions can take several forms: synergistic genetic interactions in which the effect of one gene depends on the presence or absence of other genes; gene-environment covariance in which certain genes are more likely to be found in certain environments; and gene-environment interactions in which the effect of a gene depends on the particular environment in which it is found (Falconer 1989).

These examples of complexity are not hypothetical; all have been well documented in animal studies (Crabbe et al. 1999; Falconer 1989). Studies of human somatic diseases such as cancer, diabetes, hypertension and vascular disease show that these issues cannot be ignored (Sack 1999). Because it is highly likely that mental illness and personality traits are, if anything, more complicated than somatic diseases, these mechanisms must be taken into account in analyzing the genetics of such illnesses and behaviors.

Methods of Genetic Analysis

These difficulties have led to the publication of numerous review articles discussing the strengths and weaknesses of the methods being employed (Baron 1998; Baron et al. 1990; Kidd 1993, 1997; Lander and Kruglyak 1995; Risch and Botstein 1996; Risch and Merikangas 1996). For example, linkage studies require an accurate model of the inheritance of a trait and depend on a more accurate diagnosis of each individual in the study. Association studies must avoid the problem of population stratification; the sample of individuals must be random with respect to ethnicity and race.

These reevaluations have included critiques of the statistical methods used to analyze results. One difficulty in statistical analysis arises from the use of multiple hypotheses, any one of which might give rise to an association between a gene and a behavioral trait. The greater the number of these hypotheses that are tested, the more likely it is that an association is due to such an accident. The statistical analysis of the data must correct for this situation.

The problem of multiple hypotheses arises in at least two guises in the study of the genetics of human behavior. First, even though a researcher might restrict her attention to a single chromosome in the search for a gene associated with schizophrenia, other researchers might focus on other chromosomes. Consequently, each researcher is actually testing multiple hypotheses and so must perform a statistical analysis based on a genome wide search rather than based on the single chromosome examined in the study. Second, the criteria for the characterization of a mental illness or personality trait may vary from study to study. Each choice of characterizing the trait represents a different possible hypothesis. Clearly the greater the number of possible characterization of the trait that are available, the more likely it is that one of these characterizations will result in an association between the trait and a gene. In each of these examples, a pedestrian use of statistics will result in an overly optimistic statistical estimate of the degree of confidence in the result. Statistical errors of these types probably account for the majority of the retractions and failed replications in human behavioral genetics.

Some Case Studies

In discussing the complex genetics of personality, we point out that even single-gene conditions such as cystic fibrosis (Desgeorges et al. 1994; Donat et al. 1997; Meschede et al. 1993; Parad 1996), Huntington disease (Rubinsztein et al. 1996), and Gaucher's disease (Sidransky and Ginns 1993) display remarkable complexities. In the case of cystic fibrosis, a single-gene autosomal recessive disorder, more than 500 mutations have been found in the gene associated with the disease. Different combinations of altered alleles result in different sets of symptoms some of which do not seem to be related to the classic set of symptoms for cystic fibrosis at all. And more surprisingly, given previous impressions, the same pair of altered alleles can result in cases of cystic fibrosis with dramatically different degrees of severity or even different sets of symptoms. Although it now seems probable that the environment does not play a significant role in cystic fibrosis, it appears that gene-gene interactions play an important role in the etiology of this disease.

Common multifactorial diseases such as breast cancer are of course even more complex (Couch et al. 1997; Newman et al. 1998). Even though genes, e.g., *BRCA1* and *BRCA2*, have been found whose altered forms significantly increase the probability that a woman will develop breast cancer, most women who develop the disease do not have altered forms of these genes. It seems evident, then, that in addition to the genetic interactions present in "single-gene" diseases, multifactorial diseases involve environmental influences and most likely, gene-environmental interactions (Lichtenstein et al. 2000).

Given these complexities, it is perhaps not surprising that so little progress has been made in associating genes with complex mental illnesses. One explanation for this failure that is rarely considered is that these illnesses are not in fact heritable. The evidence for heritability comes from behavior genetics familial studies involving, for example, comparisons between identical and fraternal twins. Perhaps the critics who maintained that these familial studies were suspect have been right all along (Beckwith and Alper 1998; Joseph 1998; Kamin 1974; Lewontin et al. 1984; Spitz and Carlier 1996). These critics have argued that crucial assumptions of such studies are flawed, including the assumption that both identical and fraternal twins share environments to the same degree.

The analysis of the genetics of personality traits introduces additional difficulties. Genetic alterations can clearly influence behavior. Individuals with PKU (phenylketonuria), a single-gene metabolic disease, have diminished IQ scores (Tourian and Sidbury 1983); individuals with Lesch-Nyhan disease often engage in self-mutilating behavior. But does the finding that abnormal behavior can be caused by altered genes mean that normal variations in behavior are caused by genetic variation?

In 1993, a Dutch research team studying a single family discovered a mutation that inactivated the MAO A (monoamine oxidase A) gene. This gene was immediately labeled by the media as the "criminal gene" (Brunner et al. 1993a, 1993b; Cowley and Hall 1993; Felsenthal 1994; Mestel 1994). Men in this family who carried the mutation were reported to engage in violent behavior. It is known that this mutation has a significant impact on biochemical reactions required for the normal functioning of the nervous system. Consequently, it would not be surprising that this mutation did indeed affect mental functioning and even contribute to antisocial tendencies.

The MAO A gene is not a "criminal gene" for the same reason that the gene in which mutations cause PKU is not an "intelligence gene." PKU is a rare disease contributing to only a tiny fraction of cases of mental retardation. No one has suggested that variation in intelligence in populations can be explained by mutations in this gene. Analogously, a correlation between mutations in the MAO A gene and antisocial behavior has only been found in this single family. Extreme cases of this sort are highly unlikely to contribute to the understanding of variation of such traits in the general population.

In fact, there is probably no such thing as an "aggression gene" or "criminal gene." It is certainly true that many of the people who commit violent crimes such as robbery and murder are much more aggressive than the average person and it may even be true that their aggressive behavior is influenced by their genes. However, it does not follow that differences in aggression among people can be explained by the presence or absence of mutations in a few identifiable genes. In view of what we have learned from psychology and sociology about the complexity of aggressive behavior, it is most probable that the discovery of any genes associated with certain cases of aggressive or criminal behavior will be of little value in explaining or understanding these behaviors, in general.

As with the search for genes associated with mental illness, reports of linkage studies with normal personality traits have also run into problems. In 1996, two reports appeared of an association between novelty seeking behavior and the length of a portion of the D4 dopamine receptor gene on chromosome 11 (Ebstein et al. 1996). Novelty seeking involves exploratory, thrill seeking, and excitable behavior. This behavior, which shows continuous variation, was measured by means of a psychological test. Despite the definitional issues we have raised, we will assume that the test does in fact measure a real trait called *novelty seeking*.

These studies appeared very convincing, as two independent groups had found the same gene for novelty seeking. However, soon after, other researchers reported that they were unable to replicate the findings. Moreover, one of the original two groups could not replicate the clear-cut results they had obtained previously. In fact, in order to obtain a positive linkage result, they were forced to redefine novelty seeking, restricting it to an extreme type of thrill seeking behavior (Baron 1998).

How is it possible that two independent studies reaching the same conclusion might both be wrong? As is the case in the search for genes for mental illness, the answer lies in the statistics of gene searches. Probably more than 20,000 genes are involved in the functioning of the human brain, any one of which could conceivably be associated with a trait such as novelty seeking. As a result, traditional statistical methods vastly overestimate the likelihood that an association between one of these genes and the trait is a real association rather than merely being the result of a statistical accident like finding five consecutive heads when tossing a coin.

Even if the two groups of researchers had been correct in their claim that they had found a "novelty seeking gene," the existence of this gene, taken in isolation, would not explain novelty seeking behavior. According to these researchers, the heritability of novelty seeking is only approximately 50%, and only 10% of that heritability is attributable to the novelty seeking gene. Thus this gene, even if it exists, accounts for only a very small portion of the variation in novelty seeking behavior.

Is a Science of the Genetics of Mental Illness and Personality Possible?

All science deals with complex systems. In a science such as physics or chemistry, progress is made by assuming that the essential features of a phenomenon can be understood even though the analysis is based on simplifying assumptions that eliminate much of the complexity of the problem.

In the case of a single-gene disease, the operation of the single gene acting in isolation from other genes and the environment is, in some cases, sufficient to explain the disease. However, in the case of complex diseases and behavior, genes may be involved in the behavior but may, by themselves, be of little use in explaining the behavior.

In order to explain complex diseases and behavior, new paradigms may be required (Risch and Botstein 1996). The old paradigm, which restricted attention to genetic explanations for mental illness and personality traits, has not resulted in any increased understanding of the nature of the illness or behavior. We believe that any new paradigm will need to incorporate the complexities caused by gene-environment interactions and covariances in a fundamental manner.

Genetic researchers are not ready to give up the old paradigm, arguing with justification that it is not dead yet. However, many of these same researchers are becoming more aware its limitations. The work of Lander, Kidd, Risch, and others has led to an increased appreciation of the difficulties in concluding from an experimental study that a gene is really associated with a trait (Kidd 1993; Lander and Kruglyak 1995; Uhl et al. 1997). This appreciation has already led to an increased number of papers reporting that a particular gene is *not* associated with a particular trait. Such reports of negative results are extremely valuable in assessing the degree of confidence that a gene is associated with a trait.

Genetic Fatalism and the Impact of the New Behavior Genetics

In 1993, geneticist Dean Hamer and his coworkers from the United States National Institutes of Health reported that they had found a region of the human X chromosome that was associated with male homosexual behavior in some families (Hamer et al. 1993). In a press release and elsewhere, Hamer took care to point out the limitations of the study and the likelihood that environment as well as genes play a role in homosexuality (Hamer and Copeland 1998; Hamer et al. 1993). Dr. Hamer was subsequently called to testify in the Supreme Court of the state of Colorado, where plaintiffs were asking that an anti–gay rights amendment to the state constitution be declared unconstitutional. There, after summarizing the evidence for a genetic component of sexual orientation, he "admit[ted] that sexual orientation is not completely genetic"(Bayliss 1993). Despite Hamer's cautions, the plaintiffs used the science and other arguments to "argue that homosexuality is inborn"(Bayliss 1993). Later, Hamer himself took a more deterministic position in a *Washington Post* interview: "On the one hand, having a gene is practically useful because you can argue that it's an immutable trait" (Weiss 1994, p. 12).

Most behavioral geneticists seem to take a more nuanced stance on determinism. Nevertheless, many of them have also adopted a basically deterministic position. Instead of espousing a strict sense of determinism meaning *immutability*, they present a softened view in which genes *limit* the degree of behavioral change possible. Although this limiting position is reasonable, we have no way of determining what these limits are; we do not know which environments will allow the greatest change in the manifestation of some particular behavior. Despite this lack of knowledge, both geneticists and the media often imply that these limits are quite stringent and even make policy recommendations based on these supposed limits.

For example, a paper in *Science* proposed a genetic hypothesis to explain the difference in performance between girls and boys on tests on mathematics ability (Benbow and Stanley 1980). Because of its social ramifications, this paper received widespread publicity. In their interviews with the media, the authors often expressed the view, going far beyond their scientific evidence, that girls were genetically limited in their mathematical potential and would be "better off accepting their differences" (Kolata 1980, p. 1235) Subsequent studies showed that the publicity this paper received influenced the attitudes of both parents and children toward the math ability of girls (Beckwith 1983; Fennema 1981).

One of the largest projects designed to assess the genetic contributions to human behavior and aptitudes is the study of identical twins led by Dr. Thomas Bouchard at the University of Minnesota. Published reports from this group have suggested that a wide range of traits is substantially influenced by genetics, with heritability estimates hovering around 50% (Bouchard et al. 1990). Even though heritability estimates are based on the range of existing environments, some of the researchers associated with the project seemed to assume that their findings apply to all possible environments, and that genes severely limit the range of a wide variety of human behaviors. In discussing *fearlessness,* Dr. Nancy Segal stated that "[p]arents can work to make a child less fearful, but they can't make that child brave" (Leo 1987). Segal's colleague, Dr. David Lykken, discussed the genetic limits on happiness and recommended that one "find the small things that you know give you a little high" (Goleman 1996). Both of these prescriptive statements include the recognition that genes do not impose a fixed limit to the expression of a trait. But, by suggesting how people should behave in accordance with their genotype, the authors are implicitly retaining the deterministic attitude toward genetics.

These genetic deterministic attitudes have already found their way into the legal system. In July 1996, at Woods Hole on Cape Cod, Massachusetts, 35 judges from both Federal and State courts met with 20 scientists to discuss the implications of the revolution in genetics for the legal system (Blakeslee 1996). As reported by Blakeslee, in one discussion on the ethical issues raised by the new genetics "judges asked what would happen if science demonstrated that genes controlled behavior or that bad early environments conspired with genes to turn some people inevitably into criminals—showing that free will did not exist in these situations."

This interest by the legal profession in the role of genes in criminal behavior and free will did not arise in a vacuum. The MAO A gene studies, referred to above, played a role in arousing public interest in the social implications of the findings. This interest was first stimulated by the researchers themselves in the Discussion sections of their papers, where they suggested that their findings might help explain the larger problem of aggressive behavior in society (Brunner et al. 1993a, 1993b).

A *Science* magazine reporter noting these suggestions wrote that "it might be possible to identify people who are prone to violent acts by screening for MAO A gene mutations" (Morell 1993, p. 1722). At this point, the baton passed to the mass media and then even to the courts. *Newsweek*'s article entitled "The Genetics of Bad Behavior" was illustrated with a photograph of a violent confrontation between Palestinians and Israelis (Cowley and Hall 1993). A TV news report used films of U.S. street gang violence in its report on the MAO A study (X. Breakefield, personal communication, December 1994). In a murder trial in Georgia, defense lawyers called upon Dr. Xandra Breakefield, one of the scientists involved in the study, to testify on the genetic basis of aggressive and violent behavior. We have described this sequence of events in some detail in order to demonstrate how a relatively minor genetic advance can rapidly be transmitted to the public, be misinterpreted, and then be incorporated into the social fabric.

To their credit, the scientists involved in the study have shown concern about the public representations of their reports. Dr. Breakefield was dismayed enough by the publicity to announce that she would no longer work on links between violence and genes (Breakefield 1994). Dr. Brunner's statement in a recent article that "the notion of an 'aggression gene' does not make sense " (Brunner 1995, p. 160) clearly reflected concern for the ways in which the study was interpreted by the media.

Where Do We Go From Here?

The interface between genetics and society is mediated by several different social institutions—the scientific community itself, the scientific journals, and the popular media. Each of these institutions plays a role in determining whether reports of genes for personality traits accurately reflect the significance of the research or whether they misrepresent the science and its social implications. Because this is an area of genetics that has historically influenced and continues to influence social policy and public attitudes, special caution in the research itself, in its interpretation, and in its presentation to the public is necessary.

As we have shown, some scientists have misstated the implications of their studies, have generalized from limited data and unreplicated studies, and have interpreted their results in the context of genetic determinism. Scientific journals, perhaps to enhance their status and sales, have exaggerated the importance of such findings. Finally, the media has far too frequently accepted these exaggerated claims of scientists and scientific journals and has often gone beyond these claims by broadening the social policy implications of the research.

Whereas heretofore, the publicized genetic studies have all been problematic, there is little doubt that genes will eventually be associated with personality traits and mental illnesses. However, in view of the historical record of the uses of behavior genetics research, even if such genes are found, it will be necessary to exercise great care in publicizing these discoveries.

To conclude this chapter we offer some concrete suggestions for conducting and presenting research in human behavioral genetics.

First, stricter criteria for the performance and evaluation of studies in behavioral genetics should be implemented. This requires a special awareness by the granting agencies, journal editors, and referees of both the technical issues involved and the potential social consequences of misinformation. Second, because of the complexities of analysis such as the definition of traits, the possible roles of multiple genes and gene-

326 Molecular Genetics and the Human Personality

environment interactions and the assumptions underlying statistical methods, conclusions appearing in both scientific journals and in the popular media should be worded much more cautiously than they have been in the past. The media and the public should be made aware of genetic complexity and of the tentative nature of a reported association between a gene and a behavioral trait.

Third, in all such reports, the temptation to refer to a "gene for" the particular behavior or illness should be avoided. The reader should be reminded that genes operate only in the context of an environment. As a consequence of gene-environment covariance and interactions inherent in any complex trait, it seems highly unlikely that it will be possible to assess the precise contribution of a gene to such traits in isolation from this environmental context.

This intertwining of genetic and environmental factors involved in the expression of human behavioral traits leads to our central conclusion: The social consequences that result from finding a genetic cause of a complex behavior are no different from those that result from finding an environmental one. Consequently, the question of whether our actions are determined or result from the exercise of free will cannot be transformed from a philosophical to a genetic question. Disregarding rare single-gene disorders such as the MAO A deficiency described by Brunner et al. (1993a), a genetic explanation of a behavior is no more deterministic than an environmental one. Thus, because contemporary jurisprudence is extremely wary of admitting environmental excuses for criminal behavior ("rotten social background"), for the sake of consistency it should be equally wary of admitting genetic excuses (Alper 1998). Similarly, finding a gene associated with male homosexuality has no clear bearing on the question of whether a man has any choice in his sexual orientation. In our opinion, the debate about whether society will become more tolerant of gay men if "homosexual genes" are found is based on a simplistic picture of the genetics of human behavior as well as a misunderstanding of the origins of prejudice.

The new genetic technologies and approaches hold the promise of transforming human behavior genetics into a much more solid and replicable science. The increasing recognition of the complexity of many human traits with a genetic component presents an exciting opportunity to researchers to increase their understanding of genes and the interaction of genes with the environment. There is nothing inherent in genetic knowledge to be feared. It is only the misuse and misrepresentation of genetic knowledge that should concern us.

References

Alper JS: Genes, free will and criminal responsibility. Soc Sci Med 46:1599–1611, 1998

Angier N: Grumpy, fearful neurotics appear to be short on a gene. New York Times, November 29, 1996, B1, B17

Baron M: Mapping genes for personality: is the saga sagging? Mol Psychiatry 3:106–108, 1998

Baron M, Endicott J, Ott J: Genetic linkage in mental illness: limitations and prospects. Br J Psychiatry 157:645–655, 1990

Baur E, Fischer E, Lenz F: Human Heredity. New York, MacMillan, 1931

Bayliss HJ: District court judge findings of fact, conclusions of law and judgment: Evans v Romer, 1993. Available at: http://qrd.rdrop.com/qrd/usa/legal/colorado/evans-v-romer.RULING. Accessed November 19, 1999

Beckwith J: Gender and math performance: does biology have implications for educational policy? Journal of Education (Boston University) 165:158–174, 1983

Beckwith J, Alper JS: L'apport réel des études sur les jumeaux. La Recherche 311:72–76, 1998

Benbow C, Stanley J: Sex differences in mathematical ability: fact or artifact? Science 210:1262–1264, 1980

Bishop JE: Research points toward a "gay" gene. Wall Street Journal, July 16, 1993, B1

Blakeslee S: Genetic questions are sending judges back to classroom. New York Times, July 9, 1996, C1, C9

Bouchard TJ Jr, Lykken DT, McGue M, et al: Sources of human psychological differences: the Minnesota study of twins reared apart. Science 250:223–228, 1990

Brunner HG: MAOA deficiency and abnormal behavior: perspectives on an association, in Genetics of Criminal and Antisocial Behavior (Ciba Foundation Symposium, Vol 194). Chichester, UK, Wiley, 1995, pp 155–164

Brunner HG, Nelen M, Breakefield XO, et al: Abnormal behavior associated with a point mutation in the structural gene for monoamine oxidase A. Science 262:578–583, 1993a

Brunner HG, Nelen MR, van Zandvoort P, et al: X-linked borderline mental retardation with prominent behavioral disturbance: phenotype, genetic localization, and evidence for disturbed monoamine metabolism. Am J Hum Genet 52:1032–1039, 1993b

Butler D: Eugenics scandal reveals silence of Swedish geneticists. Nature 389:9, 1997

Couch FJ, DeShano ML, Blackwood MA, et al: BRCA1 mutations in women attending clinics that evaluate the risk of breast cancer. N Engl J Med 336:1409–1415, 1997

Cowley G, Hall C: The genetics of bad behavior. Newsweek, November 1, 1993, p 57

Crabbe JC, Wahlsten D, Dudek BC: Genetics of mouse behavior: interactions with laboratory environment. Science 284:1670–1672, 1999

Desgeorges M, Kjellberg P, Demaille J, et al: A healthy male with compound and double heterozygosities for DeltaF508, F508C, and M47OV in exon 10 of the cystic fibrosis gene. Am J Hum Genet 54:384–385, 1994

Donat R, McNeil AS, Fitzpatrick DR, et al: The incidence of cystic fibrosis gene mutations in patients with congenital bilateral absence of the vas deferens in Scotland. British Journal of Urology 79:74–77, 1997

Ebstein RP, Novick O, Umansky R, et al: Dopamine D4 receptor (D4DR) exon III polymorphism associated with the human personality trait of novelty seeking. Nat Genet 12:78–80, 1996

Falconer DS: Introduction to Quantitative Genetics, 3rd Edition. London, Longman Scientific and Technical, 1989

Felsenthal E: Man's genes made him kill, his lawyers claim. Wall Street Journal, November 1, 1994, B1, B5

Fennema E: Women and mathematics, does research matter? Journal of Research in Mathematics Education 12:380–385, 1981

Gelernter J, O'Malley S, Risch N, et al: No association between an allele at the D_2 dopamine receptor gene (DRD2) and alcoholism. JAMA 266:1801–1807, 1991

Goleman D: Forget money; nothing can buy happiness, some researchers say. New York Times, July 6, 1996, C1, C9

Hamer D, Copeland P: Living With Our Genes. New York, Doubleday, 1998

Hamer DH, Hu S, Magnuson VL, et al: A linkage between DNA markers on the X chromosome and male sexual orientation. Science 261:321–327, 1993

Herrnstein RJ, Murray C: The Bell Curve. New York, Free Press, 1994

Jordan DS: Biological effects of race movements. Popular Science Monthly 87:267–270, 1915

Jordan HE: The biological status and social worth of the mulatto. Popular Science Monthly 82:573–582, 1913

Joseph J: The equal environment assumption of the classical twin method: a critical analysis. Journal of Mind and Behavior 19:325–358, 1998

Kamin L: The Science and Politics of I.Q. Potomac, MD, Erlbaum Associates, 1974

Kelsoe JR, Ginns EI, Egeland JA, et al: Re-evaluation of the linkage relationship between chromosome 11p loci and the gene for bipolar affective disorder in the Old Order Amish. Nature 342:238–243, 1989

Kevles D: In the Name of Eugenics: Genetics and the Uses of Human Heredity. Berkeley, University of California Press, 1985

Kidd KK: Associations of disease with genetic markers: déja vu all over again. Am J Med Genet 48:71–73, 1993

Kidd KK: Can we find genes for schizophrenia. Am J Med Genet 74:104–111, 1997

Kolata GB: Math and sex: are girls born with less ability? Science 210:1234–1235, 1980

Lander E, Kruglyak L: Genetic dissection of complex traits: guidelines for interpreting and reporting linkage results. Nat Genet 11:241–247, 1995

Leo J: Exploring the traits of twins. Time, January 12, 1987, p 63

Lewontin RC, Rose S, Kamin LJ: Not in Our Genes: Biology, Ideology, and Human Nature. New York, Pantheon Books, 1984

Lichtenstein P, Holm NV, Verkasalo PK, et al: Environmental and heritable factors in the causation of cancer. N Engl J Med 343:78–85, 2000

Meschede D, Eigel A, Horst J, et al: Compound heterozygosity for the deltaF508 and F508C cystic fibrosis transmembrane regulator (CFTR) mutations in a patient with congenital bilateral aplasia of the vas deferens. Am J Hum Genet 53:292–293, 1993

Mestel R: What triggers the violence within? New Scientist, February 26, 1994, pp 31–34

Morell V: Evidence found for a possible "aggression gene." Science 260:1722–1723, 1993

Muller-Hill B: Murderous Science: Elimination by Scientific Selection of Jews, Gypsies, and Others, Germany 1933–1945. Oxford, Oxford University Press, 1988

Newman B, Mu H, Butler LM, et al: Frequency of breast cancer attributable to BRCA1 in a population-based series of American women. JAMA 279:915–929, 1998

Parad RB: Heterogeneity of phenotype in two cystic fibrosis patients homozygous for the CFTR exon 11 mutation G551D. J Med Gen 33:711–713, 1996

Pato CN, Macciardi F, Pato MT, et al: Review of the putative association of dopamine D2 receptor and alcoholism: a meta-analysis. Am J Med Genet 48:78–82, 1993

Rice G, Anderson C, Risch N, et al: Male homosexuality: absence of linkage to microsatellite markers at Xq28. Science 284:665–667, 1999

Risch N, Botstein D: A manic depressive history. Nat Genet 12:351–353, 1996

Risch N, Merikangas K: The future of genetic studies of complex human diseases. Science 273:1516–1517, 1996

Robertson M: False start on manic depression. Nature 342:222, 1989

Rubinsztein DC, Leggo J, Coles R, et al: Phenotypic characterization of individuals with 30–40 CAG repeats in the Huntington disease (HD) gene reveals HD cases with 36 repeats and apparently normal elderly individuals with 36–39 repeats. Am J Hum Genet 59:16–22, 1996

Sack GH Jr: Medical Genetics. New York, McGraw-Hill, 1999

Sidransky E, Ginns EI: Clinical heterogeneity among patients with Gaucher's disease. JAMA 269:1154–1157, 1993

Spitz E, Carlier M: La Méthode des jumeaux de 1875 à nos jours. Psychiatrie de l'enfant 39:137–159, 1996

Tourian A, Sidbury JB: Phenylketonuria and hyperphenylalaninemia, in The Metabolic Basis of Inherited Disease. Edited by Stanbury JB, Wyngaarden JB, Frederickson DS, et al. New York, McGraw-Hill, 1983, pp 270–286

Uhl GR, Gold LH, Risch N: Genetic analyses of complex behavioral disorders. Proc Natl Acad Sci U S A 94:2785–2786, 1997

Watt DC, Edwards JH: Doubt about evidence for a schizophrenia gene on chromosome 5. Psychol Med 21:279–285, 1991

Weiss R: Born to be fat. Washington Post Health, December 6, 1994, pp 10–13

Wilson JG: A study in Jewish psychopathology. Popular Science Monthly 82:264–271, 1913

CHAPTER EIGHTEEN

Genes for
Human Personality Traits

Endophenotypes of Psychiatric Disorders?

Jonathan Benjamin, M.D.
Richard P. Ebstein, Ph.D.
R. H. Belmaker, M.D.

Given the difficulties inherent in the study of genes and personality traits (Chapter 1, Principles and Methods in the Study of Complex Phenotypes; Chapter 15, From Phenotype to Gene and Back; Chapter 16, Human Correlative Behavioral Genetics), we would not have proposed or persevered in this field unless we believed, and continue to believe, that it also holds great promise. In this chapter we outline our hypotheses and agenda concerning the molecular genetic study of human personality traits.

Human personality involves biological aspects, and these are partly inherited. Population genetics cannot prove the contribution of genes to an individual's characteristics, but it has convincingly shown that inter-individual differences in such characteristics are approximately 50% due to genes. The mechanisms of action of such genes (and the environment) are complex and nonlinear, but nevertheless amenable to scientific study. We suggest that some of the genes affecting personality may be heuristic "endophenotypes" for classic psychiatric disorders.

Human Personality and Behavior Are Partly Inherited

The reader who has got this far in this volume probably needs little convincing on the basic point that human personality and behavior are partly inherited. Heritabilities of normal personality traits typically range between 30% and 60%. We emphasize that *heritability* is a technical term, and it does *not* describe the quantitative contribution of genes to an individual's personality (or any other phenotype of interest); it describes the quantitative contribution of genes to *interindividual differences* in a phenotype studied in a particular population. If we study height in a population exposed to very similar environments (nutrition, exercise, and so on), the *relative* contribution of genes (i.e., heritability) to differences in this phenotype in this population may be higher than in a similar study carried out in a second population, exposed to more varied environments. Methodology also matters. Twin studies of personality traits yield heritability estimates 10% to 20% higher than studies of whole families, including adoptees. But whether heritability is as low as 20% or as high as 80%, there seems no longer room to doubt the idea that there is a substantial heritable aspect to normal personality (Loehlin 1992; Plomin 1990; Plomin et al. 1997).

Personality Is a Phenotype With Complex Genetics

Certain rare genetic disorders are caused by single-gene mutations. Whether the mode of inheritance is recessive, dominant, or X linked, these disorders are called *simple,* or *Mendelian,* after the traits studied by Gregor Mendel, the father of modern genetics. However, common diseases with genetic components, such as diabetes mellitus and myocardial infarction, are influenced (not *caused*) by more than one gene and by environment. The contribution of any single gene may be very small. Discovering the genes involved is therefore more complex, and these disorders are called *complex* genetic disorders. Quantitative phenotypes with approximately normal distributions, such as height and intelligence, probably also display complex genetics, and we propose that this is also true of personality.

As soon as more than one gene is involved, the concept of *epistasis,* or *gene-gene interactions,* also becomes important. The effect of a single gene may depend radically on the simultaneous presence or absence of another gene or genes. The word *radically* distinguishes this situation from simple, so-called additive effects of two or more genes, where each gene contributes incrementally to the phenotype. A good analogy is provided by a hand of cards in a card game. A two of clubs or diamonds may be a worthless card, but two twos (a pair in poker) are worth more than twice as much as one (synergism). The same two of clubs in a game of bridge, even when clubs are trumps, will be of little value early in the game; however, when another suit is called for, provided the player has no cards of that suit, he or she can play the two of clubs and win (negative interaction with the other suit and synergistic interaction with the contract stipulating clubs as trumps). The main point about epistasis, then, is that the leading actor in the drama is not a single gene, but a particular genetic *combination*.

Complex genetic disorders and phenotypes are probably influenced by additive and epistatic gene effects. They are also influenced by environment. Heritability estimates of only 50% are proof of the importance of nongenetic factors in personality traits. Paradoxically, one of the great difficulties of genetic researchers is the paucity of knowledge concerning nongenetic influences on personality. Were these better defined, we would be able to construct and test more explicit gene-environment hypotheses; in their absence, important genes can easily be missed because their effects are masked by environmental influences that could otherwise be allowed for. Turning to a hypothetical example, if exposure to group activities such as Boy Scouts or Girl Scouts during adolescence is a major influence on adult sociability, we might subdivide the sample in a genetic study of sociability into former participants versus nonparticipants in such activities, and then discover a gene affecting sociability only in those subjects who were also exposed to group activities in adolescence; this gene might be missed if the subjects were all lumped together.

Labels such as *complex* and *nonlinear* need not inspire scientific nihilism; even highly complex interactions may be rigorously modeled and studied. An example is a computer simulation called a *neural network* (Penny and Frost 1996). Neural networks are inspired by neurobiology and can "diagnose" myocardial infarction, "recognize" handwriting, and so on. The network is trained on a series of actual cases of the problem to be solved (typically a few hundred) until a minimum misclassification rate is reached. Neural networks function as well as experienced cardiologists, handwriting experts, etc. Although personality geneticists have not yet, to our knowledge, employed neural networks, we (Benjamin et al. 2000; Ebstein and Auerbach, Chapter 7, Dopamine D4 Receptor and

Serotonin Transporter Promoter Polymorphisms and Temperament in Early Childhood; Ebstein and Kotler, Chapter 8, Personality, Substance Abuse, and Genes) and others (Noble et al. 1998; Comings et al., Chapter 9, Role of *DRD2* and Other Dopamine Genes in Personality Traits) have begun to study interactions with the more familiar and simpler tool of analysis of variance (ANOVA). Entering two or more genetic polymorphisms as independent variables allows one to test for interactions between them. In studies of newborn babies and very young children (Ebstein and Auerbach, Chapter 7, Dopamine D4 Receptor and Serotonin Transporter Promoter Polymorphisms and Temperament in Early Childhood) longer variants of the dopamine D4 receptor (DRD4) exon III polymorphism increased approach-type behaviors only in the presence of short variants of the serotonin transporter promoter–linked polymorphism (5-HTTLPR). This finding prompted the reexamination of adult subjects previously typed for DRD4, and similar results were found in the adults (see Chapter 7, Dopamine D4 Receptor and Serotonin Transporter Promoter Polymorphisms and Temperament in Early Childhood).

Gene-gene interactions have been demonstrated in clinical disorders, both medical and psychiatric. Myocardial infarction occurs when a particular combination of atherosclerosis, turbulent blood flow, emotional excitement (Lown et al. 1973), and/or physical effort result in an acutely inadequate supply of blood to the myocardium. We restrict further discussion of this example to two *genetic* causes of just one of these factors, namely atherosclerosis. This example is taken from Templeton (1998). Apolipoprotein E (APOE) is a lipid-transport protein; it combines with lipids to form apolipoproteins. One of the primary functions of these complexes is to solubilize the lipids so that they may be transported in the blood. Defective function could conceivably affect buildup of harmful fatty deposits in coronary arteries. The APOE gene has three alleles, ε2, ε3 and ε4. The protein products of the ε2 and ε4 alleles differ by a single amino acid from that of the ε3 allele. Genetic variation at the APOE locus has been demonstrated to be predictive of coronary artery disease (CAD) (Stengard et al. 1995); individuals bearing the ε4 allele have more than double the incidence of CAD, and those homozygous for the ε3 allele have less than half the incidence of CAD, relative to the total population studied (Sing et al. 1995). Another factor influencing the risk for atherosclerosis is cholesterol levels. These are partly hereditary (and to complicate matters further, one of the genes affecting them is that for APOE itself). When cholesterol levels are considered by themselves, a family history of high cholesterol levels is associated with more than a doubling of the incidence of CAD, whereas low cholesterol levels are associated with more than a halving of the incidence of CAD (Sing et al. 1995). So we are accustomed to thinking that a high cholesterol level and the ε4 APOE allele are "bad." However, albeit individuals with the "good" ε2 allele and medium cholesterol levels have the lowest risk for CAD, individuals with the "good" ε2 allele and high cholesterol levels have the highest CAD risks of all (higher, for example, than those of individuals with high cholesterol levels and ε4 alleles). So in the context of high cholesterol levels the ε2 allele is the "bad" allele; with medium or low cholesterol levels it is a "good" allele. Individuals with ε3/ε3 genotype and high cholesterol levels have less CAD than those with other genotypes and low cholesterol levels. Even before a convincing biological explanation for these complex interactions is available, we can use increasing knowledge of these APOE–cholesterol level interactions to predict empirical risks for patients with each APOE–cholesterol level combination. *We can also exploit these interactions to construct increasingly cogent theories of atherosclerogenesis;* the more gene effects and gene-gene interactions we discover, the more we can begin to demand of our theory, and the more closely it can begin to approximate biological reality. Thus no matter how complex the interplay of events leading up to myocardial infarction, one aspect of study, namely the genetics of atherosclerosis, begins to seem tractable.

The APOE ε4 allele is associated with increased risk for Alzheimer's disease (Strittmatter and Roses 1995) as well as for atherosclerosis. Here too, the allele is neither necessary nor sufficient for expression of disease. This prompted Kamboh et al. (1995) to look for other candidate genes that may be involved in the same biological system. The gene that codes for α-antichymotrypsin (ACT) binds, like APOE, to β-amyloid peptide in the filamentous deposits found in the brains of patients with Alzheimer's disease and stimulates the formation of amyloid in plaques. Kamboh et al. found that the ACT threonine-alanine (TA) polymorphism is associated with the risk for Alzheimer's disease, in that the odds ratio for the risk of developing the disease with the AA genotype was 1.5 compared with the TT and TA genotypes (considered in isolation from the APOE genotype). The odds ratio for APOE ε4 in this study was 3.5 in heterozygotes and 11.1 in homozygotes, *in the presence of the ACT TT genotype;* with the ACT TA genotype the odds ratio declined, in ε4 heterozygotes, or increased, in ε4 homozygotes, to 2.7 and 10.1, respectively. With the ACT AA genotype it increased to 6.4 and 34.0 respectively. These two polymorphisms therefore showed both negative and positive synergistic interactions. Concerning the synergism, the authors speculated, "ACT protein containing (hydrophobic) alanine . . . may be secreted at a higher rate into plasma. . . . Elevated ACT . . . in conjunction with . . . APOE*4 . . . may induce [β-amyloid peptide] to form amyloid filaments more rapidly" (p. 488).

APOE therefore contains two lessons for psychiatric genetics. Firstly, the same polymorphism, with the same basic biological function (protein and lipoprotein binding), has pleiotropic effects (i.e., it acts both in coronary arteries and in brain). Secondly, the effects of the polymorphism, *in both illnesses,* are greatly modified by other genetic polymorphisms, but these are not necessarily the same modifying polymorphisms in the two systems.

Genes Affecting Personality: Endophenotypes for Classic Psychiatric Disorders

Concordance rates around 50% for schizophrenia in monozygotic twins leave little room for doubt that there is an important genetic component to the illness. Yet the search for a single major gene (Mendelian genetics) has frustrated even genomewide linkage approaches. The term *endophenotype* was used by Gottesman (1991) to describe a trait that may be intermediate on the chain of causality from genes to diseases. Some family relatives of affected patients also carry the endophenotype, although not the disease phenotype. This increased penetrance of the endophenotype compared with the phenotype proper is expected to help genetic studies. Cholesterol levels and myocardial infarction have been discussed in the context of gene-gene interactions. Here we point out that cholesterol levels also serve as endophenotypes for myocardial infarction. Different alleles of the APOE gene are associated with different cholesterol levels, and these in turn are associated with different risks for myocardial infarction. But numerous other factors also influence the risk for myocardial infarction. In a sense the APOE gene is a gene *for* myocardial infarction, but the relationship is closer, and therefore easier to discover, when we consider it a gene for cholesterol levels. Furthermore, we can include all family members in our analysis of this relationship, or at least all those with high cholesterol levels, not just those with myocardial infarction.

Examples of endophenotypes in psychiatry include abnormalities of eye-tracking movements (Holzman et al. 1988) and the P50 evoked potential (Freedman et al. 1997) in schizophrenic patients and their relatives. A majority of schizophrenic patients, and 45% of their first-degree relatives, show certain abnormal eye movements on electro-optical recordings. A family study of discordant twins was incompatible with simple Mendelian transmission of schizophrenia. However, when the assessment included schizophrenia and abnormal eye movements, this phenotype exhibited a pattern consistent with autosomal dominant transmission. Plainly, the combination of a gene for this characteristic and another gene(s), which together may lead to outright illness, may exhibit a more complicated transmission pattern. However, the simple inheritance of the endophenotype may permit rapid identification of at least one risk gene for schizophrenia. Schizophrenic patients also exhibit diminished inhibition of the response to the second of a pair of identical auditory stimuli, as measured by the P50 evoked potential. This may be a laboratory example of an apparent general difficulty of these patients in filtering irrelevant information. The same deficit is seen in about half of the relatives in families multiply affected with schizophrenia, including in those relatives with no clinical disorder. A linkage analysis of the P50 phenotype, utilizing existing physiological information implicating a nicotinic receptor, succeeded in linking the trait to chromosome 15 (lod score = 5.3) in nine families.

Our hypothesis is that personality traits may be heuristic endophenotypes for psychiatric geneticists. Let us imagine that a certain allele of an "introversion-extraversion" gene increases an individual's tendency to prefer to be alone by 10% compared with the commonest allele, and a rarer allele increases it by 20%. Most individuals with these alleles will still have introversion scores within the normal range, but an occasional individual who is homozygous for the rarest allele might be diagnosed with social phobia. An individual who inherits two of these introversion alleles *and* an allele that increases the risk for psychopathology in general may be more likely to have schizoid personality disorder. Now consider an individual with this genotype who also inherits a gene that contributes to unconventional thinking; he may be more liable to schizotypal personality disorder. Another individual with two of the genes affecting introversion, plus the gene affecting eccentricity, plus a gene that increases adventurousness, might become an intrepid explorer; his brother might develop schizophrenia. At the biochemical level a minor change in the dopamine transporter, reducing the amount of dopamine reuptake, might have striking consequences when paired with a minor change in a monoamine oxidase enzyme responsible for dopamine degradation. Cloninger has presented a detailed model (Cloninger 1987) of how various combinations of extreme personality traits may lead on to personality disorders.

Reports of an association between a human personality trait called *novelty seeking* and a dopamine D4 receptor (DRD4) exon III polymorphism are discussed elsewhere in this volume. The thinking behind the search for genes that might influence personality traits (Benjamin et al. 1993) was not limited to the desire to advance our understanding of normal personality alone; we in fact hypothesized (Belmaker and Biederman 1994) that such genes, once discovered, might yield new insights into the genetics and pathological chemistry of psychiatric disorders.

This idea, that individual genes might influence personality traits *and* psychopathology, would appear to be partly supported thus far by the saga of the DRD4 polymorphism (Ebstein and Belmaker 1997). The initial reports of an association between DRD4 and novelty seeking were followed by attempts at replication and also by reports of associations with attention-deficit/hyperactivity disorder (ADHD) in children (LaHoste et al. 1997), heroin abuse (Kotler et al. 1997), and Tourette's syndrome (Grice et al. 1996). Novelty Seeking, a factor on the Tridimensional Personality Questionnaire (Cloninger 1987), refers to a cluster of risk-taking, distractible, impulsive, and fickle behaviors. This behavioral tendency bears prima facie similarity to some features of ADHD and perhaps experiments with drug-taking and Tourette's syndrome; these reported associations have been replicated, especially for ADHD (e.g., Faraone et al. 1999). These associations encourage us to look afresh at our current understanding of the psychological substrates of these phenotypes (e.g., what is common to ADHD and novelty seeking?) Thus genetics and psychology can enrich each other just as genetics and physiology enrich each other in other disciplines.

An example of a different kind of connection between personality traits, genes, and pathology is the connection between cessation of smoking and a polymorphism of the dopamine transporter gene (DAT) (Sabol et al. 1999). This study replicated a previously reported association between smoking status and DAT and also employed personality testing. Lower novelty seeking was associated with the "nine" DAT allele and so was quitting smoking. The authors hypothesized that individuals with this allele have increased intracellular dopaminergic activity; this makes them less likely to seek external sources of dopamine stimulation, including novel situations and nicotine intake. This would be an example of a gene influencing a personality trait and also influencing behavioral mediation of an environmental risk for a nonpsychiatric disorder such as lung cancer.

A further contribution of replicable behavioral findings with *any* gene is that such a gene can provide the first clue on a trail ultimately leading to gene-gene combinations with large effect sizes on behavioral traits, the kind of effect that would allow for true prediction in clinical psychiatry and psychology. Just as each of the putative genes "for" schizophrenia, bipolar disorder, and so on probably has a small effect size (or none at all) when it acts alone, the same is true of the "personality" genes reported so far. The DRD4 gene, for example, explained only 4% of the variance in novelty seeking in the initial reports. A DRD4-serotonin-2C receptor polymorphism interaction, however, affected another personality trait, Reward Dependence, by about 10 standard errors of the mean in a preliminary analysis (Ebstein et al. 1997), and this interaction (with a smaller effect size) was later replicated (Kuhn et al. 1999). Such an interaction would have not have been sought without the prior reports of the DRD4 association; random searches for gene-gene interactions without good hypotheses to support them astronomically increase the problem of multiple comparisons and false-positive findings.

Concluding Remarks

Beckwith and Alper (Chapter 17, Genetics of Human Personality) rightly point out the social dangers of naive or even evil genetic theory. The past cannot be forgotten or forgiven in psychiatric genetics. The media requirement for ratings and oversimplification creates a background that harbors the potential for abuse of every published scientific discovery.

Some gene effects of personality may turn out to be mediated via banal confounding variables. The sociological literature suggesting that tall men have more friends, more self-confidence, and more social acceptance is well known. The effects of female beauty on female social status do not require proof in the literature. Genetic effects of these physical variables could appear in behavioral genetic studies as effects of genes on behavior, but knowledge of the intervening variable would allow us a much more sober assessment of the process involved.

The past abuses of environmentalism must also not be forgotten. The concept that individuals are born tabula rasa and that environment can create total equality led in some circumstances to crimes analogous to making all men equal in height by cutting off the heads of tall people. The role of dogmatic environmentalism in communism's crimes of this century is symmetrical to the role of naive geneticism in Nazi crimes. The roles, in both cases, involved aiding and abetting rather than direct causality.

It is important for a free society to accept the idea that many individual differences are innate and not easily malleable. Society is not responsible for all human faults. Although this argument has been used to try to excuse crime (the "genetic defense," see Chapter 17, Genetics of Human Personality), environmental causation has also been used to excuse crime (see *West Side Story*, "Dear Officer Krupky" [Wise and Robbins 1961]). Child-rearing can be unrealistic and perhaps pathogenic if parents overemphasize their influence and responsibility, just as child-rearing can be distorted if parents accept no responsibility.

Future molecular genetic studies should allow for a much more sober and more difficult-to-abuse body of knowledge. When the mechanism of gene effects on personality traits becomes clearer, the social meaning of the findings will be more difficult to distort. For instance, genes may affect novelty seeking via general autonomic arousal level. High novelty seeking may have a complex set of socially desirable and socially undesirable consequences such that no employer or insurance company would find value in using genotyping for unethical reasons. However, parents might find it very useful to know the genetic tendency for arousal level in their child, for example, in order to plan appropriate discipline strategies.

Einstein might not have studied relativity if he knew the consequences; the discoverers of narcotic analgesia could have hidden their discovery for fear of abuse. More likely, the scientific progress was inevitable and appropriate; open discussion is the best way to assure its ethical humanistic application. Molecular personality genetics is both equally promising and equally dangerous, but we do not have the option to close our eyes or ignore the field.

References

Belmaker R, Biederman J: Genetic markers, temperament, and psychopathology. Biol Psychiatry 36:71–72, 1994

Benjamin J, Press J, Maoz B, et al: Linkage of a normal personality trait to the color-blindness gene. Biol Psychiatry 34:581–583, 1993

Benjamin J, Osher Y, Kotler M, et al: Association between tridimensional personality questionnaire (TPQ) traits and three functional polymorphisms: dopamine receptor D4 (DRD4), serotonin transporter promoter region (5-HTTLPR), and catechol O-methyltransferase (COMT). Mol Psychiatry 5:96–100, 2000

Cloninger C: A systematic method for clinical description and classification of personality variants: a proposal. Arch Gen Psychiatry 44:573–588, 1987

Ebstein R, Belmaker R: Saga of an adventure gene: novelty seeking, substance abuse, and the dopamine D4 receptor (*D4DR*) exon III repeat polymorphism. Mol Psychiatry 2:381–384, 1997

Ebstein R, Segman R, Benjamin J, et al: 5-HT2C (HTR2C) serotonin receptor gene polymorphism associated with the human personality trait of reward dependence: interaction with dopamine D4 receptor (D4DR) and dopamine D3 receptor (D3DR) polymorphisms. Am J Med Genet 74:65–72, 1997

Faraone S, Biederman J, Weiffenbach B, et al: Dopamine D4 gene 7-repeat allele and attention deficit hyperactivity disorder. Am J Psychiatry 156:768–770, 1999

Freedman R, Coon H, Myles-Worsley M: Linkage of a neurophysiological deficit in schizophrenia to a chromosome 15 locus. Proc Natl Acad Sci U S A 94:587–592, 1997

Gottesman II: Schizophrenia Genesis: The Origins of Madness. New York, WH Freeman, 1991

Grice D, Leckman J, Pauls D, et al: Linkage disequilibrium between an allele of the dopamine D4 locus and Tourette syndrome, by the transmission disequilibrium test. Am J Hum Genet 59:644–652, 1996

Holzman P, Kringlen E, Matthysse S, et al: A single dominant gene can account for eye tracking dysfunctions and schizophrenia in offspring of discordant twins. Arch Gen Psychiatry 45:641–647, 1988

Kamboh M, Sanghera D, Ferrell R, et al: *APOE*4*-associated Alzheimer's disease risk is modified by alpha1-antichymotrypsin polymorphism. Nat Genet 10:486–488, 1995

Kotler M, Cohen H, Segman R, et al: Excess dopamine D4 receptor (D4DR) exon III seven repeat allele in opioid-dependent subjects. Mol Psychiatry 2:251–254, 1997

Kuhn K-U, Meyer K, Nothen M, et al: Allelic variants of dopamine receptor D4 (DRD4) and serotonin receptor 5HT2c (HTR2c) and temperament factors: replication tests. Am J Med Genet 88:168–172, 1999

LaHoste G, Swanson J, Wigal S, et al: Dopamine D4 receptor gene polymorphism is associated with attention deficit hyperactivity disorder. Mol Psychiatry 1:121–124, 1997

Loehlin J: Genes and Environment in Personality Development. Newbury Park, CA, Sage, 1992

Lown B, Verrier R, Corbalan R: Psychologic stress and threshold for repetitive ventricular response. Science 182:834–836, 1973

Noble E, Oskaragoz T, Ritchie T, et al: D2 and D4 dopamine receptor polymorphisms and personality. Am J Med Genet 81:257–267, 1998

Penny W, Frost D: Neural networks in clinical medicine. Med Decis Making 16:386–398, 1996

Plomin R: The role of inheritance in behavior. Science 248:183–188, 1990

Plomin R, De Fries J, McClearn G, et al: Behavioral Genetics, 3rd Edition. New York, Freeman, 1997

Sabol S, Nelson M, Fisher C, et al: Association of the dopamine transporter gene with novelty seeking and cigarette smoking behavior. Health Psychol 18:7–13, 1999

Sing C, Haviland M, Templeton A, et al: Alternative genetic strategies for predicting risk of atherosclerosis, in Atherosclerosis, Vol 10. Edited by Woodford F, Davignon J, Sniderman A. Amsterdam, Elsevier Science, 1995, pp 638–644

Stengard J, Zerba KE, Pekkanen J, et al: Apolipoprotein E polymorphism predicts death from coronary heart disease in a longitudinal study of elderly Finnish men. Circulation 91:265–269, 1995

Strittmatter W, Roses A: Apolipoprotein E and Alzheimer disease. Proc Natl Acad Sci U S A 92:4725–4727, 1995

Templeton A: The complexity of the genotype-phenotype relationship and the limitations of using genetic "markers" at the individual level. Science in Context 11:373–389, 1998

Wise R, Robbins J (dir), Lehman E (screenplay), Bernstein L, Sondheim S (music). West Side Story. Los Angeles, CA, United Artists, 1961

Index

Page numbers referring to tables and figures appear **bold**.

Acoustic startle, and animal models of anxiety, **67**

ACT threonine-alanine (TA) polymorphism, 337–338

Additive genetic variance, and IQ, 214

Affected sib-pair (ASP) method, 4, 7–8

Age, and novelty seeking, 99. *See also* Children; Infants

Aggressive behavior. *See also* Behavior; Impulsive aggression
candidate genes for, **274**
ethics of genetic research and, 320–321, 324, 326
serotonin transporter gene and, 125–126

Agreeableness, and serotonin transporter gene, 114, 116, 117, 121

Alcoholism
candidate genes for, **274**, **275**
dopamine system and, 154, 166, 169
extreme personality traits and, 100
personalities of families and, 138
serotonin system and, 235, 238

Allelic association, and IQ, 218

Alzheimer's disease, **274**, 337–338

Analysis, methods of for genetic research, 10–20, 318–319. *See also* Association analysis; Linkage analysis

Analysis of variance (ANOVA), 336

Animal models
of genetic influences on personality, 63–83
of impulsivity, 100
manipulative experiments and, 294–295
maternal effects and, 296–298

of sensation seeking, 196–197
of serotonin transporter gene and personality, 123–127

Anorexia nervosa. *See also* Eating disorders
candidate genes for, **274**
personality traits and, 37, 100

Antichymotrypsin (ACT), 337–338

Antidepressants, personality and differential response to, 38

Antisocial personality disorder, and aggression, 232, 233, 234. *See also* Personality disorders

Anxiety
animal models of, **67**, 75, 79–80
candidate genes for, **274**
heritability of, 113, 114
serotonin transporter gene and, 117, **119–120**

Anxiety disorders, and personality disorders, 37

Apolipoprotein E (APOE), 217, 336–338

Arched-backed nursing (ABN), and maternal effects in animal studies, 297–298

Arousal, and sensation seeking, 193, 194

Assessment scales, for sensation seeking, 193–196

Association analysis
forward genetics and, 278–282
methods for, 15–18
study design and, 5–6
substance abuse and novelty seeking, 99

Assortative mating, and IQ, 214

Atherosclerosis, 336–337

Attachment behavior, **275**
Attention-deficit/hyperactivity disorder
  (ADHD)
  candidate genes for, **274**
  dopamine system and, 155, 169–
    170, 202–203, 249, 251, 340
  genotype variability and, 183
  novelty seeking and, 153–154
Autism
  broad phenotype and genetic
    studies of, 46–48, 55–58
  candidate genes for, **275**
  genetic factors in, 45
  nature and boundaries of, 49–54
  spectrum of behavior, 43–44
Autism Family History Interview, 47,
  48
Avoidance learning paradigms, and
  animal models of anxiety and
  depression, 69. See also Harm
  avoidance; Schizoid avoidant
  behavior

Background noise, in human genetic
  studies, 100
Bailey, J. M., 258
Baltimore-London Autism Family
  Studies, 49, 51
Baur, Erwin, 316
Behavior. See also Aggressive
  behavior; Novelty seeking;
  Sensation seeking; Sexual
  behavior; Social behavior; Violent
  behavior
  animals models and tests of
    temperament, 65–70
  assessment of in neonates and
    infants, 138–139
  autism and spectrum of, 43–44, 46
  critical review of research on
    correlative genetics, 293–309
  dopamine system and disorders of,
    99–101
  heritability of, 334
  longitudinal studies of temperament
    differences in children and, 247–
    248
Behavioral genomics, and IQ, 222–226

Behaviorism, and personality
  differences in children, 245
Bell Curve, The (Herrnstein & Murray
  1994), 212
Bipolar disorder, **274, 275**
Blum, K., 166, 172, 173
Borderline personality disorder, 232
Boredom, and sensation seeking, 195
Bouchard, Thomas, 323
Brain
  autism and abnormalities of, 55–56
  sensation seeking and reward
    mechanisms, 152–153
  serotonin transporter gene and
    development of, 117
Brazelton Neonatal Assessment Scale,
  249
Breakefield, Xandra, 324, 325
Breast cancer, 319
Broad autism phenotype (BAP), 46–58
Brown Attention-Deficit Disorder
  Scales (BADDS), 175, **178**
Brunner syndrome, **274**
Bulimia nervosa, 37, 99–100
Buss-Durkee Hostility Inventory, 175,
  179, 236

Candidate genes, for neuropsychiatric
  diseases, **274–275**, 276, 280–282
Case-controlled studies, and
  association analysis, 15–16
Catechol O-methyltransferase (COMT),
  155–156, **157**
Cerebrospinal fluid (CSF), and
  serotonin transporter gene, 123,
  124–125
Character, and Temperament and
  Character Inventory (TCI), 35
Child Behavior Checklist, 250, **251**
Children. See also Development;
  Infants
  DRD4 and serotonin transporter
    genes and temperament, 137–146
  molecular genetics of temperament
    in, 245–252
Cholesterol levels, and atherosclerosis,
  336–337
Chromosomes 4 and 22, and IQ, 219–
  221

Chromosome 6p21, and reading
  disability, 217
Chromosome 17, and unstability of
  pericentric region, 112
Chronic unpredictable mild stress, **67**,
  70
Classification and regression trees
  (CART) methodology, and
  subgroup analyses, 20, 24
Cloninger, C. R., 145, 152, 169, 184,
  196, 339
Cognition and cognitive deficits
  autism and, 51–54
  intelligence and quantitative trait
    loci, 211–226
  personality traits and reward
    mechanisms, 152
Cognitive-behavioral therapy,
  personality as predictor of
  response to, 38
Colorado Adoption Project, 212
Communication, and autism, 52–54
Comorbidity, of personality disorders
  and psychopathology, 37–38
Complex genetic disorders, 334–335
Complex traits. *See also* Genetics;
    Gene variation
  ethics of genetic research and, 317–
    318
  methodologies for genetic study of,
    1–24
  phenotype for autism and, 55–56
  phenotype for personality and, 334–
    338
  serotonin transporter gene
    variations and, 110–113
Compliance, with recommended
  lifestyle practices, 39
Conditioned tests, and animal models
  of anxiety and depression, 66,
  68–69, 70–74
Conduct disorder
  dopamine system and, 171, 202
  genotype variability and, 183
Context dependency, and subgroup
  analyses, 20
Continuous marker density, and false
  negatives or false positives, 22

Cooperativeness, and Temperament
  and Character Inventory (TCI), 35,
  36
Coronary artery disease (CAD), 336–
  337
Correlative behavioral genetics, critical
  review of research on, 293–309
Corticotropin releasing hormone
  (CRH), and animal models of
  personality, 76
Cost, of sampling methods for genetic
  studies, 4
Cost-benefit analysis, and study
  design, 8–10
Cross-cultural differences, in Neonatal
  Behavioral Assessment Scale,
  139–140. *See also* Ethnicity
Cystic fibrosis, 278, 319

Defense Style Questionnaire (DSQ),
  172–173, 175, **180**
Dementia, and Apolipoprotein E, 217
Depression. *See also* Major depressive
    disorder; Unipolar depression
  animal models of, **67**, 70, 80–81
  negative emotionality and, 116
Determinism, and behavior genetics,
  323
Development. *See also* Children;
    Infants
  critical review of behavior genetics
    and, 301–303, 307
  heritability of intelligence and, 213–
    214
  serotonin transporter gene and
    personality traits, 117
Disinhibition, and sensation seeking,
  195
DNA pooling, and IQ QTL Project,
  219–221
Domestic abuse, and personality
  disorders, 232
Dopamine D2 receptor gene (*DRD2*),
  and personality traits, 165–184
Dopamine D3 receptor gene (*D3DR*),
  and personality traits, 100–101
Dopamine D4 receptor (*DRD4*). *See
  also* Dopamine system

Dopamine D4 receptor (*DRD4*)
(*continued*)
animal models of mood and, 76–78
attention-deficit/hyperactivity
disorder and, 155, 340
behavioral effects of in neonates,
121–122
novelty seeking and, 91–99, 138,
145, 153–154, **157**, 248–249, 321,
340, 341
sensation seeking and, 201–204
sexual behavior and, 264–266
substance abuse and, 155, 340
temperament differences in children
and, 137–146, 249–251
Dopamine D5 receptor gene (*DRD5*),
and sensation seeking, 204
Dopamine system. *See also* Dopamine
D4 receptor
personality and behavior disorders,
99–101
reward system and substance abuse,
151–152
role of in personality traits, 165–184
sexual behavior and, 257
smoking and, 340
Down syndrome, 47, 48, 50, 51, 53, 54
DSM-III-R, and classification of autism,
44
DSM-IV-TR
autistic disorder and, 43, 44
general criteria for personality
disorders and, 35
Dyslexia, 57
Dysthymia, 37–38

Eating disorders, and personality traits,
37, 99–100. *See also* Anorexia
nervosa
Ebstein, R. P., 264
Elevated plus maze, 66, **67**
Endocrinology, and longitudinal
studies of temperament in
children, 247–248
Endophenotypes, of psychiatric
disorders, 277, 333–342. *See also*
Phenotypes
Environment. *See also* Gene-
environment interactions

complex genetic disorders and, 335
influence of on IQ, 213–214
influence of on sexual behavior,
269–270
relative influence of genetic factors
on temperament and behavior,
109–110
studies of neonates and, 121
Epistasis, 334–335. *See also* Gene-gene
interactions
Ethics
behavioral genomics and studies of
intelligence, 225–226
misleading representations of
studies of correlative behavior
genetics and, 307–308
social implications of research on
genetics of personality and, 315–
326, 341–342
Ethnicity. *See also* Cross-cultural
differences; Race
DRD4 and novelty seeking, 98
social and ethical implications of
genetic research and, 315–316
Eugenics movement, 316
Evolution, and serotonin transporter
gene, 123–124
Executive function deficits, and
autism, 52, 54
Experience seeking, and sensation
seeking, 195
Extraversion, heritability of, 153, 339
Extremely concordant (EC) sib pairs,
4, 5
Extremely discordant and extremely
concordant (EDAC) sib pairs, 4,
9–10
Extremely discordant (ED) sib pairs,
4–5, 7, 8, 9–10
Extreme sib pairs (ESP), 4
Eye-tracking movements, and
schizophrenia, 338–339
Eysenck, H. J. & S. B. G., 152
Eysenck Personality Questionnaire, 64,
118, 121, 173

Factor analysis, 19
False negatives and false positives,
and study design, 7, 21–23

Family-based methods, and
    association analysis, 16
Family history studies. *See also* Parents
    of autism, 47–48
    of sexual orientation, 258–259
    of substance abuse, 100
Fearlessness, and genetic determinism,
    324
Fear-motivated behaviors, in animal
    models, 65–69, 82
Fear-potentiated startle, in animal
    models, **67**, 69
Fenfluramine, and prolactin response
    to
    impulsive aggression, 233–234
Fischer, Eugen, 316
Flinders sensitive line (FSL) and
    Flinders resistant line (FRL), of
    rats, 80–81
Folstein, S. E., 46–47
Footshock-induced freezing, **67**
Forced-swim test, and animal models
    of depression, 70
Forensics and forensic population. *See*
    Prisons and prison population
Fragile X mutation, and autism, 45
Freud, Sigmund, 193
Friendship Interview, 51, 52
Friendships, and parents of autistic
    children, 51. *See also* Social
    behavior
Functional significance, and
    polymorphisms in serotonin
    transporter gene, 237

GABA, receptor mutations and animal
    models of personality, 75–76
Geller-Seifter test, and animal tests of
    anxiety, **67**, 69
Gender
    media reports on genetic research
    and, 323
    sensation seeking and, 198
Gene action, and gene strategy, 276–
    277
Gene-environment interactions, and
    influence of serotonin transporter
    gene on personality, 123–127. *See
    also* Environment

Gene-gene interactions. *See also*
    Multiple gene interactions;
    Nonlinear genetic interactions
    complex traits and, 23, 334–335
    polygenic disorders and, 174–175
    serotonin transporter gene and
    personality, 121–122
Gene strategy, and gene action, 276–
    277
Genetic combination, 335
Genetic correlation, and IQ, 215
Genetic disorders, simple versus
    complex, 334–335. *See also*
    Polygenic disorders
Genetic engineering technology, and
    genetic manipulation of animal
    models, 74
Genetic fatalism, and ethics of
    research on behavior genetics,
    322–325
Genetics, and personality. *See also*
    Complex traits; Gene-gene
    interactions; Genotypes;
    Heritability; Phenotypes; Reverse
    genetics
    aggressive behavior and
    polymorphisms, 231–238
    animal models of, 63–83
    autism and, 43–48
    critical reviews of research on, 273–
    283, 293–309
    dopamine system and novelty
    seeking, 91–99
    DRD4 and serotonin transporter
    genes and early childhood
    temperament, 137–146
    endophenotypes of psychiatric
    disorders and, 333–342
    environmental influences on
    temperament and behavior, 109–
    128
    intelligence and cognitive ability,
    211–226
    methods for study of complex
    phenotypes, 1–24
    sensation seeking and, 193–206
    serotonin transporter gene and,
    109–128, 137–146

Genetics and personality (*continued*)
  sexual behavior and, 257–270
  social and ethical implications of
    research on, 315–326
  temperamental differences in
    children and, 137–146, 245–252
Gene variation. *See also* Complex
    traits; Genetics
  complexity of for serotonin
    transporter gene, 110–113
  genotype and personality traits,
    182–183
  neurogenetic research on learning
    and memory, 223–224
Genomic linkage disequilibrium (LD)
    scan, 17–18
Genotype
  gene variation and personality traits,
    182–183
  genotyping and study design, 5
  relationship of Neonatal Behavioral
    Assessment Scale and Infant
    Behavior Questionnaire, 144–145
  serotonin transporter gene and
    phenotype correlations, 113–121

Hamer, Dean, 248, 322–323
Hardy-Weinberg proportions, for
    genotypic frequencies, 15
Harm avoidance. *See also* Avoidance
    learning paradigms; Schizoid
    avoidant behavior
  eating disorders and, 100
  serotonin transporter gene and, 101
  Temperament and Character
    Inventory (TCI) and, 35, 36, 38
Haseman-Elston method, and linkage
    analysis, 14
Hebb, D. O., 193
Heterosis, and physiological correlates
    with DRD2, 170–171
Heritability. *See also* Genetics
  of anxiety-related traits, 113
  of autism, 45
  of extraversion, 153, 339
  of impulsive aggression and
    suicidality, 233
  of intelligence, 212

Neonatal Behavioral Assessment
    Scale and, 139–140
  of personality and behavior, 334
  simplistic assumptions in behavioral
    genetics and, 295–299
Hole board, **67**
Homicide, and antisocial personality
    disorder, 233
Homosexuality, and genetics of sexual
    orientation, 258–263, 266, 269,
    322–323, 326
Hostility, negative emotionality and
    serotonin transporter gene, 116,
    117
HTR1B, and aggressive behavior, 235–
    236, 238
Human Genome Project, 23
Huntington's disease, 278
Hyponeophobia, **67**
Hypothalamic-pituitary-adrenal (HPA)
    axis, and animal models of
    personality, 76

ICD-10, and autism, 48
Identical-by-descent (IBD) sharing,
    between sib pairs, 4, 12–13
Identity by state (IBS), and linkage
    analysis, 13
Immature defenses, and *DRD2* A1
    allele, 172–173
Immutability, and genetic
    determinism, 323
Impulsive aggression, and personality
    disorders, 231–238. *See also*
    Aggressive behavior; Impulsivity
Impulsive sensation seeking, and twin
    studies, 199
Impulsive Sensation Seeking scale
    (ImpSS), 195, 200
Impulsivity, and eating disorders, 100.
    See also Impulsive aggression
Infant Behavior Questionnaire (IBQ),
    98, 122, 139, 142–143, 144–145
Infants. *See also* Development;
    Neonates
  assessment of temperament and
    behavior in, 138–139

DRD4 and sensation seeking, 203
longitudinal studies of temperament
  differences in, 246–251
temperament and psychological
  qualities of, 121
Intelligence quotient (IQ)
  autism and, 52
  quantitative trait loci and cognitive
    ability, 211–226
Interdisciplinary research, and future
  of correlative behavioral genetics,
  309
Interindividual differences, and
  heritability of personality and
  behavior, 334
Intermittent explosive disorder, 232
Interpretation, of results of genetic
  studies of complex traits, 21–24.
  See also Simplistic assumptions
  and interpretations
Introversion, and endophenotypes, 339
Iowa Autism Family Study, 48, 49
IPC Locus of Control Inventory (IPC-
  LOCI), 175, **179**
IQ QTL Project, 217–222

Jordan, H. E., 315
*Journal of the American Medical
  Association*, 166

Kanner, Leo, 43, 46, 57
Karolinska Scales of Personality
  (KSP), 92

Latent factor analysis, 19
Learned helplessness, and animal tests
  of depression, **67**, 70
Legal profession, and research in
  behavior genetics, 324
Lenz, Fritz, 316
Lesch-Nyhan syndrome, **274**, 320
Licking/grooming (LG), and maternal
  effects in animal studies, 297–298
Lifestyle choices, and personality, 39
Light-dark transition, 66, **67**
Linkage analysis
  sexual orientation and, 259–263
  study design and, 5–6, 10–14

Linkage disequilibrium approach, and
  association studies, 279
LIPED computer program, 11
LL genotype, and impulsive
  aggression, 236, 238
Lod score method, of linkage analysis,
  11–12
Longitudinal studies, of childhood
  temperament, 246–251
Long-term potentiation (LTP), and
  abnormal fear conditioning in
  animal models, 77
Lumping strategies, and study of
  complex genetic traits, 24
Lykken, David, 324

Major affective disorder (MAD), 54
Major depressive disorder, 37–38. *See
  also* Depression

Mapping, of genes and temperamental
  differences in animal models, 81–
  83
Marital status, and frequency of sexual
  intercourse, 267
MASC method, and association
  analysis, 17–18
Maternal effects, and animal models,
  296–298
Maudsley reactive (MR) and Maudsley
  nonreactive (MNR) strains, 79, 80
Media, and misrepresentations of
  genetic studies, 307–308, 315–
  316, 323, 324–326, 341
Mellon Personality Inventory, 173
Mendel, Gregor, 334
Meta-analysis, application of to genetic
  studies, 18–19
Minnesota Multiphasic Personality
  Inventory, 99
Misleading representations, and
  correlative behavior genetics,
  307–308
Model-free methods, of linkage
  analysis, 12–13
Modified Personality Assessment
  Schedule, Revised (M-PAS-R), 49–
  51, 52

Monoamine oxidase A (MAOA) gene, and aggressive behavior, 320–321, 324, 326
Monoamine oxidase B (MAO B) sensation seeking and, 203, 206 smoking and, 204
Mood, and animal models of personality, 76–78
Multicenter genetic studies, 2
Multidimensional Personality Questionnaire, 199
Multiple gene interactions, COMT and personality, 156. *See also* Gene-gene interactions
Multiple hypotheses, and methods of genetic analysis, 318–319
Multipoint linkage analysis, 11–12
Multivariate methods, and genetic studies of complex traits, 19
Myocardial infarction, 336, 338

Narrative discourse, and autism, 53–54
Negative reinforcement model, of addiction, 151–152
Neonatal Behavioral Assessment Scale (NBAS), 93, 98, 121, 122, 139–140, 144–145
Neonates. *See also* Infants assessment of temperament and behavior in, 138–139 serotonin transporter gene and gene-gene interaction, 121–122
NEO-Five Factor Personality Inventory (NEO-FFI), 175, **177**
NEO Personality Inventory, Revised (NEO-PI-R), 50, 92, 115, 118, 121, 201, 237, 264, 304
Neural networks, and computer simulations, 335
Neurogenetics, and studies of cognitive ability, 223
Neuroticism
DRD2 A1 allele and, 173 heritability of, 153 serotonin transporter gene and, 114, 115–116, 117, 118
New York Longitudinal Study, 139

N-methyl D-aspartate (NMDA), and studies of learning and memory, 223
Noble, E. P., 170, 172
Nonlinear genetic interactions, 335. *See also* Gene-gene interactions
Nonparametric methods, of linkage analysis, 12–13
Nonrandom sampling, and study design, 7
Nonshared environment, and IQ, 214
Novelty seeking. *See also* Sensation seeking
brain reward mechanisms and, 152–153
candidate genes for, **274**
catechol *O*-methyltransferase (COMT) and, **157**
dopamine D2 receptor gene (*DRD2*) and, 173–174, 184
dopamine D4 receptor gene (*DRD4*) and, 91–99, 138, 145, 153, **157**, 196, 248–249, 321, 340, 341
Neonatal Behavioral Assessment Scale and, 142
psychopathology and, 153–154
self-report personality questionnaires and, 152–153
serotonin transporter gene and, **157**
sexual behavior and, 263–266
Temperament and Character Inventory (TCI) and, 35, 36, 38

Obesity
candidate genes for, **275**
DRD2 A1 allele and, 172
Obsessive-compulsive disorder, **274**, **275**
Oligogenic hypothesis
autism and, 55–56 complex genetic traits and, 2
One gene, one disorder (OGOD) idea, 204–205
One-stage procedure, for study design, 6
One neurotransmitter for one mechanism (ONOM) model, 205

Open field test, and animal models, **67**, 79, 196–197
Oppositional defiant disorder, 183

P50 evoked potential, and schizophrenia, 338–339
Panic, and candidate genes, **275**
Parental genetic imprinting, 296
Parents, of autistic children, 46, 50, 51, 52–54
Parkinson's disease, 99
Paroxetine, 117
Partner numbers, and sexual behavior, 263–266
Pathological gambling
  dopamine system and, 171, 202
  polygenic traits and, 183–184
Persistence
  serotonin transporter gene and, 122
  Temperament and Character Inventory (TCI) and, 35
Personality, and genetics. *See also* Temperament
  aggression and polymorphisms, 231–238
  animal models of, 63–83
  autism and, 43–58
  critical reviews of research on, 273–283, 293–309
  dopamine system and, 91–99, 137–146, 165–184
  endophenotypes of psychiatric disorders and, 333–342
  intelligence and cognitive ability, 211–226
  lifestyle choices and, 39
  as predictor of treatment response, 38–39
  psychiatrists and, 33–34, 39–40
  sensation seeking and, 193–206
  serotonin transporter gene and, 109–128, 137–146
  social and ethical implications of research on, 315–326
  structure of human, 34–35
  substance abuse and, 151–158

Personality disorders. *See also* Antisocial personality disorder
  comorbidity and, 37–38
  general criteria for, 35–37
  impulsive aggression, 231–233
Pervasive developmental disorder, not otherwise specified (PDD-NOS), 44
Pharmacological validation, and animal models of personality, 65, 66–67
Phenotypes. *See also* Endophenotypes; Genetics
  animal models of personality and, **71–73**
  autism and, 46–58
  genetic redefinition of behavioral, 282–283
  serotonin transporter gene and genotype correlations, 113–121
  study of complex genetic traits and, 1–24, 334–338
Phenylketonuria (PKU), 320
Physiology, and longitudinal studies of temperament in children, 247–248
Pleiotropy, and animal studies, 299
Polychotomization, and analysis of quantitative traits, 14, 17
Polygenic disorders. *See also* Genetic disorders
  complex genetic traits and, 2
  interaction of multiple genes in, 174–175
  single-gene disorders compared with, 167–168
Population stratification, and association studies, 279–280
Porsolt swim immobility, **67**, 70
Positional cloning, 277–278
Posttraumatic stress disorder, 169, 171
Power, and design for genetic studies of complex traits, 6–8, **9**. *See also* Predictive power
Pragmatic Language Scale, 53
Pragmatism, and personality differences in children, 245

Predictive power, and correlative behavior genetics, 300. *See also* Power

Predisposition, and identification of genes, 23

Prevalence, of autism, 44

Principal component analysis, 19

Prisons and prison population personality disorders and aggression, 232–233

violent behavior and *DRD2* allele, 171

Prolactin, and response to fenfluramine impulsive aggression, 233–234

Prozac, 267

Psychiatric disorders. *See* Psychopathology; *specific disorders*

Psychiatric hospitalization, and aggression associated with personality disorders, 232

Psychiatrists, and significance of personality, 33–34, 39–40

Psychopathology. *See also* Anxiety disorders; Attention-deficit/ hyperactivity disorder; Depression; Eating disorders; Personality disorders; Schizophrenia endophenotypes of, 333–342 novelty seeking, 153–154

Psychoticism novelty seeking and, 152–153 serotonin transporter gene and, 121

Quantification of behavior, 303–305 tests of personality and, 317

Quantitative trait loci (QTLs) intelligence and cognitive ability, 211–226 linkage analysis and, 12, 13–14 mapping of genes for emotionality in animal models, 81–83

Race, and media reports on genetic research, 315–316. *See also* Ethnicity

Reading disability, and chromosome 6p21, 217

Recurrence risk, for autism, 45

Reverse genetics, in psychiatry, 277–278

Reward dependence *DRD4* gene and, 341 Temperament and Character Inventory (TCI) and, 35, 36

Roman high-avoidance (RHA) and Roman low-avoidance (RLA) strains, 79, 80

Rutter, M., 46–47

Sample size and sampling units, and design of genetic studies of complex traits, 2, 3–4, 6–8, 24

Schizoid avoidant behavior, and *DRD2* A1 allele, 173. *See also* Avoidance learning paradigms; Harm avoidance

Schizophrenia candidate genes for, **274**, **275** characterization of traits and, 317 endophenotypes for, 338–339

Science (journal), 323

Segal, Nancy, 324

SEGPATH method, and association analysis, 14, 18, 19

Segregation test, and animal models of temperament, 78, 80

Selective sampling, and study design, 4–5

Self-directedness, and Temperament and Character Inventory (TCI), 35, 36, 38

Self-report personality questionnaires, and novelty seeking, 152–153

Self-transcendence, and Temperament and Character Inventory (TCI), 35

Sensation seeking. *See also* Novelty seeking

brain reward mechanisms and, 152–153
  dopamine D3 receptor gene and, 100–101
Separation, and animal tests of depression, **67**
Serotonin system. *See also* Serotonin transporter gene
  animal models of personality and, 74–75
  impulsive aggression and, 233–238
  sexual behavior and, 257, 267
  substance abuse and promoter region, 155
Serotonin transporter (5-HTTLPR) gene. *See also* Serotonin system
  gene-gene and gene-environment interactions in personality and behavior, 109–128
  harm avoidance and, 101
  impulsive aggression and, 237
  novelty seeking and, **157**
  sexual behavior and, 267–269
  temperament differences in children and, 137–146, 249–251
Sexual behavior, genetics of, 257–270. *See also* Behavior
Sexual orientation. *See* Homosexuality
Shy behavior, in children, 246–247
Sib pairs
  nonparametric methods of linkage analysis and, 12–13
  as sampling unit for genetic studies of complex traits, 3–4, 5, 7–8, 9–10
Significance levels, and interpretation of results of genetic studies, 21–23
Simple genetic disorders, 334
Simplistic assumptions and interpretations, of research on correlative behavior genetics, 295–307, 322. *See also* Interpretation
Single-gene disorders, polygenic disorders compared to, 167–169

Single nucleotide polymorphisms (SNPs)
  genomic linkage disequilibrium scan, 17
  quantitative trait loci and intelligence, 218–219
16 Personality Factor Inventory, 115, **116**
SLC6A4, and aggressive behavior, 235
Smoking
  dopamine system and, 154, 172, 340
  MAO B gene and, 204
Social behavior. *See also* Behavior
  animal models of anxiety and, **67**
  autism and, 52
  parents of autistic children and, 51
  withdrawal in children and, 246–247
Social phobia, 54
Society. *See* Ethics
SOLAR method, 14, 19
Somatization, and personality disorders, 37
Splitting strategies, and study of complex genetic traits, 24
Stimulation, and sensation seeking, 193, 194
Structured Interview for DSM-III-R Personality Disorder (SIDP-R), 54
Study design, for genetic studies of complex traits, 2–10
Subgroup analyses, 19–20
Substance abuse
  candidate genes for, **275**
  dopamine system and, **94–97**, 99, 201–202, 204, 340
  extremes of temperament and, 100
  genetic influences on personality and, 151–158
Suicide and suicidal behavior
  candidate genes for, **274**
  heritability of, 233
  personality disorders and, 232
  serotonin system and, 234, 236, 238

Temperament. *See also* Personality
　animal models and behavioral tests
　　of, 65–83
　DRD4 and serotonin transporter
　　genes and early childhood, 137–
　　146
　molecular genetics of differences in
　　children, 245–252
　psychological qualities of infants
　　and, 121
Temperament and Character Inventory
　(TCI), 34, 35, 36, 37, 38–39, 92,
　174, 175, **176, 181**
Thigmotaxis, and genetic mapping, 82
Thrill and adventure seeking, and
　sensation seeking, 195
Tourette syndrome
　candidate genes for, **275**
　dopamine system and, 169–170, 340
Tower of Hanoi test, 52, 53
Transmission disequilibrium test
　(TDT), and association analysis,
　16
Treatment response, personality as
　predictor of, 38–39
Tridimensional Personality
　Questionnaire (TPQ), 34, 92, 93,
　98, 99, 121, 122, 138, 152, 173,
　201, 264, 304, 340
Tryptophan hydroxylase gene (*TPH*),
　and aggressive behavior, 235,
　236–237
Tuberous sclerosis, 45
Twin studies
　of autism, 45, 46–47
　differences in intrauterine
　　environments and, 296
　of DRD4 and personality, 98–99
　ethics of behavior genetic research
　　and, 323
　of intelligence, 212

of sensation seeking, 197–201
of sexual orientation, 258
Two-stage designs, for studies of
　complex genetic traits, 6, 17
Two-way avoidance conditioning, **67**
Type I and Type II errors, and
　association studies, 279

Unconditioned tests, and animal
　models of fear-motivated
　behavior, 66–68
Unipolar depression, 112. *See also*
　Depression

Validation methods, and animal
　models of personality, 65
Variance components method, and
　linkage analysis, 14
Violent behavior. *See also* Behavior
　antisocial personality disorder and,
　233
　DRD2 allele and imprisonment for,
　171
　impulsivity and serotonin
　　transporters, 100
Virtual behaviors, 303, 305
Vogel conflict test, **67**, 69
Volunteering, and sensation seekers,
　194

Wechsler IQ test, 52
Wilson, J. G., 315
World Congress on Psychiatric
　Genetics (1995), 91

X chromosome, and sexual behavior,
　257, 259–263
Xq28 region, and sexual orientation,
　260, 261, 262–263

Zuckerman, M., 196, 263